Breast Cancer Updates

Edited by Selim Sözen and Seyfi Emir

Published in London, United Kingdom

Breast Cancer Updates
http://dx.doi.org/10.5772/intechopen.104150
Edited by Selim Sözen and Seyfi Emir

Contributors
Vijayakumar Chellappa, Ankit Jain, Kadambari Dharanipragada, Leila Martina Passerino, Nohemí Salinas-Jazmín, María Adriana Medina-Mondragón, Sofia Álvarez-Lorenzo, Rebeca Elizabeth Montalvo-Castro, Jeannie Jiménez-López, Agnieszka Jagiello-Gruszfeld, Agnieszka Mlodzinska, Poornima Pandey, Arvind Bhake, Sarah N. Bishop, Elizabeth A. Bailey, Vahid Raja, Ziba Farajzadegan, Marjan Mansourian, Khojaste Ghasemi, Mohammad Sadegh Aboutalebi, Rasool Nouri, Fariborz Mokarian, Margit Eidenberger, Massimiliano Berretta, Oreste Claudio Buonomo, Gianluca Vanni, Bianca Arianna Facchini, Debora Louzada Carvalho, Mônica de Castro Maia Senna, Thaislayne Nunes de Oliveira, Benjamin Liliav, Luis Torres-Strauss, Vishal Shah, Farah Raheem, Ana Car Peterko, Rahmah Mohammed Abed Alghazal, Ah Haggaa Ali, Eman Soliman Metwally, Philip Adewale Adeoye, Perçin Karakol, Mert Noyan Dabak, Ömer Büyükkaya, Selim Sözen, Abdullah Şişik, Hasan Erdem, Muhammed Said Dalkılıç, Mehmet Gençtürk, Merih Yilmaz, Amir Iqbal Memon, Aisha Masroor Bhatti, Ikram Din Ujjan

First published in London, United Kingdom, 2023 by IntechOpen
IntechOpen is the global imprint of INTECHOPEN LIMITED, registered in England and Wales, registration number: 11086078, 5 Princes Gate Court, London, SW7 2QJ, United Kingdom

British Library Cataloguing-in-Publication Data
A catalogue record for this book is available from the British Library

Additional hard and PDF copies can be obtained from orders@intechopen.com

Breast Cancer Updates
Edited by Selim Sözen and Seyfi Emir
p. cm.
Print ISBN 978-1-80355-930-8
Online ISBN 978-1-80355-931-5
eBook (PDF) ISBN 978-1-80355-932-2

For EU product safety concerns:
IN TECH d.o.o., Prolaz Marije Krucifikse Kozulić 3, 51000 Rijeka, Croatia,
info@intechopen.com or visit our website at intechopen.com.

Meet the editors

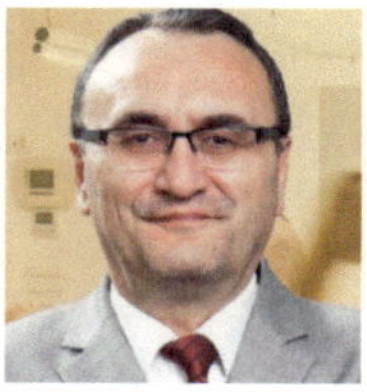

Dr. Selim Sözen is an expert in general surgery who received his medical degree from Ondokuz Mayıs University, Turkey, in 1998. From 1999 to 2004, he was an assistant doctor at Ankara Atatürk Education and Research Hospital, Turkey. From 2004 to 2013, he worked as a specialist at different government hospitals in Turkey. He joined the Department of General Surgery, Medicine Faculty, Namık Kemal University, Turkey, as an associate professor in 2013. He completed liver transplantation surgery at İnönü University, Turkey, in 2014–2015. Since 2016, Dr. Sözen has run his own surgery clinic in İstanbul, Turkey. He is a member of the Turkish Surgical Association and a review board member for several journals. He has published 105 articles in scientific journals and presented 64 poster papers at scientific congresses. His research interests include general, gastrointestinal, emergency, and trauma surgery, bacterial translocation, liver disease, and hernia surgery.

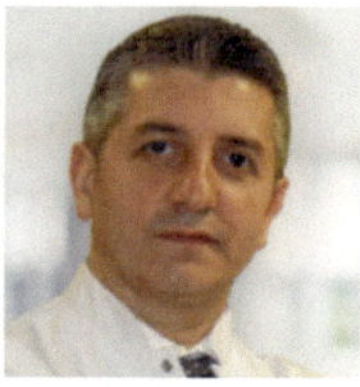

Dr. Seyfi Emir received his medical degree from Dokuz Eylul University, Turkey, in 2000. He worked as an assistant doctor at Haydarpaşa Numune Education and Research Hospital, Turkey, from 2002 to 2008. He then worked at Elazığ Education and Research Hospital, Turkey, from 2009 to 2013. He became an assistant professor in the Department of General Surgery, Medicine Faculty, Namık Kemal University, Turkey, in 2013. Since 2016, Dr. Emir has worked at Reyap Hospital, in Turkey. He is a member of the Turkish Surgical Association. His research interests include general, gastrointestinal, colorectal, obesity, and endocrine surgery.

Contents

Preface

This book presents essential knowledge and key facts about breast cancer. It is divided into two sections.

In Section 1, Chapter 1, "Obesity and Breast Cancer," Dr. Selim Sözen et al. discuss obesity and breast cancer. Chapter 2, "Epidemiology of Breast Cancer in Sub-Saharan Africa" by Dr. Adeoye Philip, examines the literature that shows higher mortality rates of women with breast cancer in less developed countries. Chapter 3, "Breast Cancer and Pregnancy: Epidemiology, Phenotypes, Presentation during Pregnancy, and Therapeutic Approaches" by Dr. Massimiliano Berretta et al., discusses how breast cancer incidence is slowly rising and how awareness of its correct management is fundamental for every physician. Chapter 4, "Breast Cancer in Brazil: Social Conditions and Access to Health Care" by Debora Louzada Carvalho et al., emphasizes the high number of deaths from breast cancer among Brazilian women. Breast cancer is the second greatest cause of mortality in women in Brazil. Chapter 5, "Breast Cancer, Gender, and Body Experience – A Qualitative Study in Argentina on the Transit of the Illness, Femininity, and Sexuality at Stake" by Leila Martina Passerino, discusses the transit of women through breast cancer by investigating the transformations in lifestyles and social behaviors that the experience of illness inaugurates. Chapter 6, "Breast Cancer in the Elderly" by Dr. Agnieszka Jagiello-Gruszfeld and Agnieszka Mlodzinska, discusses comorbidities in breast cancer, which occur much more frequently in the elderly compared to the younger population. Chapter 7, "Management of the Triple Negative Locally Advanced Breast Cancer" by Dr. Amir Iqbal Memon et al., reminds us that patients with triple-negative breast cancer (TNBC) have greater chances of disease relapse, metastasis, and limited survival. Chapter 8, "Inter-Relationship of Ki-67 and Triple-Negative Breast Cancer" by Dr. Vijayakumar Chellappa et al., discusses how higher baseline Ki-67 level, which is a marker of active cell proliferation, is found in the highly proliferating tumors in TNBC. Chapter 9, "Bcl-2 Immunoexpression in Invasive Ductal Carcinoma and Its Evaluative Correlation with Molecular Sub-Types and BR-Grade and TNM Stage" by Dr. Pandey Poornima and Arvind Bhake, discusses the molecular pathogenesis of breast cancer and the involvement of multiple gene types. Bcl-2 is an anti-apoptotic protein that is upregulated by estrogen in breast cancer patients. Chapter 10, "Correlation between Ultrasound Findings and Molecular Subtypes of Breast Cancer" by Rahma Mohammed Abed Alghazal et al., recommends that radiologists be aware of the different imaging features of different molecular subtypes of breast cancer, especially TNBC, which has the most benign-looking criteria, to achieve better lesion characterization and allow the patient to benefit from earlier non-invasive, cost-effective diagnosis and treatment. Chapter 11, "A Short Communication: Non-acid Nucleic Blood Multi-Factors Panels for Primary Breast Cancer Detection – A Systematic Review and Network Meta-Analysis" by Vahid Raja et al., compares non-acid nucleic blood multi-factor panels with mammography in terms of sensitivity, specificity, and accuracy in primary breast cancer detection (stages I, II, III, and IV). The authors systematically review studies assessing the diagnostic value of non-acid nucleic blood tumor marker panels in both healthy women and breast cancer patients (before any anticancer treatment) for the detection of primary breast cancer. Chapter 12, "Membrane-Bound Complement Regulatory Proteins in Breast Cancer: Are They Best Therapeutic Targets?" by Dr. Nohemí Salinas-Jazmín et al., discusses membrane-bound complement regulatory proteins (mCRPs) as potential targets to increase therapeutic efficacy and avoid cancer progression.

In Section 2, Chapter 13, "Minimally Invasive Surgery in Breast Reconstruction: The Past and Future," Dr. Elizabeth A. Bailey and Sarah N. Bishop discuss future applications of emerging technology and the controversies surrounding the widespread adoption of minimally invasive techniques in breast cancer and breast reconstructive surgery. Chapter 14, "Solutions in Breast Reconstruction" by Dr. Karakol Perçin et al., focuses on breast reconstruction after cancer surgery. Skin grafts and local flaps, dermal equivalents, fat transfer, and tissue expansion operations are among the options. Chapter 15, "Breast Reconstructive Options" by Dr. Benjamin Liliav and Luis Torres-Strauss, explores the various modalities of breast reconstruction available to patients. There are, generally, three components or factors that need to be considered while devising a reconstructive option for a particular patient. These are patient factors, surgeon factors, and oncologic factors. Chapter 16, "Oncoplastic Breast Conservation: A Standard of Care in Modern Breast Cancer Surgical Management" by Dr. Ana Car Peterko, suggests that mastectomy should no longer be offered as an equivalent treatment option for early-stage breast cancer patients with low-volume breast disease, irrespective of the availability of postmastectomy breast reconstruction. Chapter 17, "Physiotherapeutic Management in Breast Cancer Patients" by Dr. Margit Eidenberger, examines how breast cancer treatment can lead to various physical and long-term morbidities such as restricted shoulder joint range of motion, lymphedema, impaired muscle strength, and cancer-related fatigue. Finally, Chapter 18, "Antibody Drug Conjugates" by Dr. Farah Raheem and Vishal Shah, discusses antibody-drug conjugates (ADCs), which continue to change the treatment paradigm of breast cancer.

I thank the authors for their professional dedication and outstanding work in summarizing their clinical and research practices.

Selim Sözen
Associate Professor of General Surgery,
Sözen Surgery Clinic,
Tekirdağ, Turkey

Seyfi Emir
Assistant Professor of General Surgery,
Department of General Surgery,
Reyap Hospital,
Tekirdağ, Turkey

Section 1

Epidemiology, Social Conditions and General Information

Chapter 1

Obesity and Breast Cancer

Abdullah Şişik, Hasan Erdem, Muhammed Said Dalkılıç, Mehmet Gençtürk, Merih Yılmaz and Selim Sözen

Abstract

Obesity is associated with a higher risk of chronic diseases. Breast cancer is one of the malignancies, which has been related to obesity. Patients with a BMI more than 35 kg/m^2 had an 86% greater risk of having breast cancer than those with a normal BMI. Every 5 kg/m^2 rise in BMI has also been demonstrated to increase the risk of postmenopausal breast cancer. Obese people have poorer outcomes in terms of lymph node positivity, disease-free survival, and overall survival, according to research. Leptin, whose circulating levels rise in proportion to BMI and body fat reserves, is usually regarded as the primary driver of the intricate web that connects obesity and breast cancer. The number of studies examining the association between leptin activity and breast cancer genesis and behavior is growing. The effectiveness of bariatric surgery on lessening the risk of developing breast cancer has been proven.

Keywords: breast cancer, leptin, obesity, bariatric surgery

1. Introduction

Obesity prevalence is rapidly increasing in many developed and developing countries. Obesity is related to an increase in the risk of chronic diseases. Obesity is associated with type 2 diabetes, hypertension, cardiovascular disease, and a variety of cancers. Breast cancer is another malignancy that has been related to obesity [1, 2].

American Institute for Cancer Research (AICR) reported that 13 cancers, including postmenopausal breast cancer, colorectal cancer, endometrial/uterine cancer, esophageal adenocarcinoma, gallbladder cancer, stomach cancer, hepatocellular cancer, meningioma, multiple myeloma, ovarian cancer, pancreatic cancer, kidney cancer, and thyroid cancer, were associated with obesity [3, 4].

Breast cancer is one of the most frequently diagnosed cancers among women worldwide. It is known that breast cancer has a worse prognosis and higher mortality rates in obese women [5, 6]. Hyperinsulinemia, estrogen signaling, inflammation, and adipokine expression hypotheses have been proposed for the mechanism of action of obesity in breast cancer patients [7, 8]. At this point, the concept of adipokines is emerging. Despite being primarily produced by adipocytes, adipokines, which are endocrine, paracrine, and autocrine mechanisms produced in a variety of different cells, influence the development of malignancies in obese people [8]. Leptin, an adipokine, plays an important role in the relationship between obesity and breast cancer [9, 10].

 IntechOpen

2. Breast carcinoma

Classification of breast carcinoma is based on clinicopathological features and expression of the estrogen receptor (ER), progesterone receptor (PR), and human epidermal growth factor receptor 2 (HER2). Approximately 70% of breast cancers consist of tumors that express hormonal receptors.

Genetic profile, age at menarche and menopause, parity, age of first child, past cancer occurrence, and lifestyle are the most important risk factors for breast cancer. However, BRCA1/2 mutations account for approximately 5–10% of cases [11]. Also, obesity, metabolic syndrome, alcohol, and hypercholesterolemia are the other risk factors for breast cancer [12]. Despite all the advances in medical oncology in people with breast cancer, fatal metastases may occur even years after surgical treatment [13, 14]. Bone, lung, and brain are the primary areas of metastasis. The invasion-metastasis process takes place in successive steps. These steps are defined as local invasion, intravasation, circulation survival, attachment and extravasation in distant organ regions, creation of micrometastases, and metastatic growth [15, 16]. Failure at any step will end the metastasis process.

3. Relationship between obesity and breast cancer

3.1 Epidemiology

It is worrying that the incidence of obesity has increased rapidly all over the world, and the relationship between obesity and different types of cancer has been revealed recently. According to WHO data, the incidence of obesity in women is above 35–40%. It has been shown that patients with class 2 and class 3 (class 2: body mass index (BMI) = 35–40 kg/m^2, class 3: BMI= > 40 kg/m^2) obesity have an 86% higher risk of developing breast cancer than patients with normal BMI [17]. The impact of obesity on breast cancer risk differs according to menopausal status and disease subtypes. Current evidence suggests that while increased BMI is associated with a reduced risk of breast cancer before menopause, it is strongly associated with an increased risk after menopause [18].

As is known, postmenopausal obesity is a risk factor for hormone receptor positive breast cancer in women [19–21]. Postmenopausal breast cancer risk has also been found to be positively associated with every 5 kg/m^2 increase in BMI [22].

Class 2 and class 3 obese individuals had more negative results in terms of tumor size and metastasis. There are also studies showing that obese individuals have worse outcomes in lymph node positivity, disease-free, and overall survival [23–30]. Secondary primary cancer formation and contralateral breast cancer formation have been reported to be increased in obese individuals [31]. On the other hand, adverse effects of obesity in adjuvant therapy have been demonstrated. Less response to treatment was obtained in obese individuals in both chemotherapy and aromatase inhibitor therapy.

3.2 Physiopathogenesis

In the presence of obesity, hypertrophy and hyperplasia are seen in white adipocytes, and accordingly pathophysiological changes such as increase in free fatty acid (FFA) and triglyceride levels increase in blood sugar and increase in insulin resistance occur.

Obese adipose tissue also produces inflammatory cytokines (e.g. tumor necrosis factor alpha (TNF-α), interleukin-6 (IL-6), interleukin-1 beta (IL-1β), and TGF-β) and factors called adipokines with important local and systemic functions. The release of these molecules can profoundly affect breast cancer progression, both through a direct effect on neoplastic epithelial cells and indirect effects on the tumor microenvironment [32]. Among the adipokines, leptin, whose circulating levels rise in proportion to the amount of BMI and body fat stores, has been widely accepted as the main driver of the complex web linking obesity and breast cancer.

3.2.1 Obesity, chronic inflammation, and breast cancer

Excessive calorie intake or low calorie expenditure leads to an increase in fat compartments. This causes dysregulation in the production of steroid hormones and adipokines and causes chronic subclinical inflammation. Such changes have been associated with carcinogenesis, tumor progression, and metastasis [33]. Adipose tissue inflammation may explain the physiological link between obesity and breast cancer. Inflamed adipose tissue is characterized by infiltrating macrophages surrounding dying adipocytes, termed crown-like structures (CLS) [34]. The presence of CLS in breast adipose tissue (CLS-B) is associated with activation of NF-κB and increased levels of pro-inflammatory factors, resulting in upregulation of estradiol (E2). In conclusion, locally produced estrogens can be considered the main driver for the development of hormone-dependent breast cancer in postmenopausal women.

Adipocytes produce adiponectin and leptin, which are involved in the regulation of calorie intake and metabolism, inflammation, angiogenesis, and cell proliferation. Breast cancer cells are surrounded and affected by this microenvironment. A strong role for leptin in breast carcinogenesis has been reported with abundant evidence. It may contribute to local pro-inflammatory mechanisms, especially in obese patients. There is a positive correlation between the BMI index and leptin levels, whereas adiponectin concentrations generally decrease with more adiposity. The increased leptin-adiponectin ratio seen in obesity has been associated with neoplastic transformation and tumor progression [35].

3.2.2 Leptin and breast cancer

Leptin is a molecule involved in appetite control, hematopoiesis, osteogenesis, angiogenesis, and proliferation of different cells such as breast cells [9, 10]. Studies showing the relationship between leptin activity and breast cancer formation and cancer behavior are increasing in the literature. Leptin may act as a molecular link between obesity and breast cancer [36]. Leptin exerts its effects through the transmembrane leptin receptor (ObR) expressed in various tissues. Many studies, both clinical and experimental, have shown that the leptin/ObR axis is involved in breast cancer progression and metastasis. Breast cancer cells overexpress the leptin receptor, thus rendering them highly susceptible to the effect of the high leptin levels typically seen in obese patients [37]. Leptin exerts pleiotropic effects in breast cancer cells, including inhibition of proapoptotic signals, sensitivity to estrogens, and modulation of the tumor microenvironment, contributing to local pro-inflammatory mechanisms and promoting breast tumor growth [37–39]. Increased leptin levels in breast cancer patients have been associated with the increased risk of metastasis and reduced survival [25].

Niu et al. showed the presence of higher leptin levels in people with breast cancer than in normal individuals in their epidemiological-based meta-analysis. In addition, people with breast cancer with lymph node metastases have been shown to have higher leptin levels than those without metastatic disease [40]. It has also been shown that serum leptin levels are higher in obese breast cancer patients [41]. In postmenopausal ER-positive breast cancer patients, serum leptin levels were higher at more advanced tumor stage (pT and TNM stage) and in the presence of distant metastases [42]. Similarly, leptin concentrations were significantly associated with TNM staging, tumor size, histological grading, lymph node involvement, and metastasis in postmenopausal breast cancer cases [43, 44]. Tumor size and lymph node metastasis have also been shown to correlate with increased leptin/adiponectin serum ratio in breast cancer patients. Ishikawa et al. observed that patients with overexpression of ObR and leptin in primary breast tumors developed more distant metastases [37]. In ER-negative breast cancer patients, ObR was found to be significantly overexpressed in metastatic lymph nodes compared to primary tumors or lymph nodes from ER-positive patients [45].

3.2.3 Dietary cholesterol intake/fat intake and breast cancer risk

In general, dietary-saturated fat intake is synonymous with cholesterol intake. It is well known that saturated fat raises low-density lipoprotein (LDL) cholesterol, a leading cause of atherosclerosis and cardiovascular disease [46]. Li et al. showed a relationship between daily cholesterol consumption of more than 370 mg and the development of breast cancer. The Mediterranean diet is a good example of a low-fat diet. It is characterized by moderate alcohol intake and low consumption of red meat, with high levels of extra virgin olive oil, vegetables, fruits, plant proteins, fish and other seafood, wholegrains, nuts, and low-fat dairy products [47]. The beneficial effects of the Mediterranean diet have been noted in reducing the risk of breast cancer and breast cancer recurrence while improving overall survival [48–50]. Being overweight and obese is closely associated with the development and recurrence of breast cancer. The interaction between obesity, inflammation, and the tumor microenvironment induces tumorigenesis primarily in hormone-sensitive and postmenopausal patients. Several meta-analyses have provided evidence that obesity carries a 35–40% increased risk of relapse and death, regardless of menopause or hormone receptor status. In this context, prevention of breast cancer requires raising awareness about monitoring body weight, especially in menopausal women. This can be achieved through a low cholesterol/low-saturated fat diet and regular exercise [51].

4. Obesity surgery and its effects on breast cancer

Today, bariatric surgery is the gold standard in the treatment of morbid obesity. Many studies have shown that only diet and exercise are insufficient in the fight against morbid obesity. In recent years, the rate of bariatric surgery has been increasing significantly all over the world. Laparoscopic sleeve gastrectomy, Roux en Y gastric bypass, and One anastomosis gastric bypass are the most frequently applied methods. Acceptable and sustainable weight loss has been reported with the implementation of appropriate postoperative lifestyle changes in all surgical techniques. In addition, remissions are possible in many obesity-related diseases.

It is not difficult to predict the reduction in breast cancer risk in individuals who have undergone bariatric surgery, due to effective weight loss, reduced fat tissue in the body, and correspondingly reduced inflammation, and reduced leptin effects. At the same time, the possibility of an earlier diagnosis of possible breast cancer increases due to both the examinations performed during the operation and the reduction in the volume of the breast tissue after the operation. Lovrics et al. found in their meta-analysis that surgical treatment of obesity in women was associated with a significantly reduced risk of developing breast cancer. In the same study, it was emphasized that previous bariatric surgery was associated with a lower-stage diagnosis in breast cancer [52].

The SPLENDID study examines obesity and obesity-related cancers. The patients included in the study had an average follow-up of 6.1 years. SPLENDID results showed that bariatric surgery was associated with a 32% reduction in obesity-related cancers and a 48% reduction in overall cancer-related mortality [53].

With regard to breast cancer specifically, bariatric surgery has been observed to reduce the risk of breast cancer in postmenopausal women, particularly ER-negative breast cancer, by 64% [54–56]. Moderate reductions in ER-positive and HER2-positive breast cancer rates have been reported [57]. It has also been proven that thanks to bariatric surgery, possible later cancers are less aggressive and they are diagnosed earlier. At diagnosis of breast cancer in patients after bariatric surgery, the rate of diagnosis of stage I breast cancer increases, while stage III or IV decreases [52].

Conflict of interest

The authors declare no conflict of interest.

Author details

Abdullah Şişik[1*], Hasan Erdem[1], Muhammed Said Dalkılıç[2], Mehmet Gençtürk[1], Merih Yılmaz[1] and Selim Sözen[3]

1 Department of General Surgery, Dr. HE Obesity Clinic, Kurtköy Ersoy Hospital, Istanbul, Turkey

2 Department of General Surgery, Medical School, Marmara University, Istanbul, Turkey

3 Department of General Surgery, Sözen Surgery Clinic, Tekirdağ, Turkey

*Address all correspondence to: abdullahsisik@gmail.com

References

[1] Calle EE, Kaaks R. Overweight, obesity and cancer: Epidemiological evidence and proposed mechanisms. Nature Reviews. Cancer. 2004;**4**(8): 579-591. DOI: 10.1038/nrc1408

[2] Renehan AG, Tyson M, Egger M, Heller RF, Zwahlen M. Body-mass index and incidence of cancer: A systematic review and meta-analysis of prospective observational studies. Lancet. 2008;**371**(9612):569-578. DOI: 10.1016/S0140-6736(08)60269-X

[3] Perry RJ, Shulman GI. Mechanistic links between obesity, insulin, and cancer. Trends Cancer. 2020;**6**(2):75-78. DOI: 10.1016/j.trecan.2019.12.003 Epub 2020 Jan 14

[4] Clinton SK, Giovannucci EL, Hursting SD. The World Cancer Research Fund/American Institute for Cancer Research third expert report on diet, nutrition, physical activity, and cancer: Impact and future directions. The Journal of Nutrition. 2020;**150**(4):663-671. DOI: 10.1093/jn/nxz268

[5] Protani M, Coory M, Martin JH. Effect of obesity on survival of women with breast cancer: Systematic review and meta-analysis. Breast Cancer Research and Treatment. 2010;**123**(3):627-635. DOI: 10.1007/s10549-010-0990-0 Epub 2010 Jun 23

[6] Renehan AG, Soerjomataram I, Tyson M, Egger M, Zwahlen M, Coebergh JW, et al. Incident cancer burden attributable to excess body mass index in 30 European countries. International Journal of Cancer. 2010;**126**(3):692-702. DOI: 10.1002/ijc.24803

[7] Taubes G. Cancer research. Unraveling the obesity-cancer connection. Science. 2012;**335**(6064):28-30. DOI: 10.1126/science.335.6064.28 Erratum in: Science. 2012;335(6066):286

[8] Park J, Euhus DM, Scherer PE. Paracrine and endocrine effects of adipose tissue on cancer development and progression. Endocrine Reviews. 2011;**32**(4):550-570. DOI: 10.1210/er.2010-0030 Epub 2011 Jun 2

[9] Andò S, Barone I, Giordano C, Bonofiglio D, Catalano S. The multifaceted mechanism of leptin signaling within tumor microenvironment in driving breast cancer growth and progression. Frontiers in Oncology. 2014;**4**:340. DOI: 10.3389/fonc.2014.00340

[10] Andò S, Catalano S. The multifactorial role of leptin in driving the breast cancer microenvironment. Nature Reviews. Endocrinology. 2011;**8**(5):263-275. DOI: 10.1038/nrendo.2011.184

[11] Shah R, Rosso K, Nathanson SD. Pathogenesis, prevention, diagnosis and treatment of breast cancer. World Journal of Clinical Oncology. 2014;**5**(3):283-298. DOI: 10.5306/wjco.v5.i3.283

[12] Jones LW, Fels DR, West M, Allen JD, Broadwater G, Barry WT, et al. Modulation of circulating angiogenic factors and tumor biology by aerobic training in breast cancer patients receiving neoadjuvant chemotherapy. Cancer Prevention Research (Philadelphia, Pa.). 2013;**6**(9):925-937. DOI: 10.1158/1940-6207.CAPR-12-0416 Epub 2013 Jul 10

[13] Cardoso F, Costa A, Norton L, Cameron D, Cufer T, Fallowfield L, et al. 1st international consensus guidelines for advanced breast cancer (ABC 1). Breast.

2012;**21**(3):242-252. DOI: 10.1016/j.breast.2012.03.003 Epub 2012 Mar 16

[14] Early Breast Cancer Trialists' Collaborative Group (EBCTCG), Peto R, Davies C, Godwin J, Gray R, Pan HC, et al. Comparisons between different polychemotherapy regimens for early breast cancer: Meta-analyses of long-term outcome among 100,000 women in 123 randomised trials. Lancet. 2012;**379**(9814):432-444. DOI: 10.1016/S0140-6736(11)61625-5 Epub 2011 Dec 5

[15] Fidler IJ. The pathogenesis of cancer metastasis: The 'seed and soil' hypothesis revisited. Nature Reviews. Cancer. 2003;**3**(6):453-458. DOI: 10.1038/nrc1098

[16] Valastyan S, Weinberg RA. Tumor metastasis: Molecular insights and evolving paradigms. Cell. 2011;**147**(2):275-292. DOI: 10.1016/j.cell.2011.09.024

[17] Neuhouser ML, Aragaki AK, Prentice RL, Manson JE, Chlebowski R, Carty CL, et al. Overweight, obesity, and postmenopausal invasive breast cancer risk: A secondary analysis of the Women's Health Initiative randomized clinical trials. JAMA Oncology. 2015;**1**(5):611-621. DOI: 10.1001/jamaoncol.2015.1546

[18] Kerr J, Anderson C, Lippman SM. Physical activity, sedentary behaviour, diet, and cancer: An update and emerging new evidence. The Lancet Oncology. 2017;**18**(8):e457-e471. DOI: 10.1016/S1470-2045(17)30411-4 Epub 2017 Jul 26

[19] Munsell MF, Sprague BL, Berry DA, Chisholm G, Trentham-Dietz A. Body mass index and breast cancer risk according to postmenopausal estrogen-progestin use and hormone receptor status. Epidemiologic Reviews. 2014;**36**(1):114-136. DOI: 10.1093/epirev/mxt010

[20] Nagrani R, Mhatre S, Rajaraman P, Soerjomataram I, Boffetta P, Gupta S, et al. Central obesity increases risk of breast cancer irrespective of menopausal and hormonal receptor status in women of south Asian ethnicity. European Journal of Cancer. 2016;**66**:153-161. DOI: 10.1016/j.ejca.2016.07.022 Epub 2016 Aug 27

[21] Ahn J, Schatzkin A, Lacey JV Jr, Albanes D, Ballard-Barbash R, Adams KF, et al. Adiposity, adult weight change, and postmenopausal breast cancer risk. Archives of Internal Medicine. 2007;**167**(19):2091-2102. DOI: 10.1001/archinte.167.19.2091

[22] Renehan AG, Roberts DL, Dive C. Obesity and cancer: Pathophysiological and biological mechanisms. Archives of Physiology and Biochemistry. 2008;**114**(1):71-83. DOI: 10.1080/13813450801954303

[23] Loi S, Milne RL, Friedlander ML, McCredie MR, Giles GG, Hopper JL, et al. Obesity and outcomes in premenopausal and postmenopausal breast cancer. Cancer Epidemiology, Biomarkers & Prevention. 2005;**14**(7):1686-1691. DOI: 10.1158/1055-9965.EPI-05-0042

[24] Caan BJ, Kwan ML, Hartzell G, Castillo A, Slattery ML, Sternfeld B, et al. Pre-diagnosis body mass index, post-diagnosis weight change, and prognosis among women with early stage breast cancer. Cancer Causes & Control. 2008;**19**(10):1319-1328. DOI: 10.1007/s10552-008-9203-0 Epub 2008 Aug 28

[25] Rosenberg L, Czene K, Hall P. Obesity and poor breast cancer prognosis: An illusion because of hormone replacement therapy? British Journal of Cancer. 2009;**100**(9):1486-1491. DOI: 10.1038/sj.bjc.6605025 Epub 2009 Apr 14

[26] Majed B, Senouci K, Asselain B. Shortened survival and more metastasis recurrences among overweight breast cancer patients. The Breast Journal. 2009;**15**(5):557-559. DOI: 10.1111/j.1524-4741.2009.00785.x Epub 2009 Aug 4

[27] Fuentes-Mattei E, Velazquez-Torres G, Phan L, Zhang F, Chou PC, Shin JH, et al. Effects of obesity on transcriptomic changes and cancer hallmarks in estrogen receptor-positive breast cancer. Journal of the National Cancer Institute. 2014;**106**(7):dju158. DOI: 10.1093/jnci/dju158

[28] Copson ER, Cutress RI, Maishman T, Eccles BK, Gerty S, Stanton L, et al. POSH study steering group. Obesity and the outcome of young breast cancer patients in the UK: The POSH study. Annals of Oncology. 2015;**26**(1):101-112. DOI: 10.1093/annonc/mdu509 Epub 2014 Oct 30

[29] Osman MA, Hennessy BT. Obesity correlation with metastases development and response to first-line metastatic chemotherapy in breast cancer. Clinical Medicine Insights: Oncology. 2015;**9**:105-112. DOI: 10.4137/CMO.S32812

[30] Alarcón Rojas CA, Alvarez-Bañuelos MT, Morales-Romero J, Suárez-Díaz H, Hernández-Fonseca JC, Contreras-Alarcón G. Breast cancer: Metastasis, molecular subtypes, and overweight and obesity in Veracruz, Mexico. Clinical Breast Cancer. 2019;**19**(1):e166-e171. DOI: 10.1016/j.clbc.2018.08.003 Epub 2018 Aug 22

[31] Druesne-Pecollo N, Touvier M, Barrandon E, Chan DS, Norat T, Zelek L, et al. Excess body weight and second primary cancer risk after breast cancer: A systematic review and meta-analysis of prospective studies. Breast Cancer Research and Treatment. 2012;**135**(3):647-654. DOI: 10.1007/s10549-012-2187-1 Epub 2012 Aug 5

[32] Andò S, Gelsomino L, Panza S, Giordano C, Bonofiglio D, Barone I, et al. Obesity, leptin and breast cancer: Epidemiological evidence and proposed mechanisms. Cancers (Basel). 2019;**11**(1):62. DOI: 10.3390/cancers11010062

[33] Hursting SD, Dunlap SM. Obesity, metabolic dysregulation, and cancer: A growing concern and an inflammatory (and microenvironmental) issue. Annals of the New York Academy of Sciences. 2012;**1271**(1):82-87. DOI: 10.1111/j.1749-6632.2012.06737.x

[34] Cinti S, Mitchell G, Barbatelli G, Murano I, Ceresi E, Faloia E, et al. Adipocyte death defines macrophage localization and function in adipose tissue of obese mice and humans. Journal of Lipid Research. 2005;**46**(11):2347-2355. DOI: 10.1194/jlr.M500294-JLR200 Epub 2005 Sep 8

[35] Housa D, Housová J, Vernerová Z, Haluzík M. Adipocytokines and cancer. Physiological Research. 2006;**55**(3):233-244. DOI: 10.33549/physiolres.930848 Epub 2005 Oct 17

[36] Barone I, Giordano C, Bonofiglio D, Andò S, Catalano S. Leptin, obesity and breast cancer: Progress to understanding the molecular connections. Current Opinion in Pharmacology. 2016;**31**:83-89. DOI: 10.1016/j.coph.2016.10.003 Epub 2016 Nov 2

[37] Ishikawa M, Kitayama J, Nagawa H. Enhanced expression of leptin and leptin receptor (OB-R) in human breast cancer. Clinical Cancer Research. 2004;**10**(13):4325-4331. DOI: 10.1158/1078-0432.CCR-03-0749

[38] Delort L, Rossary A, Farges MC, Vasson MP, Caldefie-Chézet F. Leptin,

adipocytes and breast cancer: Focus on inflammation and anti-tumor immunity. Life Sciences. 2015;**140**:37-48. DOI: 10.1016/j.lfs.2015.04.012 Epub 2015 May 6

[39] Frankenberry KA, Skinner H, Somasundar P, McFadden DW, Vona-Davis LC. Leptin receptor expression and cell signaling in breast cancer. International Journal of Oncology. 2006;**28**(4):985-993

[40] Niu J, Jiang L, Guo W, Shao L, Liu Y, Wang L. The association between leptin level and breast cancer: A meta-analysis. PLoS One. 2013;**8**(6):e67349. DOI: 10.1371/journal.pone.0067349

[41] Romero-Figueroa Mdel S, Garduño-García Jde J, Duarte-Mote J, Matute-González G, Gómez-Villanueva A, De la Cruz-Vargas J. Insulin and leptin levels in obese patients with and without breast cancer. Clinical Breast Cancer. 2013;**13**(6):482-485. DOI: 10.1016/j.clbc.2013.08.001 Epub 2013 Sep 29

[42] Macciò A, Madeddu C, Gramignano G, Mulas C, Floris C, Massa D, et al. Correlation of body mass index and leptin with tumor size and stage of disease in hormone-dependent postmenopausal breast cancer: Preliminary results and therapeutic implications. Journal of Molecular Medicine (Berlin, Germany). 2010;**88**(7):677-686. DOI: 10.1007/s00109-010-0611-8 Epub 2010 Mar 26

[43] Madeddu C, Gramignano G, Floris C, Murenu G, Sollai G, Macciò A. Role of inflammation and oxidative stress in post-menopausal oestrogen-dependent breast cancer. Journal of Cellular and Molecular Medicine. 2014;**18**(12):2519-2529. DOI: 10.1111/jcmm.12413 Epub 2014 Oct 22

[44] Assiri AM, Kamel HF, Hassanien MF. Resistin, visfatin, adiponectin, and leptin: Risk of breast cancer in pre- and postmenopausal saudi females and their possible diagnostic and predictive implications as novel biomarkers. Disease Markers. 2015;**2015**:253519. DOI: 10.1155/2015/253519 Epub 2015 Mar 8

[45] Alshaker H, Krell J, Frampton AE, Waxman J, Blyuss O, Zaikin A, et al. Leptin induces upregulation of sphingosine kinase 1 in oestrogen receptor-negative breast cancer via Src family kinase-mediated, janus kinase 2-independent pathway. Breast Cancer Research. 2014;**16**(5):426. DOI: 10.1186/s13058-014-0426-6

[46] Mensink RP, Sanders TA, Baer DJ, Hayes KC, Howles PN, Marangoni A. The increasing use of Interesterified lipids in the food supply and their effects on health parameters. Advances in Nutrition. 2016;**7**(4):719-729. DOI: 10.3945/an.115.009662

[47] Schwingshackl L, Schwedhelm C, Galbete C, Hoffmann G. Adherence to Mediterranean diet and risk of cancer: An updated systematic review and meta-analysis. Nutrients. 2017;**9**(10):1063. DOI: 10.3390/nu9101063

[48] Schwingshackl L, Hoffmann G. Mediterranean dietary pattern, inflammation and endothelial function: A systematic review and meta-analysis of intervention trials. Nutrition, Metabolism, and Cardiovascular Diseases. 2014;**24**(9):929-939. DOI: 10.1016/j.numecd.2014.03.003 Epub 2014 Apr 2

[49] Hoffmann G, Schwingshackl L. Mediterranean diet supplemented with extra virgin olive oil reduces the incidence of invasive breast cancer in a randomised controlled trial. Evidence-Based Medicine. 2016;**21**(2):72.

DOI: 10.1136/ebmed-2015-110366 Epub 2016 Jan 7

[50] Skouroliakou M, Grosomanidis D, Massara P, Kostara C, Papandreou P, Ntountaniotis D, et al. Serum antioxidant capacity, biochemical profile and body composition of breast cancer survivors in a randomized Mediterranean dietary intervention study. European Journal of Nutrition. 2018;**57**(6):2133-2145. DOI: 10.1007/s00394-017-1489-9 Epub 2017 Jun 20

[51] Garcia-Estevez L, Moreno-Bueno G. Updating the role of obesity and cholesterol in breast cancer. Breast Cancer Research. 2019;**21**(1):35. DOI: 10.1186/s13058-019-1124-1

[52] Lovrics O, Butt J, Lee Y, Lovrics P, Boudreau V, Anvari M, et al. The effect of bariatric surgery on breast cancer incidence and characteristics: A meta-analysis and systematic review. American Journal of Surgery. 2021;**222**(4):715-722. DOI: 10.1016/j.amjsurg.2021.03.016 Epub 2021 Mar 18

[53] Aminian A, Wilson R, Al-Kurd A, Tu C, Milinovich A, Kroh M, et al. Association of Bariatric Surgery with Cancer Risk and Mortality in adults with obesity. Journal of the American Medical Association. 2022;**327**(24):2423-2433. DOI: 10.1001/jama.2022.9009

[54] Ashrafian H, Ahmed K, Rowland SP, Patel VM, Gooderham NJ, Holmes E, et al. Metabolic surgery and cancer: Protective effects of bariatric procedures. Cancer. 2011;**117**(9):1788-1799. DOI: 10.1002/cncr.25738 Epub 2010 Nov 29

[55] Schauer DP, Feigelson HS, Koebnick C, Caan B, Weinmann S, Leonard AC, et al. Bariatric surgery and the risk of cancer in a large multisite cohort. Annals of Surgery. 2019;**269**(1):95-101. DOI: 10.1097/SLA.0000000000002525

[56] Wiggins T, Antonowicz SS, Markar SR. Cancer risk following bariatric surgery-systematic review and meta-analysis of National Population-Based Cohort Studies. Obesity Surgery. 2019;**29**(3):1031-1039. DOI: 10.1007/s11695-018-3501-8

[57] Heshmati K, Harris DA, Rosner B, Pranckevicius E, Ardestani A, Cho N, et al. Association of Bariatric Surgery Status with reduced HER2+ breast cancers: A retrospective cohort study. Obesity Surgery. 2019;**29**(4):1092-1098. DOI: 10.1007/s11695-018-03701-7

Chapter 2

Epidemiology of Breast Cancer in Sub-Saharan Africa

Philip Adewale Adeoye

Abstract

Breast cancer has increasingly become a disease of high morbidity and mortality globally, and in the sub-Saharan African region in particular. Therefore, there is a need to review the current status of breast cancer in the region in the last decade. Though Africa has one of the lowest incidence rates, it has the highest mortality rate globally. There have been reported inter- and intra-country variations in breast cancer morbidity and mortality in the region, with East Africa having the largest incidence rate increase, while southern Africa experiences the lowest increase between 2008 and 2012. Histology remains the commonest modality of diagnosis in sub-Saharan Africa; with invasive ductal cancers being the commonest among patients. Novel genes have also been popular among certain populations, in the presence of the more popular BRACA genes. Adverse outcomes reported include physical and mental health outcomes, which have been linked to some health behaviours. There has been varying modalities of treatments across the region. Therefore, there is a need for better organized and improved screening/diagnostics service accessibility in resource-constrained settings in sub-Saharan Africa. There should also be increased awareness creation among African populations about the availability of treatment facilities and modalities in their communities.

Keywords: breast cancer, morbidity, mortality, incidence, adverse outcomes, novel genes, sub-Saharan Africa

1. Introduction

Breast cancer is the most common cancer among women and one of the most important causes of death among them. Breast cancer (BC) is the most frequently diagnosed cancer in women worldwide with 2.3 million new cases in 2020 and the fifth leading cause of cancer mortality, with 685,000 deaths [1, 2]. It ranks first for incidence in the vast majority of countries (159 of 185 countries) and mortality in 110 countries, and it accounts for 11.7% of all incident cancer cases – just ahead of new lung cancer cases [2]. It is the leading cause of cancer-related morbidity and mortality among women; accounting for 24.5% of all incident cancer cases and 15.5% of cancer-related mortality [2]. Incidence rates are 88% higher in transitioned countries than in transitioning countries (55.9 and 29.7 per 100,000, respectively), with the highest incidence rates (>80 per 100,000) in Australia/New Zealand, Western Europe

(Belgium has the world's highest incidence), Northern America, and Northern Europe and the lowest rates (<40 per 100,000) in Central America, Eastern and Middle Africa, and South-Central Asia [1, 2]. High and very high HDI countries have 55.9 incidence ASR per 100,000 females compared to 29.7 incidence ASR per 100,000 females globally [2]. Furthermore, China has the highest proportion of incident cases of breast cancer, globally; accounting for 49.3%, 49.9%, and 48.6% of total incidence rates overall, males and females, respectively [2]. The burden of breast cancer has been projected to reach over 3 million incident cases and 1 million deaths every year by the year 2040 [1].

Generally, the global burden of breast cancer is reported to be an age-standardized incidence rate of 43.3 per 100,000 women per year and an age-standardized mortality rate of 12.9 per 100,000 women per year. The more developed countries significantly have a higher incidence rate (74.1 per 100, 000 women per year) and mortality rate (14.9 per 100,000 women per year) compared to the less developed countries with an incidence rate of 31.3 per 100,000 women per year and mortality rate of 11.5 per 100,000 women per year [3]. High and very high HDI countries have a 12.8 mortality ASR per 100,000 females compared to a 15.0 mortality ASR per 100,000 females globally [2]. While Western Europe has the highest incidence of breast cancer (90.7 incidence ASR per 100,000 women); the West African region and Melanesia have the highest mortality (22.3 and 27.5 ASR per 100,000 women, respectively) [2]. Furthermore, China has the highest proportion of breast cancer-related mortality rates, globally; accounting for 58.3%, 60.6%, and 55.5% of total mortality rates overall, males and females, respectively [2].

Incidence rates of breast cancer are rising fast in transitioning countries in South America, Africa, and Asia as well as in high-income Asian countries where rates are historically low [2]. Dramatic changes in lifestyle, sociocultural, and built environments brought about by growing economies and an increase in the proportion of women in the industrial workforce have had an impact on the prevalence of breast cancer risk factors—the postponement of childbearing and having fewer children, greater levels of excess body weight and physical inactivity—and have resulted in a convergence toward the risk factor profile of western countries and narrowing international gaps in breast cancer morbidity [4].

Incidence and death rates have increased over the last three decades due to long-standing higher reproductive and hormonal risk factor profiles (such as early age at menarche, later age, at menopause, advanced age at first birth, fewer number of children, less breastfeeding, menopausal hormone therapy, oral contraceptives, diethylstilbestrol), behavioral risk factors (alcohol intake, smoking, excess body weight, physical inactivity, insufficient vitamin supplementation, intake of processed food, excessive exposure to artificial light, exposure to chemicals and other drugs), higher prevalence of breast cancer-associated genes, better cancer registration, and cancer detection [4–7]. The non-modifiable factors include female sex, older age, family history, ethnicity/race, genetic mutation, pregnancy and breastfeeding, menstrual period and menopause, the density of breast tissue, previous history of breast cancer, noncancerous breast diseases and previous radiation therapy [7]. The incidence rate of breast cancer varies greatly with race and ethnicity and is higher in developed countries [2, 4, 6].

Literature has shown that the mortality rate of breast cancer is higher in less developed regions [2, 6]. women living in transitioning countries have 17% higher mortality rates compared with women in transitioned countries (15.0 and 12.8 per 100,000, respectively) because of high fatality rates, with the highest mortality rates found in Melanesia, Western Africa, Micronesia/Polynesia, and the Caribbean (Barbados has the world's highest mortality) [2]. A 5 -year survival variation analysis for breast cancer has now been said to be close to 90% in the US and Australia; while as low as 40% in South Africa according to a CONCORD-3 study of cancer survival in 71 countries [8].

There is thus a need to review the epidemiology of breast cancer in the last decade; examine gaps and proffer recommendations to aid the prevention and control of breast cancer in sub-Saharan Africa.

1.1 The burden of breast cancer in sub-Saharan Africa

Breast cancer is the leading diagnosed cancer and the second most common cause of cancer mortality in sub-Saharan Africa. Sub-Saharan Africa has the highest age-standardized incidence rate of 17.3 per 100,000 women per year, globally; with the Southern Africa region and West African region having the highest age-standardized incidence rate of 38.9 and 38.6 per 100,000 women per year in sub-Saharan Africa, respectively. However, the Northern Africa region has the highest incidence rate of 43.2 ASR incidence in the whole of Africa [3]. Country-specific prevalence shows that there is a 15.3%, 4.6% and 3.3% prevalence of breast cancer in the Central African Republic, Rwanda and Sierra Leone, respectively [9, 10]. Mauritius and Nigeria have been said to be the countries with the highest incidence in Africa at 64.2 and 50.4 ASR incidence per 100,000 repetitively [3].

The 5-year age-standardized relative survival in 12 sub-Saharan African countries was 66% for cases diagnosed during 2008 through 2015, sharply contrasting with 85% to 90% for cases diagnosed in high-income countries from 2010 through 2014 [8]. A multi-country estimate of 3-year survival of breast cancer patients was 50% [95%CI: 48, 53] between 2014 and 2017 [11]. Western African region has the highest mortality rate of 20.1 ASR mortality per 100,000; with central African region having the least mortality rate of 14.9 ASR mortality globally. However, Nigeria has the highest mortality rate in Africa with 25.9 ASR mortality per 100,000 [3]. This is, nonetheless, higher than the world average of 12.9 ASR mortality [3].

Population-specific variations in 3-year mortality rates have also been reported across sub-Saharan Africa; with a survival range of 90% among white women to 56% in black Namibian women; and in South Africa where survival ranges from 76% among mixed-race women to 59% in black women [11]. Country-specific variation in 3-year mortality shows a 44–47% survival rate in Uganda and Zambia compared to the 36% survival rate in Nigeria [11].

The population-specific 5-year survival ASR was as low as 5% [95%CI: 1.9, 11.3] in Uganda (Kyadondo) and as high as 80% [95%CI: 22.2, 96.8] and 93.7% [95%CI: 75.5, 98.5] in Namibia and Mauritius, respectively [12]; comparable to 55% in the US state of Connecticut and 57% in Norway during the late 1940s, 48 3 decades before the introduction of mammography screening and modern therapies [2]. Survival also varies within countries in sub-Saharan Africa. For example, in Zimbabwe 3-year relative survival rate in the capital (Harare) is 56.7% [95%CI: 48.2, 64.6] compared to 21.6% [95%CI: 8.2, 39.8] reported in Bulawayo [12].

These variations can be said to be due to the level of access to early diagnosis and prompt treatment of breast cancer cases across the continent; with up to 22% survival increase in Nigeria, Uganda and Zambia [11]. Further explanation for the variations between countries may also be a result of their level of human development index (HDI). For example, though Mauritius (a country with a very high HDI) has the highest incidence rate of breast cancer in Africa [3]; it also has the highest survival rate compared to Zimbabwe (medium HDI) with a lower survival rate [12]. This shows that though, Mauritius detects more breast cancer patients; most of whom were able to survive beyond the 5-year survival period – which can be due to improved access to prompt diagnosis and early treatment for a better outcome.

Because organized, population-based mammography screening programs may not be cost-effective or feasible in low-resource settings [13], efforts to promote early detection through improved breast cancer awareness and clinical breast examination by skilled health providers [14], followed by timely and appropriate treatment, are essential components to improving survival. A recent study conducted in 5 sub-Saharan African countries estimated that 28% to 37% of breast cancer deaths in these countries could be prevented through an early diagnosis of symptomatic disease and adequate treatment, with a fairly equal contribution of each [11]. The Breast Health Global Initiative has established a series of evidence-based, resource-stratified guidelines that support phased implementation into real-world practice [15].

2. The distribution of breast cancer in sub-Saharan Africa

Globally, while Africa has one of the lowest age-standardized breast cancer incidence rates (36.2 per 100,000 women per year) after Asia (29.1 per 100,000 women per year); it has the highest mortality rate of 17.3 per 100, 000 compared to other regions of the world. However, the mortality rate is highest (20.1 per 100,000 women per year) in the West African sub-region [3]. Majority of breast cancer patients in sub-Saharan Africa are women [16–18]. A recent systematic review reported that 97% [95%CI: 97–98] of all breast cancer cases in Africa are seen in Females [16]. About 18% prevalence has been reported among male Ethiopians; which is likely the highest in the region among breast cancer patients [16]. Oftentimes, many of these breast cancer rates are obtained from institutional-based records or registries across sub-Saharan Africa; with varying reports across the sub-continent.

More than half (58%) of breast cancer patients were diagnosed before the age of 50 [16]. The median and peak ages have also been reported in some studies. The peak age of incidence of 47.8%, 52.5%, 57.4%, 57.5% and 57.9% between the 3rd and 5th decades among patients in Rwanda, Lagos-Nigeria, Southern Ethiopia, Central African Republic and Northwest Amhara regions of Ethiopia, respectively [9, 17, 19–21]. Similar report was observed among breast cancer patients in Adis Ababa Ethiopia with 63.1% at the same peak range [22]. Almost two-thirds of breast cancer patients are below 50 years old in Burkina Faso [23]. Gabretsadik A et al, in a seven-year (2013–2019) review, reported a median age of 38 years among patients in Southern Ethiopia [21]. Ouedraogo SY et al, Balekouzou et al. and Sayed et al. reported a mean age of 45.79 years, 45.85 years, 47.5 years and 47.8% among patients with breast cancer in Burkina Faso, Central African Republic, Kenya and Rwanda [9, 18, 19, 23]. Fatiregun reported a mean age of 49.6 (±11.2) years among breast cancer patients in Lagos, Nigeria [20]. However, a population-based study revealed a much lower average age of 33.4 (± 1.25) in Burkina Faso [24]. This shows that institutional-based studies might present a higher age level compared to the population-based study and give an illusion of higher average age of patties with breast cancer. Thus, studies must indicate the study setting to contextualize the study findings.

It was also observed that the number of cases diagnosed or reported is dependent on the distance of communities from the health facilities offering screening, diagnosis and treatment. For example, Gabretsadik et al. reported a higher number of cases in zones and districts closest to the tertiary hospital in Hawassa city; with the number of cases observed to thin out as the distance increases away from this specialist University hospital. It can be said that, unless a population-based survey is done, the true incidence/prevalence and distribution of breast cancer in communities in sub-Saharan Africa may be unknown and estimates from institutions will be affected by Berksonian Bias [21].

2.1 African trends on breast cancer

Some of the most rapid increases are occurring in sub-Saharan Africa. Between the mid-1990s and the mid-2010s, incidence rates increased by >5% per year in Malawi (Blantyre), Nigeria (Ibadan), and Seychelles and by 3% to 4% per year in South Africa (Eastern Cape and Zimbabwe (Harare) [25]. Between 2008 and 2012, East Africa experienced the largest incidence rate increase of 36.5% from 19.30 ASR in 2008 incidence to 30.4 ASR in 2012. However, the incidence remains highest in the North African region at 43.2 ASR; with southern Africa having the lowest increase of 2% from 38.2 ASR incidence in 2008 to 38.9 ASR incidence in 2012 [3]. In southern Ethiopia, there has been an increasing incidence of breast cancer between 2013 and 2019 according to institutional records. It has increased from 12.3% in 2013 to 19.0% in 2019 [21]. Nigeria has continuously shown increases in incident rates from 13.7 ASR between 1960 and 1969 to 50.4 ASR between 2000 and 2012 and has been projected to 84.2 ASR between 2013 and 2050 [3]. In Central African Republic, the average prevalence rate has been on the increase; with breast cancer prevalence just above 10% in 2003 and just above 15% in 2015 among breast cancer patients; after dropping from 20% in 2014 [9].

Mortality rates in sub-Saharan African regions have increased simultaneously and rank now the world's highest, reflecting weak health infrastructure and subsequently poor survival outcomes. Between the same periods, East Africa also showed the largest increase of 26% mortality from 11.4 ASR in 2008 to 15.6 ASR in 2012. Southern Africa has the least mortality rate reduction of 24.5%; with a reduction from 19.3 ASR mortality in 2008 to 15.5 ASR mortality in 2012 [3]. This has been said to be due to the human development index of the country and stage at diagnosis. For example, low HDI (HR: 2.3 [95%CI: 1.4, 3.7]; $p = 0.001$) and medium HDI (HR: 1.9 [95%CI: 1.2, 3.1]; $p = 0.01$) countries are more likely to have higher odds of breast cancer-related mortality compared to African HDI countries. Patients in late stages at presentation have higher odds (HR: 2.5 [95%CI: 1.8, 3.3]; $p < 0.001$) of breast cancer-related deaths compared to those who presented at the early stage of the disease [12].

2.2 Determinants/risk factors of breast cancer reported in the last decade

Various factors have been associated with the development of breast malignancies across sub-Saharan Africa in the last decade. Body size has been associated with the development of breast cancer. A recent study from Ghana, by Brighton LA et al, reported that increasing body size increased the likelihood of breast cancer (slightly heavy body size – OR: 1.30 [95%CI: 1.04, 1.62] and heavy body size – OR: 1.50 [95%CI: 1.11, 2.02]) among patients with suspicious lesions of breast cancer [5]. Level of education has also been associated with the development of breast cancer among Populations in the region. The higher the level of education, the higher the likelihood of the development of breast cancer. Also from the same Ghanaian study, those with at least secondary school education (more than basic education) are significantly more likely to develop breast cancer compared to those without formal education.

(OR:1.50 [95%CI: 1.21, 1.87]; $p < 0.01$) [5]. The number of births has also been said to reduce the likelihood of breast cancer. multiparous women (at least 5 orders) are significantly less likely to develop breast cancer compared to nulliparous Ghanaian patients (parity ≥5 - OR: 0.71 [95%CI: 0.52,0.97]; $p < 0.01$) [5].

3. Types of breast cancer

These are often obtained from clinical, histopathological and genomic diagnoses. Availability and accessibility of these are, however, varying in sub-Saharan Africa. This had affected presentation, reportage, early screening and diagnosis and treatment of breast cancer in the region. In many countries, breast cancer is still commonly confirmed by histology (85%); and 6% cytological confirmed; while 9% were clinically confirmed in many sub-Saharan African countries [11]. Fine needle aspiration (FNAC) and biopsy remain the commonly reported means of diagnosis; as it stands at 60% and 37.9%, respectively in Ethiopia [21].

About half (52.5%) of all suspicious breast lesions have been reported to be malignant; with 36% being benign conditions in some African populations [5]. Invasive ductal cancers appear to be the commonest among African populations accounting for more than half of all reported breast cancers [9, 17–19, 21]. This is congruent with globally reported histological type reported globally; which has been reported to be 40–80% [7]. It ranges between 55.3% in Southern Ethiopia and 84.2% in Kenya [18, 21]. Tumor behavior reported includes moderately differentiated in 31.7% of cases and poorly differentiated in 27.7% of cases in Southern Ethiopia. Only 13.6% were reported to be well-differentiated among Ethiopian patients [21].

Molecularly, BRACA 1 and BRAC 2 remains the commonest molecular gene for breast cancer in African populations. Each accounts for 5.6%, respectively, in sub-Saharan Africa the populations. Other reported genes include ATM (1.5%), PALB2 (1%), BARD1 (0.5%), CDHI (0.5%) and TP53 (0.5%) [26]. This is in line with the global commonly reported genes of 45–87% of BRACA 1, and 50–85% for BRACA 2 [7]. Novel variants of these genes have been reported to predominate in certain sub-Saharan African regions. This includes the PIK3CA genes and the TP53 genes; which account for 39.09% and 12.78%, respectively in Burkina Faso [23].

Most cases of breast cancer in the last decade have presented with unilaterally located left breast cancer across sub-Saharan Africa [9, 16, 19, 21, 27]. The highest prevalence of bilateral breast cancer was reported at 8% [95%CI: 6, 12] in Nigeria [16]. Country-specific prevalence of left breast cancer has been reported across the sub-region. For example, Gabretsadik A et al. and Kramer and Colleagues; Ouedrago SY et al. and Uyisenga JP et al. reported that 54%, 52.2%, 51% and 50% of most breast cancer cases are on the left breast among Southern Ethiopian, Rwanda, South African patients and Burkinabe patients [19, 21, 23, 27]. Balekouzou A et al. reported that the left breast is more commonly affected compared the right (12% versus 4%, respectively) among patients in Central African Republic [9].

4. Common breast cancer outcomes

Krammer et al. reported that 75% of patients reported the presence of any pain or disability while only 9% experienced severe pain and disability among South African patients [27]. It was further reported that the presence of the tumor on the right side (OR: 0.31 [95%CI: 0.10, 1.03];p < 0.05); being a Caucasian (OR: 0.21 [95%CI: 0.05, 0.82]; p < 0.05); not being on chemotherapy (OR: 0.39 [95%CI: 0.18, 0.83]; p < 0.05); had axillary lymph node dissection (OR: 0.48 [0.23, 0.98]; p < 0.05) and older age (OR: 0.93 [95%CI: 0.93, 0.98];p < 0.01) are significantly less likely to report cancer-related pains compared to others of differing corresponding attributes [27]. Also, reported is that those not on chemotherapy are significantly less likely to experience disabilities compared to those treated with chemotherapy (OR: 0.37 [95%CI: 0.18, 0.77]; p < 0.01) [27].

It was also reported that 36.6% of South Africans with breast cancer in the Western Cape have depression [28]. However, a lower prevalence of depression (25%) was reported similar population in Addis Ababa, Ethiopia [22]. This has been said to be due to body change stress; in which a higher body change stress significantly predicts depression ($\beta = 0.38$; $p = 00$) among breast cancer patients [28]. It has also been said to be due to perceived social support; in which a lower perceived social significantly predicts depression ($\beta = -0.30$; $p = 0.01$) among breast cancer patients [28].

Also reported is 34.3% psychological distress among South African patients with breast cancer [28]. This has been said to be due to body change stress; with a higher body change stress significantly associated with higher psychological distress ($\beta = 0.37$; $p = 0.00$) [28]. It has also been said to be due to perceived social support; with lower perceived social support significantly associated with higher psychological distress ($\beta = -0.27$; $p = 0.02$) among breast cancer patients [28].

Anxiety disorders were also reported as outcomes of breast cancer among patients in sub-Saharan Africa in the sources reviewed over the last decade. For example, Fatiregun OO et al. reported that 19% of breast cancer patients have anxiety disorders; with mixed anxiety and depressive disorder accounting for 44.7%. Predictors for anxiety disorder among this population include the absence of a history of breast cancer (OR: 3.5 [95%CI: 1.2, 7.0];p = 0.006) and early stage of breast cancer (OR: 1.56 [95%CI: 1.12, 2.17]; p = 0.009) [20].

Almost three-quarters (71.03%) of patients with breast cancer have drug-related problems among patients with breast cancer in Gondar, Ethiopia: with 48.6% reporting adverse drug reactions, with 45.8% need for additional drug therapy and 32.7% non-adherence [17]. Comorbidity and the non-use of neoadjuvant chemotherapy have been associated with the development of drug problems among breast cancer patients. Degu A and Kebede K reported that those with comorbidity are three times more likely to develop drug-related problems compared to those who do not have comorbidities among breast cancer patients in Gondar, Ethiopia [17]. Those on neoadjuvant are significantly less likely to have drug-related problems compared to those on other regimens [17].

5. Preventive behaviors and factors associated

5.1 Late and delayed presentation

Most patients often present at a late stage during the course of the disease; with two-thirds (67%) of all African patients presenting at the advanced stage of breast cancer; albeit, 50% seen at stage 3 and 17% seen at stage 4. The highest level of advanced or late presentation is in West Africa; which stands at 67% [16]. A close estimate of a multi-country study of 8 sub-Saharan countries reported an overall late-stage presentation of 64.8%; with the highest (91.7%) among the countries studied being reported in Harare-Zimbabwe and the lowest (42.6%) reported in Seychelles [12]. Similar report has been reported from cancer registries across Africa; and 18% of which are already metastatic at the time of diagnosis. (Joko-Fu WY et al, 2020) Other estimates have reported that 77% of all staged cases were stage III/IV at diagnosis [29]. In Southern Ethiopia, 66.5% of all diagnoses were made at advanced stages (3 and 4) of the disease [21]. Among patients with breast cancer in Rwanda, the diagnosis was made in about half (52.9%) at stage 3 [19]. In Kenya, almost two-thirds (61.6%) of breast cancer patients have stages 3 and 4 when the diagnosis was made [18]. In Lagos-Nigeria and Addis Ababa-Ethiopia, about half (54% and 51.9%, respectively) of the diagnosis was made at stages 3 and 4 among similar patients [20, 22]. However, half (51.7%) of patients have their diagnosis made at stage 2 in Western Cape, South Africa [28]. In contrast, only 19.48% of breast cancer cases were diagnosed at stage 3 among patients in Cape Town, South Africa [27].

The delayed presentation was also reported in the reviewed literature. Only 25% presented within the first 3 months, and 30% within 1 year, of the onset of symptoms among breast cancer patients in Khartoum-Sudan [30]. In the Central African Republic, only 30% presented within the first year of the onset of symptoms among breast cancer patients in Khartoum-Sudan [9]. Also, in Sierra Leone and Rwanda, 66.7% and 88.6% respectively, presented after 12 months among participants in population-based surveys [10].

Many factors have been said to be responsible for delayed or late presentation for screening and treatment for breast cancer among sub-Saharan African populations. A prior diagnosis of breast cancer has been shown to increase the odds of delayed presentation; with those diagnosed within at least 3 months with higher odds of late presentation compared to those diagnosed more recently (3–12 months – OR: 9.6 [95%CI: 9.55, 9.75]; $p < 0.00$ and >12 months –OR: 9.3 [95%CI: 9.33, 9.33]; $p < 0.00$) among breast cancer patients in Khartoum, Sudan. The fear of mastectomy/chemotherapy is the commonest reason for delays among Sudanese breast cancer patients [30].

5.2 Non-presentation and use of traditional healers

About 43% and 26.7% of Burkinabe women either do nothing or visit traditional healers, respectively, about their breast-related conditions. Medical advice is only sought in 30% of the cases [24].

5.3 Low utilization of screening services

Early diagnosis has been said to improve survival; with a 3-year relative survival of 78% (95%CI: 71.6–83.3) among those diagnosed at the early stages of cancer compared with 40.3% (95%CI: 34.9–45.7) relative survival when the diagnosis is made at advanced (III and IV) stages of the disease [12]. However, the use of mammography and other screening modalities is very low in sub-Saharan Africa for screening and aiding the diagnosis of breast cancer. This hovers between 3.61% of community-based Ghanaian women and a quarter (23.7%) screening level among community-based women of reproductive age in Namibia.[3132] Other levels of utilization between these two ends include 5.2% breast cancer screening in the Ivory coast [31]; with 13.4% mammography screening among the south African general women population [32]; mammography screening of 15.5% among older women in South Africa [33]; and 18.6% mammography screening rate among patients in Southern Ethiopia [21].

Several factors have been found to explain the limited use of mammography services. This includes ethnicity, age, level of education, marital status, residence, type of employer, country of residence, wealth index, number of living children, possession of household items of worth, health insurance coverage, level of physical activity and presence of chronic diseases and regular visitation of health facility [31].

Older age is a strong predictor of mammography screening among African women. Phaswana-Mafuya N and Peltzer K reported that older middle-aged (40–49 years) and elderly (60–69 years) significantly increases the likelihood of mammography screening compared to the early middle ages (30–39 years) among South African women; and likelihood increases with age among this population (40–49 years – OR: 2.39 [95%CI: 1.54, 3.69] and 60–69 years – OR: 2.70 [95%CI: 2.70, 8.10]; $p < 0.001$) [32]. Also, Older women of the reproductive age group (25–49 years) are significantly more likely to access breast cancer screening compared to younger women of the reproductive age group (35–49 years – OR: 1.73 [95%CI: 1.56, 1.91]; $p < 0.001$; 25–34 years – OR: 1.41 [95%CI: 1.29, 1.54]; $p < 0.001$) [31]. However, Calys-Tagoe BNL et al. reported that older age is a negative predictor of mammography use. Those that are at least 70 years are significantly less likely to have used mammography screening services compared to younger women in Ghana (≥ 70 years – OR: 0.42 [95%CI: 0.19, 0.93]; $p < 0.05$) [34].

Also, Ethic group has been said to be an important index of access to mammography services. Calys-Tagoe BNL et al. reported that those of the majority ethnic group are significantly more likely to use mammography services compared to other ethnic groups among Ghanaian women (Akan – OR: 3.41 [95%CI: 1.88, 6.16]; $p < 0.001$) [34]. This was corroborated by Phaswana-Mafuya N and Peltzer K reported that whites, colored and Asian south Africans were significantly more likely to have mammography services compared to black South African women; with whites having the highest odds of mammography access (whites – OR: 5.06 [95%CI: 3.36, 7.60]; colored – OR: 2.87 [95%CI: 1.87, 4.41] and Indian/Asian 2.52 [95%CI: 1.47, 4.32]) [32]. Further insight was provided by Pelztzer K and Phaswana-Mafuya N as they reported that older adult white ad Indian/Asian adult women are significantly more likely to have used mammography compared to older adult Black South African women. (Asian/Indian – OR: 4.08 [95%CI: 1.71, 9.71]; $p < 0.01$; whites - OR: 3.33 [95%CI: 1.54,7.19]; $p < 0.01$) [33]. In this wise, Asian/Indians have higher odds compared to whites which might have been due to the variation in the availability of social support as this demography of south Africans with the highest access to mammography services aged.

An increasing level of education has been said to increase the odds of mammography screening among Sub-Saharan African populations. Phaswana-Mafuya N and Peltzer K reported that south African women with at least grade 8 were reported to be significantly more likely to access mammography services compared to grades 0–7 (grade 8 – OR: 2.25 [95%CI: 1.34, 3.78; $p < 0.01$; grade ≥ 12 – OR: 2.72 [95%CI: 1.55, 4.77]; $p < 0.001$) [32]. In fact, Pelztzer K and Phaswana-Mafuya N reported that any level of access to education is a strong predictor of mammography use among older adult south African women compared to those with no formal education. (primary education – OR: 2.76 [95%CI: 2.31, 5.85]; $p < 0.01$; at least secondary education – OR: 3.81 [95%CI: 1.88, 7.74]; $p < 0.001$) [33]. Sub-Saharan Africans with at least a formal education are significantly more likely to do breast cancer screening compared to those with no formal education, and the odds of breast cancer screening increase with the level of education. (Primary – OR: 1.77 [95%CI: 1.56, 2.01]; $p < 0.01$; at least secondary – OR: 2.33 [95%CI: 2.05,2.66]; $p < 0.001$) [31].

Ever being in a partnered relationship is a significant predictor of breast cancer screening among African populations compared to single African populations (married/living with partner – OR: 1.13 [95%CI: 1.04, 1.22]; $p = 0.003$; widow/divorce/separated – OR: 1.15 [95%CI: 1.03, 1.28]; $p = 0.01$) [31].

Country of residence is a significant determinant of mammography services use among African populations. Namibians, Burkinabe and Kenyans are significantly more likely to use mammography services compared to Ivoirians; with Namibians having the highest odds of breast cancer screening among the studied African countries (Namibia – OR: 3.3 [95%CI: 2.90, 3.83]; $p < 0.001$; Burkina Faso – OR: 1.58 [95%CI: 1.32, 1.89]; $p < 0.001$; Kenya – OR: 1.92 [95%CI: 1.67, 2.21]; $p < 0.001$) [31].

Place of residence has been shown to determine the use of mammography services among African populations. Phaswana-Mafuya N and Peltzer K reported that rural informal residents are significantly less likely to have used mammography services compared to urban formal dwelling South African women. (Rural informal – OR: 0.40 [95%CI: 0.24, 0.72]; $p < 0.01$) [32].

Employment status is also a significant predictor of mammography utilization. Ghanaian women who are self-employed and those in the informal sectors are less likely to use mammography services compared to others in the civil service (self-employed – OR: 0.21 [95%CI: 0.11, 0.42]; $p < 0.000$; informal - OR: 0.26 [95%CI: 0.12, 0.57]; $p < 0.001$) [34].

Possession of household items of worth has also been said to determine breast cancer screening. Possession of television was reported to increase the likelihood of breast cancer screening among African populations compared to those who do not (possession of TV – OR: 1.17 [95%CI: 1.08, 1.27]; $p < 0.001$) [31].

Socioeconomic status has been said to be a significant predictor of mammography services utilization. Pelztzer K and Phaswana-Mafuya N reported that south African older adult women with a high wealth index are twice more likely to use mammography services compared to those with a low wealth index (high wealth index – OR: 2.18 [95%CI: 1.00, 4.76]; $p < 0.05$) [33].

Lifestyle behaviors have also been an important determinant of the use of mammography services. Phaswana-Mafuya N and Peltzer K reported that south African women who reported moderate-vigorous physical activity significantly have higher odds of mammography services utilization compared to the physically inactive south African women (moderate-vigorous physical activity – OR: 1.55 [95%CI: 1.12; 2.13]; $p < 0.01$) [32].

The presence of chronic diseases has also been said to be a strong predictor of mammography service use. South African women with chronic diseases are significantly more likely to use mammography services compared to those with none (at least one chronic disease – OR: 1.49 [95%CI: 1.08, 2.05]; $p < 0.05$) [32]. Similar outcomes were reported among older South African women by the same authors (at least 2 chronic conditions – OR: 1.92 [95%CI: 1.01, 3.63]) [33].

Access to medical aid has also been said to be a strong predictor of mammography services use. South African women with medical aid were twice significantly more likely to use mammography services compared to south African women who have no medical aid [32]. This was further corroborated by the same authors among Older south African women; where older south African women with health insurance are twice significantly more likely to use mammography services compared to those who are not covered by health insurance (health insurance – OR: 2.71 [95%CI: 1.57, 4.66]; $p < 0.001$) [33].

Health facility visitation has also been said to be associated with breast cancer screening among women of reproductive age group; with those who frequently visited health facilities reporting higher odds of mammography services use compared with those who do not (OR: 1.37 [95%CI: 1.28, 1.45]; $p < 0.001$) [31].

6. Common modalities of treatment

Traditionally, breast cancer is commonly treated through chemotherapy, immunotherapy, hormonal therapy, biological therapy, radiotherapy and surgery [7]. Reported modalities of treatment in the last decade reported that chemotherapy, hormonal therapy and surgery remain the mainstay of management in many settings in sub-Saharan Africa in the last decade. Overall, breast cancer patients had surgery; with an overall mastectomy prevalence of 71% [95%CI: 51, 88]; with beast conserving surgery at 1% [95%CI: 0–2]. Chemotherapy was used in the treatment of 83% [95%CI: 64, 96]; and 77% received hormonal therapy for their treatments in the region [16]. However, country-specific treatment modalities have been reported at varying rates and types across sub-Saharan Africa.

Gabretsadik reported the use of chemotherapy, surgery and hormonal therapy in southern Ethiopia; where Doxorubicin, cyclophosphamide and paclitaxel every 3 weeks for 8 cycles are used for the treatment of stage 1–3) was reported in 59% of cases; doxorubicin and cyclophosphamide every 3 weeks for 6 cycles was reported in 41% of cases and modified radical mastectomy was reported in 35.1% of cases [21]. Also, hormonal therapy has been reported for premenopausal men and women; in which Tamoxifen use was reported in 76.7% of cases. For hormonal therapy for post-menopausal women in which anastrozole after surgery has been reported in 23.3% of cases. Chemotherapy alone, chemotherapy plus surgery and chemotherapy, surgery and hormonal therapy are reported in 65%, 20% and 35%, respectively [21].

Degu A and Kebede K reported different regimens used in the management of breast cancer patients in Gondar, Ethiopia. The commonest regimen was an Adriamycin-Cyclophosphamide combination (Adjuvant and Neoadjuvant, 43% and 22% respectively) and Tamoxifen (Adjuvant and Neoadjuvant, 30% and 8%, respectively) [17].

Kramer and colleagues reported the use of modified radical mastectomy surgery among 73.35% of patients; Axillary lymph node dissection in 78.23%; chemotherapy in 72.78%; hormonal therapy in 70.49% of cases and radiotherapy in 63.32% of cases. Similarly, different combinations of these modalities of treatment were also reported: wide local excision and radiotherapy in 95.24%; modified radical mastectomy and chemotherapy in 88.44% of cases; wide local excision and chemotherapy in 78.85% of cases and modified radical mastectomy and radiotherapy in 57.65% of cases among south African patients [27]. Similarly higher utilization rates of different modalities have been reported from the Central African Republic; where it was reported that 95.4% had surgery; and 91.4% having had chemotherapy and a lower 30.4% having had radiotherapy in the course of breast cancer treatments among patients [9].

Almost similar modalities of treatment were reported among Patients in Burkina Faso where 72.9% and 74.4% had chemotherapy and surgery, respectively. However, a lower proportion (28.6%) of these patients had radiotherapy [23]. Similar reports were observed in Addis Ababa-Ethiopia, where 83.9% had chemotherapy, and 88.1% had had surgery; with 7.9% and 11.4%, having had radiotherapy and hormonal therapy, respectively [22]. Lower utilization has however been reported in Lagos-Nigeria where 50% had chemotherapy; 28.5% have had a combination of chemotherapy and surgery; with 12.5% have had chemotherapy and radiotherapy, and 9.0% had radiotherapy only [20].

7. Strategies to prevent the growing burden of NCDs in sub-Saharan Africa

Establishing primary prevention programs for breast cancer remains a challenge. Nevertheless, efforts to decrease excess body weight and alcohol consumption and to encourage physical activity and breastfeeding may have an impact on stemming the incidence of breast cancer worldwide. Population-wide breast cancer screening programs aim to reduce breast cancer mortality through early detection and effective treatment [2]. Reports have indicated that women who participated in breast cancer screening programs have a lower risk of dying from breast cancer compared with the corresponding risk from nonparticipants [2, 35].

There should be early diagnosis and prompt treatment to prevent and control breast cancer globally, specifically in sub-Saharan Africa. The WHO recommends organized, population-based mammography screening every 2 years for women at average risk for breast cancer aged 50 to 69 years in well-resourced settings [13]. The American cancer society (ACS) recommends that generally, women should have the opportunity to begin yearly screening for women between 40 and 44 years. This should continue as long as they are in good health and have a life expectancy of at least 10 years. ACS strongly recommends that women with an average risk of breast cancer should begin mammography screening beginning at age 45. Those between 45 and 54 years should be screened annually and those at least 55 years should be screened biennially or whenever an opportunity comes up [36]. Clinical breast examination is not directly effective in reducing breast cancer mortality among average-risk women at any age according to guidelines and recent systematic reviews [14, 36].

Mammographic screening, however, has limitations, such as overdiagnosis and overtreatment [2, 37, 38]. There are opportunities to improve the cost-effectiveness and benefit-to-harm ratio of screening by adopting a risk-stratified screening strategy using existing and evolving risk prediction models [2, 37]. Therefore offering breast cancer only to women with higher risk can improve the cost-effectiveness of screening, maintains the benefits and reduce overdiagnosis [37]. Ongoing screening trials are evaluating the clinical acceptability, cost and utility of risk-stratified screening programs in the general population [2, 39, 40].

The establishment and funding of cancer registries is a veritable tool in the prevention and control of breast cancer in sub-Saharan Africa as it can generate recent, accurate data on the incidence, survival, treatment and outcomes in nations/populations hosting such registries [41, 42]; as revealed in some reports reviewed in this update [8, 12, 25]. Though there are cancer registries in only 54% of the 46 countries in sub-Saharan Africa; improved budgeting and infrastructure will improve the availability of data on cancer diagnosis, treatment, follow-up and survival [41, 43]; which can help in the estimation of cancer burden in sub-Saharan Africa and improve the policy and practice of the national cancer control programs which can improve the healthcare for patients with breast cancer in the years to come [41]. However, due to resource constraints in many countries of sub-Saharan Africa, hospital-based cancer registries can be established which can be a source of information on breast cancer (and other cancers) for the population-based cancer registries [43].

Finally, there is a need to ameliorate the financial burden of cancer prevention and care in sub-Saharan Africa; especially among the high-risk population and the vulnerable [42]. This is because the majority of healthcare financing in sub-Saharan Africa is out-of-pocket which places catastrophic healthcare expenditure on patients and caregivers [44, 45]. There is therefore the need increase include cancer screening and care in universal healthcare programs and policies of governments in sub-Saharan Africa [42].

8. Conclusion

Breast cancer has increasingly become a disease of global public health importance, and in particular in sub-Saharan Africa. It has been projected to increase to over 3 million by the year 2040. This might have been due to improved detection rates, awareness, and treatments globally; especially in higher-income countries. There appears to be an intra- and inter-country variation in breast cancer detection rates and mortality in sub-Saharan Africa. BRACA genes still appear to be commonly reported; though, some populations have commonly reported novel genes more than the former genes. Better organized screening programs, the establishment of a well-functioning cancer registry, and improved access and utilization of mammography and treatment services in resource-constrained regions can improve early presentation, reduce adverse breast cancer-related outcomes (including mortality) and help reduce future sub-Saharan African burden of breast Africa and the world.

Author details

Philip Adewale Adeoye
Department of Community Medicine, Jos University Teaching Hospital, Jos, Plateau State, Nigeria

*Address all correspondence to: philipadeoye@gmail.com

References

[1] Arnold M, Morgan E, Rumgay H, Mafra A, Singh D, Laversanne M, et al. Current and future burden of breast cancer: Global statistics for 2020 and 2040. Breast. 2022;**66**:15-23. Available from: https://www.ncbi.nlm.nih.gov/pmc/articles/PMC9465273/pdf/main.pdf

[2] Sung H, Ferlay J, Siegel RL, Laversanne M, Soerjomataram I, Jemal A, et al. Global Cancer Statistics 2020: GLOBOCAN estimates of incidence and mortality worldwide for 36 cancers in 185 countries. CA: A Cancer Journal for Clinicians. 2021;**71**(3):209-249. DOI: 10.3322/caac.21660

[3] Azubuike SO, Muirhead C, Hayes L, McNally R. Rising global burden of breast cancer: The case of sub-Saharan Africa (with emphasis on Nigeria) and implications for regional development: A review. World Journal of Surgical Oncology. 2018;**16**(1):63. Available from: https://www.ncbi.nlm.nih.gov/pmc/articles/PMC5863808/pdf/12957_2018_Article_1345.pdf

[4] Metcalfe KA, Poll A, Royer R, Llacuachaqui M, Tulman A, Sun P, et al. Screening for founder mutations in BRCA1 and BRCA2 in unselected Jewish women. Journal of Clinical Oncology. 2010;**28**(3):387-391. DOI: 10.1200/jco.2009.25.0712

[5] Brinton LA, Gaudet MM, Gierach GL. Breast cancer. In: Thun M, Linet MS, Cerhan JR, Haiman CA, Schottenfeld D, editors. Cancer Epidemiology and Prevention. 4th ed. New York: Oxford University Press; 2017. pp. 861-888. Available from: https://academic.oup.com/book/25326/chapter-abstract/192394313?redirectedFrom=fulltext

[6] Momenimovahed Z, Salehiniya H. Epidemiological characteristics of and risk factors for breast cancer in the world. Breast Cancer. 2019;**11**:151-164. Available from: https://www.ncbi.nlm.nih.gov/pmc/articles/PMC6462164/pdf/bctt-11-151.pdf

[7] Łukasiewicz S, Czeczelewski M, Forma A, Baj J, Sitarz R, Stanisławek A. Breast cancer-epidemiology, risk factors, classification, prognostic markers, and current treatment strategies-An updated review. Cancers. 2021;**13**:4287. Available from: https://www.ncbi.nlm.nih.gov/pmc/articles/PMC8428369/pdf/cancers-13-04287.pdf

[8] Allemani C, Matsuda T, Di Carlo V, Harewood R, Matz M, Nikšić M, et al. Global surveillance of trends in cancer survival 2000-14 (CONCORD-3): Analysis of individual records for 37 513 025 patients diagnosed with one of 18 cancers from 322 population-based registries in 71 countries. Lancet (London, England). 2018;**391**(10125):1023-1075. Available from: https://www.ncbi.nlm.nih.gov/pmc/articles/PMC5879496/pdf/nihms940842.pdf

[9] Balekouzou A, Yin P, Pamatika CM, Bishwajit G, Nambei SW, Djeintote M, et al. Epidemiology of breast cancer: Retrospective study in the Central African Republic. BMC Public Health. 2016;**16**(1):1230. Available from: https://www.ncbi.nlm.nih.gov/pmc/articles/PMC5142143/pdf/12889_2016_Article_3863.pdf

[10] Ntirenganya F, Petroze RT, Kamara TB, Groen RS, Kushner AL, Kyamanywa P, et al. Prevalence of breast masses and barriers to care: Results from a population-based survey in Rwanda

and Sierra Leone. Journal of Surgical Oncology. 2014;**110**(8):903-906. DOI: 10.1002/jso.23726

[11] McCormack V, McKenzie F, Foerster M, Zietsman A, Galukande M, Adisa C, et al. Breast cancer survival and survival gap apportionment in sub-Saharan Africa (ABC-DO): A prospective cohort study. The Lancet Global Health. 2020;**8**(9):e1203-e1212. Available from: https://www.ncbi.nlm.nih.gov/pmc/articles/PMC7450275/?report=printable

[12] Joko-Fru WY, Miranda-Filho A, Soerjomataram I, Egue M, Akele-Akpo M-T, et al. Breast cancer survival in sub-Saharan Africa by age, stage at diagnosis and human development index: A population-based registry study. International Journal of Cancer. 2020;**146**(5):1208-1218. Available from: https://www.ncbi.nlm.nih.gov/pmc/articles/PMC7079125/pdf/IJC-146-1208.pdf

[13] World Health Organization. WHO Position Paper on Mammography Screening. Geneva: World Health Organization; 2014. p. 82. DOI: 10665/137339/?sequence=1

[14] Ngan TT, Nguyen NTQ, Van Minh H, Donnelly M, O'Neill C. Effectiveness of clinical breast examination as a "stand-alone" screening modality: An overview of systematic reviews. BMC Cancer. 2020;**20**(1):1070. Available from: https://www.ncbi.nlm.nih.gov/pmc/articles/PMC7653771/pdf/12885_2020_Article_7521.pdf

[15] Duggan C, Dvaladze A, Rositch AF, Ginsburg O, Yip C-H, Horton S, et al. The Breast Health Global Initiative 2018 Global Summit on Improving Breast Healthcare Through Resource-Stratified Phased Implementation: Methods and overview. Cancer. 2020;**126**(10):2339-2352. Available from: https://www.ncbi.nlm.nih.gov/pmc/articles/PMC7482869/pdf/nihms-1584159.pdf

[16] Olayide A, Isiaka A, Ganiyu R, Samuel O, Halimat A, Julius O, et al. Demographic pattern, tumor size and stage of breast cancer in africa: A meta-analysis. Asian Pacific J Cancer Care. 2021;**6**(4):477-492. Available from: http://waocp.com/journal/index.php/apjcc/article/view/711/1831

[17] Degu A, Kebede K. Drug-related problems and its associated factors among breast cancer patients at the University of Gondar Comprehensive Specialized Hospital, Ethiopia: A hospital-based retrospective cross-sectional study. Journal of Oncology. 2021;**27**(1):88-98

[18] Sayed S, Moloo Z, Wasike R, Bird P, Oigara R, Govender D, et al. Is breast cancer from Sub Saharan Africa truly receptor poor? Prevalence of ER/PR/HER2 in breast cancer from Kenya. Breast. 2014;**23**(5):591-596. Available from: https://www.thebreastonline.com/action/showPdf?pii=S0960-9776%2814%2900116-7

[19] Uyisenga JP, Butera Y, Debit A, Josse C, Ainhoa CC, Karinganire E, et al. Prevalence of histological characteristics of breast cancer in rwanda in relation to age and tumor stages. Horm Cancer. 2020;**11**(5-6):240-249. DOI: 10.1007/s12672-020-00393-3.pdf

[20] Fatiregun OA, Olagunju AT, Erinfolami AR, Fatiregun OA, Arogunmati OA, Adeyemi JD. Anxiety disorders in breast cancer: Prevalence, types, and determinants. Journal of Psychosocial Oncology. 2016;**34**(5):432-447. DOI: 10.1177/1078155220914710

[21] Gebretsadik A, Bogale N, Negera DG. Epidemiological trends of breast cancer in Southern Ethiopia:

A Seven-Year Retrospective Review. Cancer Control. 2021;**28**:1073. DOI: 10.1177_10732748211055262.pdf

[22] Wondimagegnehu A, Abebe W, Abraha A, Teferra S. Depression and social support among breast cancer patients in Addis Ababa, Ethiopia. BMC Cancer. 2019;**19**(1):836. Available from: https://www.ncbi.nlm.nih.gov/pmc/articles/PMC6712811/pdf/12885_2019_Article_6007.pdf

[23] Ouedraogo SY, Zoure AA, Zeye MMJ, Kiendrebeogo TI, Zhou X, Sawadogo AY, et al. BRCA1, BRCA2, TP53, PIK3CA, PTEN and AKT1 genes mutations in Burkina Faso breast cancer patients: Prevalence, spectrum and novel variant. Molecular Genetics and Genomics. 2022;**297**(5):1257-1268. Available from: https://www.researchgate.net/profile/Moutanou-Modeste-Judes-Zeye/publication/361477823_BRCA1_BRCA2_TP53_PIK3CA_PTEN_and_AKT1_genes_mutations_in_Burkina_Faso_breast_cancer_patients_prevalence_spectrum_and_novel_variant/links/62b3fefadc817901fc74b747/BRCA1-

[24] Ströbele L, Kantelhardt EJ, Traoré Millogo TFD, Sarigda M, Wacker J, Grosse Frie K. Prevalence of breast-related symptoms, health care seeking behaviour and diagnostic needs among women in Burkina Faso. BMC Public Health. 2018;**18**(1):447. Available from: https://www.ncbi.nlm.nih.gov/pmc/articles/PMC5883529/pdf/12889_2018_Article_5360.pdf

[25] Joko-Fru WY, Jedy-Agba E, Korir A, Ogunbiyi O, Dzamalala CP, Chokunonga E, et al. The evolving epidemic of breast cancer in sub-Saharan Africa: Results from the African Cancer Registry Network. International Journal of Cancer. 2020;**147**(8):2131-2141. DOI: 10.1002/ijc.33014

[26] Adedokun B, Zheng Y, Ndom P, Gakwaya A, Makumbi T, Zhou AY, et al. Prevalence of inherited mutations in breast cancer predisposition genes among women in Uganda and Cameroon. Cancer Epidemiology, Biomarkers & Prevention. 2020;**29**(2):359-367. Available from: https://www.ncbi.nlm.nih.gov/pmc/articles/PMC7007381/pdf/nihms-1546820.pdf

[27] Kramer N, Ramjith J, Shamley D. Prevalence of shoulder morbidity after treatment for breast Cancer in South Africa. Support Care Cancer. 2019;**27**(7):2591-2598. Available from: https://www.academia.edu/download/66880086/thesis_hsf_2018_kramer_nicole.pdf

[28] Kagee A, Roomaney R, Knoll N. Psychosocial predictors of distress and depression among South African breast cancer patients. Psychooncology. 2018;**27**(3):908-914. Available from: https://www.chicom.be/sites/default/files/kagee_et_al-2018-psycho-oncology.pdf

[29] Jedy-Agba E, McCormack V, Adebamowo C, Dos-Santos-Silva I. Stage at diagnosis of breast cancer in sub-Saharan Africa: A systematic review and meta-analysis. The Lancet Global Health. 2016;**4**(12):e923-e935. Available from: https://www.ncbi.nlm.nih.gov/pmc/articles/PMC5708541/pdf/nihms919368.pdf

[30] Salih AM, Alfaki MM, Alam-Elhuda DM, Nouradyem MM. Factors delaying presentation of sudanese breast cancer patients: An analysis using Andersen's Model. Asian Pacific Journal of Cancer Prevention. 2016;**17**(4):2105-2110. Available from: https://koreascience.kr/article/JAKO201621650893947.pdf

[31] Ba DM, Ssentongo P, Agbese E, Yang Y, Cisse R, Diakite B, et al.

Prevalence and determinants of breast cancer screening in four sub-Saharan African countries: A population-based study. BMJ Open. 2020;**10**:e039464. Available from: https://www.ncbi.nlm.nih.gov/pmc/articles/PMC7552834/pdf/bmjopen-2020-039464.pdf

[32] Phaswana-Mafuya N, Peltzer K. Breast and cervical cancer screening prevalence and associated factors among women in the South African General Population. Asian Pacific Journal of Cancer Prevention. 2018;**19**(6):1465-1470. Available from: https://www.ncbi.nlm.nih.gov/pmc/articles/PMC6103566/pdf/APJCP-19-1465.pdf

[33] Peltzer K, Phaswana-Mafuya N. Breast and cervical cancer screening and associated factors among older adult women in South Africa. Asian Pacific Journal of Cancer Prevention. 2014;**15**(6):2473-2476. Available from: http://journal.waocp.org/article_28943_5116620c9c844158e95adfa201f07fe1.pdf

[34] Calys-Tagoe BNL, Aheto JMK, Mensah G, Biritwum RB, Yawson AE. Mammography examination among women aged 40 years or older in Ghana: Evidence from wave 2 of the World Health Organization's study on global AGEing and adult health multicountry longitudinal study. Public Health. 2020;**181**:40-45. DOI: 10.1016/j.puhe.2019.11.022

[35] Tabár L, Dean PB, Chen TH-H, Yen AM-F, Chen SL-S, Fann JC-Y, et al. The incidence of fatal breast cancer measures the increased effectiveness of therapy in women participating in mammography screening. Cancer. 2019;**125**(4):515-523. Available from: https://www.ncbi.nlm.nih.gov/pmc/articles/PMC6588008/pdf/CNCR-125-515.pdf

[36] Oeffinger KC, Fontham ETH, Etzioni R, Herzig A, Michaelson JS, Shih Y-CT, et al. Breast cancer screening for women at average risk: 2015 guideline update from the American Cancer Society. JAMA. 2015;**314**(15):1599-1614. Available from: https://www.ncbi.nlm.nih.gov/pmc/articles/PMC4831582/pdf/nihms775387.pdf

[37] Pashayan N, Morris S, Gilbert FJ, Pharoah PDP. Cost-effectiveness and benefit-to-harm ratio of risk-stratified screening for breast cancer: A Life-Table Model. JAMA Oncology. 2018;**4**(11):1504-1510. Available from: https://www.ncbi.nlm.nih.gov/pmc/articles/PMC6230256/?report=printable

[38] Michalopoulos D, Duffy SW. Estimation of overdiagnosis using short-term trends and lead time estimates uncontaminated by overdiagnosed cases: Results from the Norwegian Breast Screening Programme. Journal of Medical Screening. 2016;**23**(4):192-202. DOI: 10.1177_0969141315623980.pdf

[39] Antoniou A, Anton-Culver H, Borowsky A, Broeders M, Brooks J, Chiarelli A, et al. A response to "Personalised medicine and population health: Breast and ovarian cancer". Human Genetics. 2019;**138**:287-289. Available from: https://www.ncbi.nlm.nih.gov/pmc/articles/PMC8207533/pdf/nihms-1065448.pdf

[40] Gierach GL, Choudhury PP, García-Closas M. Toward risk-stratified breast cancer screening: Considerations for changes in screening guidelines. JAMA Oncology. 2020;**6**:31-33. Available from: https://www.ncbi.nlm.nih.gov/pmc/articles/PMC8170848/pdf/nihms-1703288.pdf

[41] Omonisi AE, Liu B, Parkin DM. Population-based cancer registration in Sub-Saharan Africa: Its role in research and cancer control. JCO Global Oncology. 2020;**6**:1721-1728. Available

from: https://www.ncbi.nlm.nih.gov/pmc/articles/PMC7713579/pdf/GO.20.00294.pdf

[42] Ngwa W, Addai BW, Adewole I, Ainsworth V, Alaro J, Alatise OI, et al. Cancer in sub-Saharan Africa: A Lancet Oncology Commission. The Lancet Oncology. 2022;**23**(6):e251-e312. DOI: 10.1016/S1470-2045(21)00720-8

[43] Curado MP. Importance of hospital cancer registries in Africa. Ecancermedicalscience. 2019;**13**:948. Available from: https://www.ncbi.nlm.nih.gov/pmc/articles/PMC6722112/pdf/can-13-948.pdf

[44] The Lancet Oncology. Strengthening cancer control in Africa gathers momentum. The Lancet Oncology. 2022;**23**(11):1343. Available from: https://www.thelancet.com/action/showPdf?pii=S1470-2045%2822%2900644-1

[45] Songwe V. Strategies for financing Africa's health sector. Brookings—Africa in focus. 2022. Available from: https://www.brookings.edu/blog/africa-in-focus/2022/02/03/strategies-for-financing-africas-health-sector/ [Accessed: November 29, 2022]

Chapter 3

Breast Cancer and Pregnancy: Epidemiology, Phenotypes, Presentation during Pregnancy, and Therapeutic Approaches

Massimiliano Berretta, Oreste Claudio Buonomo, Gianluca Vanni and Bianca Arianna Facchini

Abstract

Breast cancer (BC) represents the most frequent cancer worldwide, with almost 2.26 million new diagnoses recorded in 2020, and is the most common malignant neoplasia diagnosed during pregnancy. Pregnancy-related Breast Cancer (PrBC), indeed, is diagnosed in 1 in 2000–4000 pregnant women every year in Europe. PrBC is frequently characterized by unfavorable biological marks that, along with the late diagnosis, the limited imaging applicable, and the often-suboptimal treatments necessary to protect the fetus, could possibly lead to a worse prognosis in this population of patients. Babies born from mothers treated for cancer during pregnancy have been followed during a long-term follow-up and have showed cognitive and physical functions not different from the general population, but more studies are needed. Taking into consideration the complexity of the disease, a multidisciplinary approach is crucial to define the best therapeutical path.

Keywords: breast, cancer, pregnancy, PrBC, BC

1. Introduction

Breast cancer (BC) represents the most frequent cancer worldwide with almost 2.26 million new diagnoses recorded in 2020. Despite the progress made throughout the years to identify new anticancer drugs aiming to improve BC patients' prognosis, it still represents the first cause of cancer-related death in women [1].

BC represents one of the most frequent cancers in women in their reproductive age, with nearly 7% of all BC being diagnosed under 40 years of age [2].

It is well known that, BC being a frequently hormone-related malignancy, its onset may be induced by a higher exposure to estrogens, as may happen with physiological hormones in early menarche, older age at menopause, first pregnancy after the age of 30 and nulliparity, or with the exposure to external sources of hormones, during hormone replacement therapy or due to oral contraceptives.

Other risk factors are represented by personal and family history of BC, dense breast tissue, and lifestyle-based risk factors [3, 4].

Pregnancy represents a protective factor against BC [5], and even the age of the woman at the first pregnancy seems to play a crucial role in preventing the onset of this disease, pregnancy being considered protective if under 30 years of age [6, 7].

2. Pregnancy-related breast cancer epidemiology

Cancer occurs in around one in 1000 pregnancies, with BC being the most frequent, followed by cervical cancer, lymphoma, ovarian cancer, leukemia, colorectal cancer, and melanoma [8], reflecting cancer epidemiology in women in their reproductive years. In Europe, Pregnancy-related Breast Cancer (PrBC), indeed, is diagnosed in 1 in 2000–4000 pregnant women every year [9], representing approximately 0.2–2.6% of all breast cancer cases, and its incidence is probably bound to increase due to the progressively older age of women at the first pregnancy.

The terms PrBC and Pregnancy-associated breast cancer (PABC) have been used for a long time as synonyms, but a recent, more precise definition has allowed to distinguish the two entities: While PrBC includes only BC cases that are diagnosed during pregnancy, PABC also includes cases of BC diagnosed in the post-partum phase, till 1 year after delivery [10].

Risk factors for PrBC seem to be consistent with the general population, and no specific pregnancy-related risk factors have been identified. Women with BRCA mutations have a higher risk of developing PrBC. As these cancer cases are often diagnosed in particularly young women, genetic counseling should be considered [11, 12].

3. Presentation

Clinical presentation of PrBC is similar to BC in non-pregnant women, the palpation of a mammalian lump frequently being the first symptom. Nipple discharge, cutaneous lesions, or palpable lymph-nodes could also occur. The breast tissue physiological modifications that happen during pregnancy, such as engorgement and increased density, along with the young age of the patient and pregnancy itself, often lead to an underestimation of the symptoms and delayed diagnosis. Indeed, women during pregnancy have a 2.5 higher risk of being diagnosed at a higher stage, causing a worse prognosis [13].

4. Biology

Some studies suggest that PrBC biology has no significant difference from non-pregnant patients' BC [14]. Notwithstanding, the hormonal modifications that occur in a pregnant woman with their growth-promoting effect suggest a possible lead to more aggressive forms of BC [15]. In fact, PrBC seems characterized by a lower expression of hormone receptors, with a higher rate of aggressive forms such as triple-negative or HER2-positive forms [16]. Moreover, several studies have shown that these types of tumors seem to be marked by unfavorable molecular characteristics, for instance, a high expression of cancer targets as PD1/PD-L1, RANK ligand, and IGF, and show a lower prevalence of tumor-infiltrating lymphocytes [17]. A recent study has aimed to identify specific genomic alterations in PrBC, demonstrating through a whole genome sequencing a higher rate of mismatch repair deficiency mutational signature, besides other mutations such as in the mucin gene family [18]. The expression of several other oncogenes could be altered, such as MYC, SRC, FOS, JUN, and KLF1 [19].

These biological marks, along with the late diagnosis, could possibly lead to a worse prognosis in this population of patients, further worsened by the limited staging exams applicable and suboptimal therapies that have to be administered to protect the fetus.

Further studies are needed to clarify the biology of this particular kind of cancer.

5. Diagnosis

Clinical examination represents the first step of the diagnostical process but needs to be always followed by imaging and biopsy. It is well known that ionizing radiations are dangerous during pregnancy due to their teratogen effect on the fetus. This makes the diagnosis and staging more complex, often leading to suboptimal results. **Table 1** summarizes allowed and forbidden diagnostical examinations during pregnancy.

Every breast lump that persists for more than 2 weeks should be investigated, even though around 80% of them result in benign lesions [20].

Breast ultrasound (US) represents the first choice when a mammalian lump during pregnancy is detected, it being non-invasive and safe for the fetus, thanks to the absence of ionizing radiations. It allows, on the one hand, to identify benign lesions that have no need to be studied with further exams and that represent the most common lesions identified during pregnancy and, on the other hand, to detect suspicious lesions that may need a biopsy [21]. US can be used to explore local lymph nodes and identify suspicious nodes that might need fine needle aspiration or biopsy.

Mammography with abdominal shield can be safely administered in these patients at every gestational age [22], but possible limitations related to parenchymal modifications during pregnancy must be considered. Contrast-enhanced breast MRI,

Diagnostical test	1st Trimester	2nd Trimester	3rd Trimester
Breast Ultrasound	✓	✓	✓
Abdomen Ultrasound	✓	✓	✓
*Chest X-Ray**	✓	✓	✓
*Mammography**	✓	✓	✓
Whole body MRI	×	✓**	✓**
Contrast-enhanced breast MRI	×	×	×
CT-scan	×	×	×
PET-scan	×	×	×
Bone scintigraphy	×	×	×
Biopsy	✓	✓	✓

✓ *Allowed;* × *Forbidden; *Abdominal shield must be used; **In selected cases only*

Table 1.
Allowed and forbidden diagnostical examinations in each pregnancy trimester.

instead, should be avoided due to the capacity of gadolinium to cross the hemato-placentar barrier and to the lack of data assessing its safety for the fetus [23]. The combination of mammography and breast US has a high detection rate, comparable to contrast-enhanced breast MRI, which can safely be avoided during pregnancy [24].

When a suspect lesion is identified, biopsy represents the gold standard. The pathologist should always be informed of the pregnancy status to better analyze the biotic sample.

The stage, according to American Joint Committee on Cancer (AJCC), should always be assessed. Abdominal and pelvis ultrasound and chest X-ray with abdominal shield are the first-choice imaging exams during pregnancy, while computed tomography, bone scintigraphy, and PET scan should be avoided due to the higher rate of ionizing radiation [25]. If strictly necessary, diffusion-weighted whole-body MRI without gadolinium might be an option in case of advanced disease or metastases after the first trimester [26].

6. Therapy

Cancer during pregnancy has for a long time been mistreated because of the lack of evidence about the efficacy and safety of the various available treatments in this peculiar population. By now, it is known that it should be treated as BC in non-pregnant women according to the stage and molecular asset, following some precautions to minimize the risks for the fetus (**Table 2**).

6.1 Surgery

Surgery is feasible at any time during pregnancy, considering that the majority of anesthetics has been demonstrated to be safe during pregnancy [27]. However, there is a slight risk of miscarriage, especially in the first trimester [26]. The preferred approach should be decided following the same guidelines for non-pregnant women, preferably after discussion by a multidisciplinary team due to the complexity of the decisions. Seen as though adjuvant radiotherapy must always be postponed after delivery, mastectomy might be discussed with the patient, especially for diagnosis done in the first trimester. Despite the limited data available on the matter, some studies suggest the feasibility and safety of conservative surgery during pregnancy [28]. Patients with PrBC who desire conservative surgery must be informed of the possible higher risk of local recurrence caused by a delay in the adjuvant radiotherapy treatment [29, 30].

Treatment	1st Trimester	2nd Trimester	3rd Trimester
Surgery	✓	✓	✓
Radiotherapy	×	×	×
Chemotherapy	×	✓	✓
Endocrine therapy	×	×	×
Target therapy	×	×	×
Immunotherapy	×*	×*	×*

✓ *Allowed;* × *Forbidden; *Further studies are needed to assess security during pregnancy.*

Table 2.
Allowed and forbidden treatments in the three pregnancy trimesters.

Concomitant breast reconstruction after mastectomy does not seem to increase the mother-fetus morbidity and can be taken into consideration; the physiological breast tissue modifications during and after pregnancy, although, could lead to a delay in the procedure [28]. There is still no univocal approach regarding sentinel lymph node biopsy during pregnancy: On the one hand, American Society of Clinical Oncology (ASCO) does not suggest this procedure [31]; on the other hand, National Comprehensive Cancer Network (NCCN) guidelines and European Society of Medical Oncology (ESMO) support the procedure when considered necessary. Although further studies are needed, the procedure is considered safe for both mother and fetus if Technetium-99 m (99mTc) colloid solution injection is administered [32], preferably using the one-day protocol, injecting the drug in the morning of the surgery day [33]. Due to the high risk of anaphylactic, a potentially life-threatening reaction, blue dye and isosulfan blue should be avoided [34], while methylene blue should be avoided especially in the first trimester because of its teratogenic effect [35].

6.2 Radiotherapy

As stated above, radiotherapy should always be postponed to after delivery because of the several toxicities that can be caused to the fetus during pregnancy, such as intrauterine growth restriction, mental retardation, risk of childhood cancer, and fetal death [26].

6.3 Chemotherapy

Chemotherapy represents a fundamental weapon in treating BC. Its possible risks for the fetus strictly depend on the gestational age. During the first trimester, chemotherapy is always contraindicated, due to its high risk of miscarriage and congenital malformations (about 14% of cases) [36–38]. If chemotherapy is strictly necessary at this time of pregnancy, its interruption may be discussed with the patient [39]. After the first trimester, the risk of congenital malformations for the fetus drops to 3%, almost equal to the general population. For this reason, chemotherapy can be considered during the second and third trimester [26].

An fetal examination with US should be performed before and periodically during the treatment.

Chemotherapy regimens must be decided according to the tumor stage and biology, as in non-pregnant women. Anthracycline regimens have been known for years to be safe in pregnant women [40–43] and should be preferred. Regimens based on anthracyclines and taxanes appear to be safe during the two last trimesters of pregnancy [44, 45]. When taxanes are indicated, weekly paclitaxel should be preferred to docetaxel every 3 weeks because of its better tolerated toxicity profile and of the no need for steroid premedication or granulocyte colony stimulating factor (GCSF) [26].

The administration of dose dense regimens is still controversial: Although some data show the safety of this approach [46], further studies are needed before it becomes clinical practice.

Chemotherapy dose should be based on body surface area as in non-pregnant women, although some possible pharmacokinetics alterations must be taken into consideration [47].

The interruption of chemotherapy should not be over 35th week of pregnancy, to permit a 3-week washout before delivery [26], reducing possible surgical complications caused by hematological toxicity.

6.4 Endocrine therapy

Endocrine therapy is contraindicated at every trimester of pregnancy. Many studies demonstrated a clear teratogenic effect of tamoxifen in animal models [48, 49] and its relationship with major and minor congenital malformations in humans [50]. Notwithstanding a possible teratogenic effect in animal models, there are still no sufficient data available for aromatase inhibitors during pregnancy [51].

6.5 Target therapy

Trastuzumab, an anti-HER2 monoclonal antibody, has become, during the last few years, the standard of care in Her 2 positive adjuvant, neoadjuvant, and metastatic settings, representing a practice-changing drug. Being a type G Immunoglobulin, it is capable to trespass the blood placenta barrier from the second trimester to the due date. It interferes with the organogenesis process and causes oligo- and/or anhydramnios, as well as unknown long-term consequences on the fetus [33]. For this reason, it is contraindicated during every gestational age. Seen as though these complications have been shown only in the case of trastuzumab administration after the second trimester, incidental trastuzumab administration during the early stage of pregnancy (first trimester) does not necessarily require pregnancy interruption [52].

In the last few years, new anti-HER2 agents have become a part of our clinical practice, as Pertuzumab, trastuzumab-emtasine (T-DM1), or trastuzumab-deruxtecan (TDX). There are no data available on their safety during pregnancy.

6.6 Immunotherapy

Immunotherapy with anti-PD1/PD-L1 monoclonal antibodies has its peculiar role in the treatment of BC, especially in the triple negative forms. Some preclinical studies demonstrated a higher risk of late miscarriage and birth mortality if administered during pregnancy in animal models, probably caused by the non-acquisition of immune tolerance against the fetus [53, 54]. Hence, it is contraindicated till further studies about its security are conducted.

6.7 Supportive care

Most of the supportive care drugs used in non-pregnant women can safely be administrated even during pregnancy. Steroids should be avoided during the first trimester due to the risk of congenital malformations. They can be administered in the second and third trimester, preferably using methylprednisolone and hydrocortisone that are metabolized in the placenta and do not seem to reach the fetus [33]. Ondansetron can be safely administered, as well as H2 antagonists; there are no sufficient data about anti-NK1 agents [16]. Granulocyte-colony stimulating factors (G-CSFs) have shown no significant fetal toxicities in the only retrospective analysis that has analyzed their safety during pregnancy, but further studies may be needed [55].

7. Fetal outcome

As stated above, during the second and third trimester, chemotherapy can be safely administered. Nevertheless, it may be connected to an increased risk of complications for the fetus, such as intrauterine growth restriction (7–9 up to 22%) or premature rupture of membranes (17–27%) [41, 56].

Mother and fetus should be strictly monitored before, during, and after the oncologic treatment, and after delivery, the placenta should be sent for histological exam, to assess if any BC cells are detected [57]. Moreover, a multidisciplinary approach is fundamental in this population of patients: Only the cooperation between all the figures involved (Oncologist, Surgeon, OBG-YN, Radiologist, Psychologist) can lead to the best approach for each patient.

Babies born from mothers treated for cancer during pregnancy have been followed during a long-term follow-up and have shown cognitive and physical functions not different from the general population, but more studies are needed [17].

8. Conclusions

PrBC incidence is slowly rising; thus, the awareness of its correct management is fundamental for every physician. It should be treated following non-pregnant BC guidelines, applying the abovementioned precautions to limit the possible risks for the fetus. There is no evidence of increased OS after pregnancy interruption; hence, this possibility must be discussed with the patient only in select cases, for instance, when the immediate start of chemotherapy is mandatory. Taking into consideration the complexity of the disease, a multidisciplinary approach is crucial to define the best therapeutical path.

Author details

Massimiliano Berretta[1*], Oreste Claudio Buonomo[2], Gianluca Vanni[2] and Bianca Arianna Facchini[3]

1 Department of Clinical and Experimental Medicine, University of Messina, Messina, Italy

2 Breast Unit, Department of Surgical Science, PTV Policlinico Tor Vergata University, Rome, Italy

3 Department of Precision Medicine, University of Campania 'Luigi Vanvitelli', Naples, Italy

*Address all correspondence to: berrettama@gmail.com

References

[1] Xia C, Dong X, Li H, Cao M, Sun D, He S, et al. Cancer statistics in China and United States, 2022: Profiles, trends, and determinants. Chinese Medical Journal. 2022;**135**(5):584-590. DOI: 10.1097/CM9.0000000000002108

[2] Ghiasvand R, Adami HO, Harirchi I, Akrami R, Zendehdel K. Higher incidence of premenopausal BC in less developed countries; myth or truth? BMC Cancer. 2014;**14**:343

[3] Goodarzi E, Beiranvand R, Naemi H, Rahimi Pordanjani S, Khazaei Z. Geographical distribution incidence and mortality of breast cancer and its relationship with the Human Development Index (HDI): An ecology study in 2018. WCRJ. 2020;**7**:e1468. DOI: 10.32113/wcrj_20201_1468

[4] Caputo R, Cianniello D, Giordano A, Piezzo M, Riemma M, Trovò M, et al. Gene expression assay in the management of early breast cancer. Current Medicinal Chemistry. 2020;**27**(17):2826-2839. DOI: 10.2174/0929867326666191205163329

[5] Kelsey JL, Gammon MD, John EM. Reproductive factors and breast cancer. Epidemiologic Reviews. 1993;**15**:36-47

[6] Lambe M, Hsieh CC, Chan HW, Ekbom A, Trichopoulos D, Adami HO. Parity, age at first and last birth, and risk of BC: A population-based study in Sweden. Breast Cancer Research and Treatment. 1996;**38**:305-311

[7] MacMahon B, Cole P, Lin TM, Lowe CR, Mirra AP, Ravnihar B, et al. Age at first birth and breast cancer risk. Bulletin of the World Health Organization. 1970;**43**(2):209-221

[8] De Haan J, Verheecke M, Van Calsteren K, Van Calster B, Shmakov RG, Mhallem Gziri M, et al. Oncological management and obstetric and neonatal outcomes for women diagnosed with cancer during pregnancy: A 20-year international cohort study of 1170 patients. The Lancet Oncology. 2018;**19**:337-346

[9] Parazzini F, Franchi M, Tavani A, Negri E, Peccatori FA. Frequency of pregnancy related cancer. International Journal of Gynecological Cancer. 2017;**27**(3):613e9

[10] Amant F, Lefr_ere H, Borges VF, Cardonick E, Lambertini M, Loibl S, et al. The definition of pregnancy-associated breast cancer is outdated and should no longer be used. The Lancet Oncology 2021;**22**(6):753e4. 10.1016/S1470-2045(21)00183-2

[11] Johannsson O, Loman N, Borg A, Olsson H. Pregnancy-associated breast cancer in BRCA1 and BRCA2 germline mutation carriers. Lancet. 1998;**352**(9137):1359e60

[12] Cardoso F, Kyriakides S, Ohno S, et al. Early breast cancer: ESMO clinical practice guidelines for diagnosis, treatment and follow-up. Annals of Oncology. 2019;**30**(8):1194e220

[13] Zemlickis D, Lishner M, Degendorfer P, Panzarella T, Burke B, Sutcliffe SB, et al. Maternal and fetal outcome after breast cancerin pregnancy. American Journal of Obstetrics and Gynecology. 1992;**166**(3):781-787

[14] Amant F, von Minckwitz G, Han SN, Bontenbal M, Ring AE, Giermek J, et al. Prognosis of women with primary breast cancer diagnosed during

pregnancy: Results from an international collaborative study. Journal of Clinical Oncology. 2013;**31**:2532-2539

[15] Schedin P. Pregnancy-associated breast cancer and metastasis. Nature Reviews. Cancer. 2006;**6**:281-291

[16] Poggio F, Tagliamento M, Pirrone C, Soldato D, Conte B, Molinelli C, et al. Update on the management of breast cancer during pregnancy. Cancers (Basel). 2020;**12**(12):3616. DOI: 10.3390/cancers12123616

[17] Peccatori FA, Lambertini M, Scarfone G, Del Pup L, Codacci-Pisanelli G. Biology, staging, and treatment of breast cancer during pregnancy: Reassessing the evidences. Cancer Biology & Medicine. 2018;**15**(1):6-13. DOI: 10.20892/j.issn.2095-3941.2017.0146

[18] Nguyen B, Venet D, Azim HA, Brown D, Desmedt C, Lambertini M, et al. Breast cancer diagnosed during pregnancy is associated with enrichment of non-silent mutations, mismatch repair deficiency signature and mucin mutations. NPJ Breast Cancer. 2018;**4**:23

[19] Korakiti A-M, Moutafi M, Zografos E, Dimopoulos M-A, Zagouri F. The genomic profile of pregnancy-associated breast cancer: A systematic review. Frontiers in Oncology. 2020;**10**:1773

[20] Collins JC, Liao S, Wile AG. Surgical management of breast masses in pregnant women. The Journal of Reproductive Medicine. 1995;**40**(11):785e8

[21] Sood R, Rositch AF, Shakoor D, Ambinder E, Pool K-L, Pollack E, et al. Ultrasound for breast cancer detection globally: A systematic review and meta-analysis. Journal of Global Oncology. 2019;**5**:1e17. DOI: 10.1200/JGO.19.00127

[22] Vashi R, Hooley R, Butler R, Geisel J, Philpotts L. Breast imaging of the pregnant and lactating patient: Imaging modalities and pregnancy-associated breast cancer. AJR. American Journal of Roentgenology. 2013;**200**:321-328

[23] Ray JG, Vermeulen MJ, Bharatha A, Montanera WJ, Park AL. Association between MRI exposure during pregnancy and fetal and childhood outcomes. Journal of the American Medical Association. 2016;**316**(9):952-961

[24] Candelaria RP, Huang ML, Adrada BE, Bassett R, Hunt KK, Kuerer HM, et al. Incremental cancer detection of locoregional restaging with diagnostic mammography combined with whole-breast and regional nodal ultrasound in women with newly diagnosed breast cancer. Academic Radiology. 2017;**24**(2):191e9

[25] Wang PI, Chong ST, Kielar AZ, et al. Imaging of pregnant and lactating patients: Part 2, evidence-based review and recommendations. AJR. American Journal of Roentgenology. 2012;**198**:785-792

[26] Peccatori FA, Azim HA Jr, Orecchia R, Hoekstra HJ, Pavlidis N, Kesic V, et al. Cancer, pregnancy and fertility: ESMO clinical practice guidelines for diagnosis, treatment and follow-up. Annals of Oncology. 2013;**24**(Suppl. 6):vi160-vi170

[27] Cohen-Kerem R, Railton C, Oren D, Lishner M, Koren G. Pregnancy outcome following non-obstetric surgical intervention. American Journal of Surgery. 2005;**190**:467-473

[28] Toesca A, Gentilini O, Peccatori F, Azim HA Jr, Amant F. Locoregional treatment of breast cancer during pregnancy. Gynecological Surgery. 2014;**11**:279-284

[29] Hershman DL, Wang X, McBride R, Jacobson JS, Grann VR, Neugut AI. Delay in initiating adjuvant radiotherapy following breast conservation surgery and its impact on survival. International Journal of Radiation Oncology, Biology, Physics. 2006;**65**:1353-1360

[30] Chen Z, King W, Pearcey R, Kerba M, Mackillop WJ. The relationship between waiting time for radiotherapy and clinical outcomes: A systematic review of the literature. Radiotherapy and Oncology. 2008;**87**:3-16

[31] Lyman GH, Temin S, Edge SB, Newman LA, Turner RR, Weaver DL, et al. Sentinel lymph node biopsy for patients with early-stage breast cancer: American society of clinical oncology clinical practice guideline update. Journal of Clinical Oncology. 2014;**32**:1365-1383

[32] Azim HA Jr, editor. Managing Cancer during Pregnancy. Cham, Switzerland: Springer International Publishing; 2016

[33] Loibl S, Schmidt A, Gentilini O, Kaufman B, Kuhl C, Denkert C, et al. Breast cancer diagnosed during pregnancy: Adapting recent advances in breast cancer Care for pregnant patients. JAMA Oncology. 2015;**1**:1145

[34] Cimmino VM, Brown AC, Szocik JF, et al. Allergic reactions to isosulfan blue during sentinel node biopsy—A common event. Surgery. 2001;**130**:439-442

[35] Amant F, Loibl S, Neven P, Van Calsteren K. Breast cancer in pregnancy. Lancet. 2012;**379**:570-579

[36] Leslie KK, Koil C, Rayburn WF. Chemotherapeutic drugs in pregnancy. Obstetrics and Gynecology Clinics of North America. 2005;**32**:627-640

[37] Cardonick E, Iacobucci A. Use of chemotherapy during human pregnancy. The Lancet Oncology. 2004;**5**:283-291

[38] National Toxicology Program NTP Monograph. Developmental E ects and pregnancy outcomes associated with cancer chemotherapy use during pregnancy. NTP Monograph. 2013;**2**:i-214

[39] Beadle BM, Woodward WA, Middleton LP, Tere e W, Strom EA, Litton JK, et al. The impact of pregnancy on breast cancer outcomes in women <35 years. Cancer. 2009;**115**:1174-1184

[40] Cardonick E, Dougherty R, Grana G, et al. Breast cancer during pregnancy: Maternal and fetal outcomes. Cancer Journal. 2010;**16**:76-82

[41] Loibl S, Han SN, von Minckwitz G, et al. Treatment of breast cancer during pregnancy: An observational study. The Lancet Oncology. 2012;**13**:887-896

[42] Hahn KM, Johnson PH, Gordon N, et al. Treatment of pregnant breast cancer patients and outcomes of children exposed to chemotherapy in utero. Cancer. 2006;**107**:1219-1226

[43] Peccatori FA, Azim HA Jr, Scarfone G, et al. Weekly epirubicin in the treatment of gestational breast cancer (GBC). Breast Cancer Research and Treatment. 2009;**115**:591-594

[44] Tehrani OS. Systemic treatments in pregnancy-associated breast cancer. Advances in Experimental Medicine and Biology. 2020;**1252**:115-124

[45] Alipour S, Omranipour R, editors. Advances in Experimental Medicine and Biology. Vol. 1252. Cham, Switzerland: Springer International Publishing; 2020. pp. 115-124

[46] Cardonick E, Gilmandyar D, Somer RA. Maternal and neonatal outcomes of dose-dense chemotherapy for breast cancer in pregnancy. Obstetrics and Gynecology. 2012;**120**:1267-1272

[47] Van Calsteren K, Verbesselt R, Ottevanger N, et al. Pharmacokinetics of chemotherapeutic agents in pregnancy: A preclinical and clinical study. Acta Obstetricia et Gynecologica Scandinavica. 2010;**89**:1338-1345

[48] Barthelmes L, Gateley CA. Tamoxifen and pregnancy. Breast. 2004;**13**:446-451

[49] Halakivi-Clarke L, Cho E, Onojafe I, Liao DJ, Clarke R. Maternal exposure to tamoxifen during pregnancy increases carcinogen-induced mammary tumorigenesis among female rat offspring. Clinical Cancer Research. 2000;**6**:305-308

[50] Buonomo B, Brunello A, Noli S, Miglietta L, Del Mastro L, Lambertini M, et al. Tamoxifen exposure during pregnancy: A systematic review and three more cases. Breast Care. 2020;**15**:148-156

[51] Tiboni GM. Aromatase inhibitors and teratogenesis. Fertility and Sterility. 2004;**81**:1158-1159

[52] Zagouri F, Sergentanis TN, Chrysikos D, Papadimitriou CA, Dimopoulos MA, Bartsch R. Trastuzumab administration during pregnancy: A systematic review and meta-analysis. Breast Cancer Research and Treatment. 2013;**137**(2):349-357

[53] Luppi P. How immune mechanisms are affected by pregnancy. Vaccine. 2003;**21**:3352-3357

[54] Hepner A, Negrini D, Hase EA, Exman P, Testa L, Trinconi AF, et al. Cancer during pregnancy: The oncologist overview. World Journal of Oncology. 2019;**10**:28-34

[55] Dale DC, Cottle TE, Fier CJ, Bolyard AA, Bonilla MA, Boxer LA, et al. Severe chronic neutropenia: Treatment and follow-up of patients in the severe chronic neutropenia international registry. American Journal of Hematology. 2003;**72**:82-93

[56] Van Calsteren K, Heyns L, De Smet F, Van Eycken L, Gziri MM, Van Gemert W, et al. Cancer during pregnancy: An analysis of 215 patients emphasizing the obstetrical and the neonatal outcomes. Journal of Clinical Oncology. 2010;**28**:683-689

[57] Pavlidis N, Pentheroudakis G. Metastatic involvement of placenta and foetus in pregnant women with cancer. In: Cancer and Pregnancy. Berlin, Heidelberg: Springer; 2008. pp. 183-194

Chapter 4

Breast Cancer in Brazil: Social Conditions and Access to Health Care

Mônica de Castro Maia Senna, Thaislayne Nunes de Oliveira and Debora Louzada Carvalho

Abstract

Breast cancer is the most predominant type among Brazilian women, ranking second position within the causes of mortality in the female population. According to the National Cancer Institute (INCA) estimates, for each year of the triennium 2023–2025, 73.610 new cases are expected. Although it is not subject to primary prevention, breast cancer tends to have a satisfactory prognosis and greater chances of cure if identified early. The high mortality rates indicate, however, that access to early diagnosis and to treatments is a flawed aspect of the country. The chapter addresses the main social conditions that affect the high rates of morbidity and mortality, emphasizing aspects both related to the provision of health care services and some social characteristics of women that mark the inequalities which make health care difficult. It also discusses aspects related to health policies and access barriers toward breast cancer control.

Keywords: breast cancer, social conditions, access to health, health care

1. Introduction

Breast cancer is currently the most common female cancer type in the world [1]. According to the International Agency for Research on Cancer [2] in 2020, there were more than 2.26 million new cases of breast cancer and almost 685,000 deaths from this cancer type worldwide. It means that breast cancer accounted for more than 10% of new cancer cases overall and it was the main cause of cancer death in women, corresponding to almost 7% of all cancer deaths in that year.

There is not only a single cause for the incidence of breast cancer, although genetic, behavioral aspects (such as excessive alcohol consumption), and populational aging are related to a greater predisposition to the disease. Thus, differently from other types of neoplasms, breast cancer is not subject to primary prevention [3, 4]. Nevertheless, the early identification of the disease and adequate access to treatment are admittedly important for better prognosis and higher chances of cure [2] providing a secondary level of prevention under the terms of Leavell and Clark [3].

Differentials in mortality by breast cancer among women from low and middle-income countries, express the iniquities related to access to health care, compared to the ones from high-income countries, as indicated by the IARC [5], showing the deep imbrications of the health social determinants for the course of the disease.

The analysis by Pinho and Coutinho [6] points out that the incidence of breast cancer cases is more present in poor countries. In rich countries, such as The United States, Canada, United Kingdom, Netherlands, Denmark, and Norway, although the incidence of breast cancer is high and growing, the mortality number shows a decrease, referring to the investment in screening, prevention, and early detection of the illness. Data provided by the All Together Against Cancer (Todos Juntos Contra o Cancer) movement, state that poor people have six times more chances of dying after oncological surgery. The institution has presented the results of a survey made in 82 countries and noticed that the tumor location can raise the mortality number. In order to make comparative purposes, it is necessary to consider the singularities of each country, both in the predicted health models and in the strategies that lead to cancer control.

Baquet and Commiskey [7] indicate that there are racial differences for women in the United States in relation to incidences, mortality, and survival taxes of breast carcinoma. They also point out that social and economic factors inside racial/ethnic groups can be considered risk factors, not only for cancer mortality and survival but also as determinants of incident rates. Gorey et al. [8] compare diagnosed women with mammary neoplasm in two different locations; one in Canada and the other in the United States, both with a low socioeconomic status population. It was identified that in Canada, the survival rate is 15 years higher than in the United States. The authors point out that this difference can be related to greater access to health services in Canada, resulting in a prolonged survival time.

Van Maaren et al. [9] identified connections between the socioeconomic status and survival of patients with breast cancer to be more pronounced among young patients in Netherlands. It is also enhanced that the risk of recurrence in 10 years was lower in the strata with higher purchasing power, indicating that the risk factors for breast cancer, in adherence to adjuvant treatment and recurrent treatment can possibly play an important role in this association between socioeconomic level and a higher survival prognosis.

In Norway, a country with universal health care assistance and national treatment guidelines, it was observed that the specific survival of young patients with breast cancer has improved, likely due to advances in diagnosis and treatment. However, it was noticed that survival highly increased in patients with higher income and education, but there was little survival gain for the ones with low education and income. In this respect, Trewin et al. [10] point out how important socioeconomic status is for the specific survival of young patients with breast cancer, even in countries with universal medical assistance.

In Brazil, a country marked by deep social inequalities, breast cancer remains with very high incidence and mortality rates. For the triennium 2023–2025, 73.610 new cases of breast cancer are estimated each year, and an age-adjusted mortality rate is calculated by the population in the order of 14.23 deaths per 100,000 women in 2018 [1, 11]. Currently, breast cancer is the type of cancer that presents the highest number of deaths among women and the second leading cause of death in the Brazilian female population.

Given this situation, the chapter addresses some of the main social conditions that have contributed to the persistence of high mortality rates from breast cancer in

Brazil. It is based on the understanding that barriers to accessing quality health services make it difficult to diagnose and treat in a timely manner, with impacts on the quality of life and the chances of cure and survival of women affected by the illness.

It should be noted that access barriers are understood as characteristics that may obstruct access and use of health services by potential users, as proposed by Travassos and De Castro [12]. The authors indicate that the mere service offer does not guarantee access to it and point out that geographic, financial, organizational, and informational barriers, among others, directly interfere with facilitating or hindering healthcare access. Based on the understanding that social inequalities in health conditions and access to health networks are a direct expression of the social structure in which we live, Travassos and De Castro [12] state that even if there are changes in the characteristics of the health system that alter significantly the social inequalities in access and use of health services, these, by themselves, are not capable of intervening in health conditions.

From this perspective, the focus given to the issue of breast cancer in this chapter values two central axes. The first one concerns social inequalities that affect the process of illness and the search for health services, particularly, those aspects related to the female condition and socioeconomic factors. The second axis considers the way in which health services are organized, which raises the need to also take into account the trajectory of public policy aimed specifically at cancer control in the country. The considerations made in the chapter were based on bibliographic research, a documental survey, and analysis of secondary data.

2. Breast cancer as a social process: a gender perspective

Studies such as Gorey's [8] point to a correlation between the women with breast cancer survival rate and socioeconomic conditions. Although the incidence of breast cancer affects women from different social classes, the prognosis differs between social strata, with higher mortality among poorer women. In this sense, among the social factors associated with breast cancer mortality are poverty, low education, and lack or difficulties in accessing health services.

Albrecht et al. [13] identified the association between a low level of education and an advanced stage of breast cancer, pointing out that women with less education are more prone to late diagnosis compared to those in strata with higher income and higher levels of education. Similarly, when investigating the association between race/ethnicity and 10-year survival with breast cancer, Nogueira et al. [14], concluded that there is a racial disparity in breast cancer survival, to the disadvantage of black women, who are also generally poorer.

Health conditions are directly related to the inequities existing in the capitalist system, which affect social groups in different ways, according to their insertion in the market. Thus, "people in disadvantaged social conditions seek [health] services when their health status is most severe and they receive care in services less suited to their needs" [12]. It is worth pointing out that Brazil is characterized by immense social inequalities, largely associated with its historical formation marked by slavery and by its subordinate and peripheral insertion in global capitalism.

A study conducted by the Brazilian Institute of Geography and Statistics indicated that in 2018 the average monthly income from work of the richest 1% of the population was 34 times higher than that of the poorest half of the population, and the Gini index was 0.542 [15]. The social inequalities are also expressed in terms of race/ethnicity: blacks are the ones that comprise 75% of the population in the country's extreme poverty situation, being 72% slum dwellers and 64% unemployed [16], in addition to being the main victims of violence and violation of rights. Brazil also presents high levels of gender wage inequality; women receiving lower salaries than men, occupying few leadership positions, working in multiple shifts, and suffering various forms of violence and harassment.

In this sense, the gender approach is relevant for understanding the phenomenon of breast cancer as a social process. The concept of gender is an analytical category historically and socially constructed from feminist struggles. It expresses a primary form of power and domination in social relations constitution, which is made from the perceived differences between the sexes [17]. At the same time, thanks especially to the contribution of black feminists and the concept of intersectionality proposed by them [18], it is important to recognize that these relations of power and domination are intertwined with others, such as race and social class, as structuring social reality.

A cross-sectional study to identify the sociodemographic profiles of women diagnosed as breast cancer from the hospital in a state in Brazil records 715 patients undergoing treatment between 2010 and 2013. The cluster analysis was used to delineate the profiles from the variables: age, color of the skin, education, and cost of treatment. The association between profiles and intervals was investigated using multinomial logistic regression, being observed even after winning barriers to access to the oncology unit profiles of social vulnerability had a longer wait for treatment [19].

Therefore, it should be considered that the family role permanence and naturalization of caring for children and household chores put women with cancer in a position of what we call "disadvantage," especially when there is a change from their condition of caregiver to someone who needs to be cared for [20]. Under the same perspective, Nogueira and Silva [21] emphasize that the woman who is the head of the family, with no support network, has little or no social protection, deals with objective barriers that make breast cancer prevention, detection, and treatment difficult or even impossible.

In a study carried out in Brazil with women who access public health services, it was identified that the probability of being alive was lower for those in advanced stages. However, the authors point out that studies have shown disparities in the survival of women with breast cancer in relation to socioeconomic status. In this sense, women with lower socioeconomic status have worse survival rates. It is also reinforced that the difficulty of accessing the diagnosis increases the probability of death from breast cancer [22].

The close correlation between the illness process and living conditions, the precariousness of work relations, and the absence of social protection constitute barriers to access and adherence to treatment, which has been expressed in the identification of the disease in its most advanced stages and has increased mortality. Thus, an element to be considered in this aspect is what Carloto and Gomes [23] understands as the "feminization of poverty." The authors resort to the notion of social and technical division of labor to identify its organization between men and women in the social structure, in such a way that an arrangement of skills and attributions are associated with the female gender and another arrangement of functions granted to the male gender are socially configured.

Another study points out that low education was identified as a risk factor for the increased possibility of mortality even in the early stages of breast cancer [24]. In the sexual division of labor, women occupy subordinate and socially discredited roles. They are limited in terms of their participation in the labor market due to the roles they are assigned in care and social reproduction. Such inequalities are naturalized by society and disregard the conflicts that permeate the construction of women in their condition as subjects. At the same time, that condition masks the difficulties faced by women not only in their socialization processes but also in their interpersonal relationships, which becomes worse with illness.

Women are submitted daily to double and/or triple shifts. It is sure that the responsibility for household chores falls on them, making gender asymmetries evident. Women are often expected to care for others and paid work. This is associated with the low standard of public social protection in Brazil and the responsibility for the care is left almost exclusively to the family itself, and within the family, more specifically to the women [25].

Portella [20] draws attention to the fact that when a woman becomes ill, the historically constructed place of caregiver undergoes changes, impacting both her social function, her body image, and interpersonal relationships as well. The author states that aspects related to how women deal with their bodies and with socially constructed conceptions of care, influence how they choose to care for themselves.

The author also points out that the absence of public social support mechanisms that cover the care function performed by women, especially the poorest ones, ends up hindering and influencing access to exams and treatments, contributing to advanced staging and, therefore, lower chances of a satisfactory prognosis, recovery from the illness, and real chances of cure.

3. Breast cancer, social policies, and health care services

The health system in Brazil presents a hybrid format, consisting of a public and universal subsystem (Sistema Único de Saúde—SUS) and a private subsystem, in addition to its own regime for military personnel. Instituted by the 1988 Federal Constitution, which recognized health as a universal right and a responsibility of the State, SUS offers a set of actions to the entire Brazilian population that range from those related to prevention and health promotion to highly complex procedures, such as transplants, for example. It is, therefore, a group of actions that cover Primary Health Care, medium and high complexity services. It also adopts a model of cooperative federalism in which the Union, states, and municipalities have shared responsibilities for the management, financing, and provision of health actions.

Thus, the SUS is composed of a network of public, philanthropic, and private services contracted with public resources from fiscal taxes. The private subsystem, on the other hand, is mostly constituted by health plans and insurance, financed directly by the insured themselves (out of pocket) or by the employing companies, in part or in full. It is evident that the hybrid character of the Brazilian health system expresses its enormous segmentation and inequalities in access to services. According to Barros and Sousa [26], despite being recognized as a universal and equal right, the SUS still faces inequities resulting from "factors such as misinformation, associated with differences in education, or even deformation in certain public policies, in some of which privileges and discrimination are still present." The authors also point out the low percentage of public spending on health, especially if compared to other universal health systems. Data compiled by IBGE, for the year 2019, show that public spending corresponded to only 3.8% of GDP, compared to 5.8% of private spending. In contrast, more than 70% of the Brazilian population, or about 150 million people, depend exclusively on the SUS [27].

In the case of private health insurance, the same IBGE [27] survey indicated that 26% of the population had a health plan for medical care. The coverage of these health plans is concentrated in urban areas, especially in the state capitals and in the Southeast and South regions of the country. The data indicate that in Brazil, there are differentials in relation to education, income per capita, and race, with greater coverage in population segments with higher education and income and among the white population. Liedke et al. carried out a study looking for differences between women diagnosed with breast cancer who have health insurance and those who access public services in Brazil. The authors identified that patients with public health coverage had more advanced diseases at diagnosis [28].

In relation to breast cancer care, the first health measures date back to the 1920s, provided by philanthropic institutions. At that time, the number of diagnosed cancer cases in Brazil was low, being the highest disease incidence and mortality rates in the country related to the group of infectious-parasitic diseases. The governmental actions to control cancer were punctual, in general, associated with personal initiatives or those of medical professionals [29]. Inflections in this model began to take shape in the 1940s, with the implementation of the National Cancer Service, largely the result of the mobilization of the Cancer Leagues organized under the leadership of medical professionals. According to Teixeira [29], the implementation of this service made it possible for the breast cancer issue to enter the Brazilian public health agenda, with the Central Institute and the National Campaign against Cancer as its bases for action. Regarding breast cancer specifically, the role played by the Social Pioneers Foundation, created in 1957 with the purpose of providing medical and educational assistance to the poor population, deserves to be highlighted. In association with this foundation, a cancerology hospital unit was created to provide outpatient care for the prevention and early detection of gynecological and breast cancer and to constitute, at the same time, a research center dedicated to the prevention of female cancer. However, following the hegemonic medical model in the country, the care provided was characterized by the predominance of individual actions, curative nature, and centered on hospital care [30].

Breast cancer control achieved greater visibility in Brazil since the 1980s when the country was undergoing important social, economic, and political reforms associated with the context of re-democratization after two decades of an authoritarian political regime. Such visibility can be credited to the recognition of the increasing number of cases and deaths from breast cancer in the country. Two government initiatives are worth mentioning here. One is the comprehensive attention to women's health program, implemented in 1983, which innovates by expanding the attention to women's health beyond the pregnancy-puerperal cycle and introducing the concept of comprehensiveness. The other prominent initiative is the creation, in 1986, of the Oncology Program (Pro-Onco), from the National Cancer Institute, which arose as a technical-administrative structure of the extinct National Campaign to Fight Cancer [30].

Next, we had the consolidation of the SUS in the 194 Article of the 1988 Federal Constitution. In addition, the beginning of the 1990s watched the legislation implementation that deals with the institutionalization of SUS, Laws No. 8.080/90 and No. 8.142/90. In the late 1990s, under the SUS structure, the *Viva Mulher* Program was implemented as the first national public health initiative aimed specifically at the control of female cancers, especially breast cancer. The program objective was to reduce mortality and the physical, psychological and social repercussions of cervical and breast cancer by offering services for prevention and detection at the early stages of the disease and for the treatment and rehabilitation of women. However, Porto et al. [31] explain that despite the progress made by this program, very little has effectively advanced in terms of health care.

The scenario changed in the 2000s. The first specific national policy for cancer in Brazil was instituted in 2005, in line with the parameters recommended by the World Health Organization, in view of the high rates of new cases and mortality from the illness worldwide. The National Policy for Oncological Care (PNAO) affirmed cancer as a public health issue and structured the oncological care services network to be implemented in a decentralized manner in the states and municipalities, in accordance with guidelines established by SUS [32]. In the same year, the Action Plan for the Control of Cervical and Breast Cancer (2005–2007) was drawn up, based on six strategic guidelines, namely: increase in the coverage of the target population; quality assurance; strengthening of the information system; development of training; social mobilization strategy; and advancement of research. According to Oliveira [32], at this moment, the greatest focus is given to early detection, for which indicators and goals for mammography and screening of the disease are agreed upon by the different federated entities. In the wake of these measures, other initiatives were adopted to encourage the early detection of breast cancer. Among them, we can cite the publication of Law No. 11.664/2008, which aims to ensure mammograms for women over 40 years, as well as referral to services of greater complexity for diagnostic complementation and treatment, when necessary. Later, some other legislations were created, including the structuring of specific programs and systems, such as the Breast Cancer Information System (SISMAMA), and the Cancer Information System (SISCAN), among others, through which they implied changes in the access to information on prevention and focus on the control of the disease in a positive way, especially in the surveillance actions of the disease.

Moreover, the discussion of breast malignancy was reaffirmed through the action plan launched in 2011, the National Plan for the Diagnosis and Treatment of Cervical and Breast Cancer, which aimed to increase mammographic exams, especially to intensify prevention and assistance to women. Then, the National Program of Quality in Mammography (PNQM) was instituted. And, later, the publication of Ordinance No. 189/2014 established financial incentives to fund referral services for breast cancer diagnosis. These measures are essential for us to think about the priority of cancer through sensitivity and encouragement of measures to prevent and control the disease.

In this sense, there is a need to discuss health prevention and promotion and the relevance of social determinants and their impacts on the number of new cases in Brazil and worldwide is evident. Significant advances have been identified since the early 2000s; Castro [33] elucidates the change in the public policy scenario in this period, starting with the government of then—President Luiz Inácio Lula da Silva. There is evidence of an expansion of social policies, enabling, a broadening of the mechanism of social protection and promotion. It is noteworthy that through international pressure, the WHO signatory countries were directed to intensify measures to prevent and control cancer.

It should be noted that, in 2013, Brazil published Ordinance No. 874/2013 establishing the National Policy for Cancer Prevention and Control in the Health Care Network for People with Chronic Diseases within the SUS, replacing the previous policy of 2005. With this, it is identified an intensification in the creation of strategic measures that should focus on the risks and aggravations of the disease. With research on the documentary collection shown by INCA, it is clear that most of these sources allocated for cancer consist of diagnosis, but there is a high expenditure on the treatment that, being of high complexity, requires the use of imported technologies [34].

Despite the undeniable advances those mentioned measures represent, the mortality rate for breast cancer among Brazilian women remains high and growing. Since the SUS creation, there has been a significant investment in Primary Health Care, expanding the health services supplies. Primary Care is responsible for preventive clinical examinations. However, diagnostic confirmation, which requires access to mammography, ultrasound, and biopsy tests, is performed at other care levels, which is a bottleneck in the SUS. The delay in scheduling these diagnostic tests and the low quality of the images are some of the factors that end up delaying the diagnosis. And once the diagnosis is confirmed, the woman with cancer faces new difficulties, now to access treatment in a timely manner. These aspects end up contributing to access to services when the breast cancer stage is already advanced, thus reducing the chances of cure.

The study conducted by Oliveira [32] showed differences in the time taken by women with breast cancer to access diagnosis and treatment between those with and without health insurance, in a disadvantageous condition for the latter. Similarly, Cabral et al. [34] concluded that women in situations of greater social vulnerability had a longer interval between diagnosis and initiation of treatment, regardless of the degree of illness staging.

To address this situation, since 2020, Federal Law No. 13,896/2019, won through the mobilization of civil society organizations, guarantees that the necessary tests to confirm the diagnosis must be performed within a maximum of 30 days, with immediate initiation of treatment.

However, the implementation of this law was faced with the arrival of the COVID-19 pandemic, at which time health actions were primarily focused on pandemic control. A study conducted in two Brazilian states showed that there was a decrease in the number of cancer-diagnosed cases due to several factors such as anxiety, stress, and social isolation associated with the restriction in access to routine tests and prevention for breast cancer diagnosis, imposed by the pandemic [35]. It is noteworthy, that during the COVID-19 pandemic, many services were affected, including oncology services, with restrictions and decreased patient flow.

Benites et al. [36] in a literature review article identified studies that reported the adaptations in breast cancer treatments performed. Considering that the interruption of cancer treatment can generate even more damage, health professionals have created alternatives for its non-interruption, seeking to avoid the patients going to hospitals and staying there for a long period of time.

The research by Mendes [37] calls attention to the "invisible patient," the one who suffered the most from the health care paralysis for chronic conditions as a side effect of COVID-19, with non-assistance caused by access restrictions or people's fear of seeking health services. As a result, chronic conditions tend to become unstable and increase in severity, cause deaths, and have a high economic and financial impact on health care systems.

4. Final marks

In Brazil, social inequalities contribute to result not only to worse health conditions but also to health care services access and use inequalities. The multifaceted profile of the social issue of cancer, closely related to the insertion of these women in the world, their family and work relationships, is an aspect that undoubtedly hinders adherence to treatment, especially considering that the illness from breast cancer has repercussions in different ways and in different spheres of women's lives and permeates the gender issue.

The double and/or triple working day, the precariousness of work relations, and the context of restrictive social policies amplify the situation of social vulnerability, without minimum protections for their sustenance and that of their families, besides being factors that notoriously hinder adherence to treatment. Besides the clinical issue, breast cancer also comprises implications involving feminine insertion in the scope of work, family, gender relations, and socioeconomic compromising, among others.

In what specifically refers to the health policy, the Brazilian Unified Health System advocates access universalization, comprehensive integrality, social equity, management and provision decentralization, hierarchization of services, and social participation. It is an example of a policy whose effective implementation presupposes the reorganization of health practices and, consequently, the care model transformation and health care services organization. Focusing on comprehensive care, it is necessary to prioritize intersectoral actions articulating the individual aspects present in the social demands of the user and the family, in order to find social answers via public social policies.

In this sense, it is possible to recognize that the Brazilian health model has changed in a positive way with the creation and implementation of the SUS. Indeed, SUS has remodeled the profile of health care provision, especially in decentralizing the health care management toward the states and municipalities.

It is worth mentioning that the policy institutionalization process has not occurred without conflicts and a set of challenges, particularly the guarantee of the comprehensiveness, continuous care, and quality of services offered. Thus, despite recognizing these advances, it is still necessary to identify that there are limits and daily challenges that weaken the consolidation of the SUS in its essence. Including, new challenges continue to reverberate in current days and are unique to this context, especially due to the reality of the service offered along with the pandemic COVID-19.

In this context, illness raises issues that problematize the debate about health as a right, which refers not only to universal health care access, but also to the quality, nature, and viability of these services provided to women for access to diagnosis and treatment. It is understood that the health-disease process is a social product and cancer is no exception to this rule. In this scenario, the barriers to access to health services lead to higher mortality rates, since, as analyzed, timely diagnosis and adequate treatment make it possible to increase the chances of cure and increase survival.

However, the latest estimated numbers of new cases and the number of deaths from breast cancer remain high. It can be seen that the social vulnerability of the population has great relevance not only because of the pathology severity but also because of the mentioned factors' complexity. This complexity is historically present in the daily life of each individual woman and tends to interfere with timely access to diagnosis, treatment, prognosis, and recovery from the illness.

Author details

Mônica de Castro Maia Senna[1,2,3], Thaislayne Nunes de Oliveira[2,4,5]
and Debora Louzada Carvalho[2,6]*

1 Public Health, Brazil

2 Department of Social Work, Fluminense Federal University, Niterói, Rio de Janeiro, Brazil

3 CNPq, Brazil

4 Multiprofessional Residency Program in Oncology in Universitary Hospital Antônio Pedro, Brazil

5 Army Central Hospital, Rio de Janeiro, Brazil

6 Cancer Hospital II, National Cancer Institute, Rio de Janeiro, Brazil

*Address all correspondence to: louzada.debora@gmail.com

References

[1] Brasil. Instituto Nacional de Câncer José Alencar Gomes da Silva. Estimativa 2023: incidência de câncer no Brasil. Rio de Janeiro: INCA; 2022. Available from: https://www.gov.br/inca/pt-br/assuntos/cancer/numeros/estimativa

[2] Organização Mundial da Saúde. International Agency for Research on Cancer. Breast Cancer. Genebra: WHO; 2020. Available from: https://www.iarc.who.int/cancer-type/breast-cancer/

[3] Leavell HR, Clark EG. Preventive Medicine for the Doctor in his Community: an Epidemiologic Approach. 2nd ed. New York: McGraw-Hill; 1965. p. 589

[4] Starfield B, Hyde J, Gérvas J, Heath I. The concept of prevention: a good idea gone astray? Journal of Epidemiology and Community Health. 2008;**62**(7):580-583. DOI: 10.1136/jech.2007.071027

[5] Organização Mundial da Saúde. Relatório da OMS sobre câncer: estabelecendo prioridades, investindo com sabedoria e cuidando de todos. Genebra: WHO; 2020. p. 149. Available from: apps.who.int/iris/handle/10665/330745;jsessionid=2722B5EBF3812CFF2E489833DF9EE9A8

[6] Pinho VFS, Coutinho ESF. Variáveis associadas ao câncer de mama em usuárias de unidades básicas de saúde. Cadernos de Saúde Pública. 2007;**23**(5):1061-1069. DOI: 10.1590/S0102-311X2007000500008

[7] Baquet CR, Commiskey P. Socioeconomic factors and breast carcinoma in multicultural women. Cancer. 2000;**88**(5):1256-1264. DOI: 10.1002/(SICI)1097-0142(20000301)88:5+<1256::AID-CNCR13>3.0.CO;2-3

[8] Gorey KM et al. Income and long-term breast cancer survival: comparisons of vulnerable urban places in Ontario and California. The Breast Journal. 2010;**16**(4):416-419. DOI: 10.1111/j.1524-4741.2010.00922.x

[9] Van Maaren MC et al. Socioeconomic status and its relationwith breast cancer recurrence and survival in young women in the Netherlands. Cancer Epidemiology. 2022;**77**:e102118. DOI: 10.1016/j.canep.2022.102118

[10] Trewin CB, Johansson ALV, Hjerkind KV, et al. Stage-specific survival has improved for young breast cancer patients since 2000: but not equally. Breast Cancer Research and Treatment. 2020;**182**:477-489. DOI: 10.1007/s10549-020-05698-z

[11] Brasil. Instituto Nacional de Câncer José Alencar Gomes da Silva. Estimativa 2020: incidência de câncer no Brasil. Rio de Janeiro: INCA; 2019. Available from: www.inca.gov.br/sites/ufu.sti.inca.local/files//media/document//estimativa-2020-incidencia-de-cancer-no-brasil.pdf

[12] Travassos C, De Castro MSM. Determinantes e desigualdades sociais no acesso e na utilização de serviços de saúde. In: Giovanela L, et al., organizators. Políticas e sistemas de saúde no Brasil. Rio de Janeiro: Ed. FIOCRUZ; 2008. pp. 215-243

[13] Albrecht CAM et al. Breast cancer mortality among patients attending a cancer hospital, Vitoria, ES. Revista Brasileira de Epidemiologia. 2013;**16**(3):582-591. DOI: 10.1590/S1415-790X2013000300003

[14] Nogueira MC, et al. Disparidade racial na sobrevivência em 10 anos

para o câncer de mama: uma análise de mediação usando abordagem de respostas potenciais. Cadernos de Saúde Pública 2018.;34(9):e00211717. DOI:10.1590/0102-311X00211717. ISSN 1678-4464

[15] Brasil. Instituto Brasileiro de Geografia e Estatística. Pesquisa Nacional por Amostra de Domícilios Contínua. Rio de Janeiro: IBGE; 2019. Available from: https://www.ibge.gov.br/estatisticas/sociais/trabalho/9171-pesquisa-nacional-por-amostra-de-domicilios-continua-mensal.html?=&t=destaques

[16] Brasil. Instituto Brasileiro de Geografia e Estatística. Desigualdades sociais por raça ou cor no Brasil. Estudos e Pesquisas: Informação Demográfica e Socioeconômica. 2019;**41**:1-12. Available from: https://biblioteca.ibge.gov.br/visualizacao/livros/liv101681_informativo.pdf

[17] Scott J. Gênero: uma categoria útil para a análise histórica. Lobo GL, translator. Educação & Realidade. 1995. Available from: https://seer.ufrgs.br/index.php/educacaoerealidade/article/view/71721

[18] Crenshaw K. Demarginalizing the intersection of race and sex: a black feminist critique of antidiscrimination doctrine, feminist theory and antiracist politics. University of Chicago Legal Forum. 1989;**189**:139-167. Available from: http://chicagounbound.uchicago.edu/uclf/vol1989/iss1/8

[19] Cabral ALLV, Giatti L, Casale C, et al. Vulnerabilidade social e câncer de mama: diferenciais no intervalo entre o diagnóstico e o tratamento em mulheres de diferentes perfis sociodemográficos. Revista Ciência & Saúde Coletiva. 2019;**24**(2):613-622. DOI: 10.1590/1413-81232018242.3167201626

[20] Portella MGR. A invisibilidade do papel de gênero no cuidado de mulheres com câncer de mama no município de Niterói [master's thesis]. Niterói: Programa de Pós-Graduação em Saúde Coletiva. Universidade Federal Fluminense; 2019. p. 132

[21] Nogueira ACC, Silva LB. Saúde, gênero e serviço social: contribuições sobre o câncer e saúde da mulher. VÉRTICES 2009;11(1/3):7-17. Available from: http://essentiaeditora.iff.edu.br/index. php/vertices/article/viewArticle/8

[22] Höfelmann DA et al. Sobrevida em dez anos e fatores prognósticos em mulheres com câncer de mama em Joinville, Santa Catarina, Brasil. Revista Ciência & Saúde Coletiva. 2014;**19**(6):7-17. DOI: 10.1590/1413-81232014196.03062013

[23] Carloto CM, Gomes AG. Geração de renda: enfoque nas mulheres pobres e divisão sexual do trabalho. Service Social. 2011;**105**:131-145. DOI: 10.1590/S0101-66282011000100008

[24] Herndon JE II, Kornblith AB, Holland JC, Paskett ED. Effect of socioeconomic status as measured by education level on survival in breast cancer clinical trials. Psycho-Oncology. 2013;**22**(2):315-323. Available from:. DOI: 10.1002/pon.2094

[25] Costa SG. Proteção social, maternidade transferida e lutas pela saúde reprodutiva. Revista Estudos Feministas. 2002;**10**(2):301-323. Available from:. DOI: 10.1590/S0104-026X2002000200003

[26] Barros FPC, Sousa MF. Equidade: seus conceitos, significações e implicações para o SUS. Saúde e Sociedade. 2016;**25**(1):9-18. DOI: 10.1590/S0104-12902016146195

[27] Brasil. Instituto Brasileiro de Geografia e Estatística. Pesquisa Nacional

de Saúde. Rio de Janeiro: IBGE; 2019. Available from: https://www.ibge.gov.br/estatisticas/sociais/saude/9160-pesquisa-nacional-de-saude.html?=&t=resultados

[28] Liedke PER et al. Outcomes of breast cancer in Brazil related to health care coverage: a retrospective cohort study. Cancer Epidemiology, Biomarkers & Prevention. 2014;**23**(1):126-133. DOI: 10.1158/1055-9965.EPI-13-0693

[29] Teixeira L. O controle do câncer no Brasil na primeira metade do século XX. História, Ciências, Saúde – Manguinhos. 2010;**17**(suppl 1):13-31. DOI: 10.1590/S0104-12902016146195

[30] Costa AM. A organização da atenção ao câncer de mama nos municípios: estudo de um sistema local de saúde [master's thesis]. Niterói: Programa de Pós-Graduação em Política Social. Universidade Federal Fluminense; 2014. p. 134

[31] Porto MAT, Teixeira LA, Silva RCF. Aspectos históricos do controle do câncer de mama no Brasil. Revista Brasileira de Cancerologia. 2010;**59**(3):331-339. DOI: 10.32635/2176-9745.RBC.2013v59n3.496

[32] Oliveira TN. Proteção social dirigida às mulheres com câncer de mama: um estudo exploratório [master's thesis]. Niterói: Programa de Pós-Graduação em Política Social. Universidade Federal Fluminense; 2017. p. 130

[33] Castro JA. Política social e desenvolvimento no Brasil. Economies et Societes. 2012;**21**(spe):1011-1042. DOI: 10.1590/S0104-06182012000400012

[34] Cabral ALLV et al. Vulnerabilidade social e câncer de mama: diferenciais no intervalo entre o diagnóstico e o tratamento em mulheres de diferentes perfis sociodemográficos. Revista Ciência & Saúde Coletiva. 2019;**24**(2):613-622. DOI: 10.1590/1413-81232018242.31672016

[35] Duarte TC et al. Diagnosis of breast câncer and COVID-19: incidence analysis in the states of Bahia and Rio Grande do Norte. RSD. 2022;**11**(2):e59611226283. DOI: 10.1590/1413-81232018242.31672016

[36] Benites ALCR, Gonçalves AJT, Mendes DG, Silva MCCN, Silvério ACP. Impacts of the COVID-19 pandemic on breast cancer treatment: chemo therapy and endocrine therapy. RSD 2022;11(7):e34211729906. DOI: 10.33448/rsd-v11i7.29906

[37] Mendes EV. O lado oculto de uma pandemia: a terceira onda da Covid-19 ou o paciente invisível. 1st ed. Brasília: CONASS; 2020. p. 92. Available from: https://www.conass.org.br/biblioteca/o-lado-oculto-de-uma-pandemia-a-terceira-onda-da-covid-19-ou-o-paciente-invisivel/

Chapter 5

Breast Cancer, Gender, and Body Experience – A Qualitative Study in Argentina on the Transit of the Illness, Femininity, and Sexuality at Stake

Leila Martina Passerino

Abstract

The chapter examines the transit of women through breast cancer by investigating the transformations in lifestyles and social behaviors that the experience of illness inaugurates. From the perspective of gender studies, we investigate the political technologies that operate on corporeality and the cultural matrices from which we signify, live, and account for this transit. These are experiences that, far from being reduced to singular events, have social roots. In particular, we focus on how the experience of illness acts as a regulating device for the notions of femininity and sexuality in play. This is produced by a reconfiguration of the gaze for oneself and for others, especially when going through certain treatments implies that the illness is "manifested" or becomes "public." With this aim in mind, we look at the different strategies that women adopt, as well as the vicissitudes and shared discomforts that occur in the face of the emergence of the diagnosis and the treatments. The results presented here are the result of research carried out in the Metropolitan Area of Buenos Aires (AMBA) in Argentina during the period 2015–2020, based on in-depth interviews with women between the ages of 25 and 75 who have been diagnosed with breast cancer.

Keywords: breast cancer, gender, femininity, sexuality, social behaviors

1. Introduction

This production is part of a qualitative research developed in the Metropolitan Area of Buenos Aires (AMBA) in Argentina during the period 2015–2020, from the development of in-depth interviews with women who have been diagnosed with breast cancer, aged between 25 and 75 years. We have used the study of biographical forms [1–3] to analyze the experience of women from their narratives and through the technique of in-depth interviews.

We start from the assumption that the experience of women diagnosed with breast cancer is not merely an individual and private aspect, but is always the effect of social norms and ways of feeling. We question the biomedical nomination of the disease as a mere diagnosis, reduced to a sociodemographic or "biological" reference as an attribute or organic condition. In this direction and drawing on critical gender studies, mainly post-structuralism, we reflect on the processes of gendered subjectivation as a gendered and situated experience in specific ways of becoming ill [4–6]. Bodies live within the productive constraints of certain regulatory, gendered schemes that function as norms of intelligibility [7, 8]. We are therefore questioning how a disease whose clinical, epidemiological, and therapeutic aspects put social mandates weighing on women is perceived. Hence, the question revolves around the principles of social regulation of corporeality that are at stake in this experience and its derivations and implications, in the transformations and sensitivities it produces, where the materiality of bodies is inseparable from the norms that regulate their materialization and significance.

The chapter explores how the experience of illness acts as a regulatory device for the notions of femininity and sexuality in play. This is produced by a reconfiguration of the gaze for oneself and for others, especially when going through certain treatments implying that the illness is "manifested" or becomes "public." With this aim in mind, we will examine the different strategies that women adopt, as well as the vicissitudes and shared discomforts that occur when faced with the emergence of the diagnosis and the treatments, particularly with regard to the transformations related to the visibility at stake and aspects related to sexuality. This approach focuses on the social networks involved in the experiences and thus differs from other studies, predominantly from the field of psychology, on sexuality and corporeality [9–13].

2. Bodily transformations and illness: visibility for others and for oneself

Going through cancer, mainly as a result of treatment, brings with it physical changes. Chemotherapy tends to cause hair loss, but also skin changes and swelling: hormone therapy, weight changes, and menopausal symptoms. Surgery, depending on the type and medical guidelines, may involve a mastectomy; that is, the entire mammary gland is removed—including the nipple-areola complex—or a quadrantectomy, in which part of the mammary gland is preserved. This may be in addition to interventions in the axilla or emptying of the axillary lymph node chain, which may coexist with the abovementioned surgeries.

The way these body changes are handled varies. For some women, these transformations go very deep, producing a significant threat to subjectivity and femininity. Thus, a whole operation is set up to "invisibilising" the transition through the disease using resources such as wigs, hats, and makeup. For other women, on the other hand, it may be about aspects that, although not considered ideal, are not entirely problematic, without experiencing them with anguish, loss, and dismay. Many of them make visibility a reason to be able to talk about the subject.

In this process, we are interested in exploring the meanings, the negotiations, the ways in which women deal with the transformations, emphasizing how certain ways of seeing are configured, as signifying processes that produce ways of experiencing illness and which are governed by this external horizon and beyond the world. John Berger [14] is categorical about the centrality of the gaze, especially with regard to the cultural constitution of female subjectivity, as a central problematic axis in his work. In her photographic studies, she has upheld the historical female position in the gender order, characterized and positioned as an object for vision: "A woman must continually contemplate herself. She must be accompanied almost constantly by the image she has of herself (...) From her earliest childhood she has been taught to observe herself continuously. And so she comes to regard the observer and the observed in her as two constituents, but always distinct, elements of her own identity as a woman" [14]. Throughout modern history, it has not been women who actively look, know, and judge but those who are observed, even by themselves. This exercise on oneself can be challenged by going through the treatments, promoting a subjective work, of bodily processing, in the face of the present transformations.

The fear of not knowing how to feel is part of the disruptive process that a surgical intervention exposes and which implies for women a singular type of work, lived intensely and from every detail. It is not only a question of being exposed to one's own fears, or at least not as the origin of them, but of dealing with them vis-à-vis the cultural legacy that permeates our being-in-the-world and our ways of seeing.

From a feminist reading, Lynda Nead [15] has historically investigated the place given to women in the field of the nude in art. She argues that this has been coextensive with the medical field, two fundamental discourses from which the body has been subjected to scrutiny and judged, regulated, and contained. In recent decades, she notes, there has been an intensification of the links between "good" femininity and physical health, "Desirable femininity has been constructed specifically in terms of both health and beauty" [15]. In the same vein, Georges Vigarello [16] does genealogical work on the history of beauty and points to the close link between beauty and health as contemporary gender regulatory ideals. If beauty was once only the privilege of a few women, in the democracies of the inter-war period, it is promoted by the increasingly refined idea that beauty is constructed [16]. The use of cosmetics, fashion, and surgical expertise, above all, guarantees the possibility of intervention. "Pure" surgery is reinvented by another, born in the First World War, "reparative" surgery. The one that should erase the scars, go unnoticed, hide any mark that could make the gaze "there" an undesirable place. Women's bodies gradually become the object of an increasing amount of knowledge and techniques aimed at beautification under the premise of a voluntarist body-object, in which there is no such thing as an ugly woman, but one who neglects herself: "This triumph of the voluntary body displaces the relationship with authority, just as it displaces the relationship with oneself (...) The order that is given ceases to be truly vertical, it plays more with guilt, involving the subject and her responsibility" [16].

This notion of the voluntarist body, but from a reading that articulates power in the processes of negotiation of visibility, allows us to reflect on the political technologies that act on bodies, as processes that are not necessarily conscious, the norm is acted upon, in Judith Butler's terms. Technologies that operate as generated power devices, as María Celia Labandeira [17] expresses, the effect of a specific dynamic of power relations from which we can understand the normativities inscribed on bodies in relation to what is expected, what is healthy, what is beautiful. In Vigarello's line of argument, not looking good is akin to perceiving oneself as ill. In this operation, wigs, makeup, and surgeries are located as *gender technologies* [18] that act on corporealities and from which it is possible to model this visibility of oneself for others after breast cancer treatments. Technologies are part of a sum of social technologies of institutionalized discourses, epistemologies, and critical practices, as much as of everyday life [18].

The negotiation of visibility, its modulations, must be considered here as a process which, as we have already noted, presupposes effort and work on oneself, on how to approach an experience that not only makes the body but also exposes it publicly.

However, beyond the voluntarism that makes this visible corporeality, in a certain way a project, we must consider that the alternatives have been barred by possibilities of access. A generalized reading that takes into account the operating intersectionality allows us here to understand that this performance of norms is part of a process that is biased by access to resources as elements that inevitably participate in the ways of experiencing the illness.

At the beginning of this section, we considered how hair loss following chemotherapy treatment is one of the circumstances that express the emergence of the disease for women. The loss of hair, even if it is a temporary effect of chemotherapy, is an event that many women experience with great anguish. Wigs, scarves, and turbans are undoubtedly elements that help to mitigate the associated feelings of discomfort. For women undergoing chemotherapy, shaving their hair is an almost obligatory step in an attempt to anticipate a more painful outcome, the loss of hair "by locks." It is also a matter of using it with a certain degree of comfort since, for most women, the use of a wig was "something annoying," "itchy," "hot," "heavy," an unhappy artifact, which in the case of synthetic wigs was exacerbated. The wig is mainly used for others and for oneself, when these bodily transformations cannot be dealt with, when one wishes to conceal one's transit in the home—for example, under the gaze of one's children—or to go unnoticed by others in public, in order to avoid giving explanations, to avoid feeling pitied, or to avoid looks of terror and fear. To sleep, they often wear scarves, and to be inside their homes, caps, hats, or turbans, devices are also used when the wig is not accessible or is "uncomfortable" in contact with the skin that is already extremely sensitive due to the drugs used for chemotherapy.

The negotiation of visibility, its modulations, must be considered here as a process that, as we have already noted, presupposes effort and work on oneself, on how to approach an experience that not only makes the body but also exposes it publicly. However, beyond the voluntarism that makes this visible corporeality, in a certain way a project, we must consider that the alternatives have been barred by possibilities of access. A generalized reading that takes into account the operating intersectionality allows us here to understand that this performance of norms is part of a process that is biased by access to resources as elements that inevitably participate in the ways of experiencing the illness.

In the accounts, the use of these artifacts prevails despite the discomfort they cause. It is in this direction that we included the artifacts as gender technologies, devices for the normalization of bodies, which produce discomfort but which operate satisfactorily mitigating other even greater misfortunes, linked to the ways of experiencing the visibility of going through the treatments. In the same direction, the analysis of breast surgery can be included, although it acquires a different subjectivity insofar as the ways of dealing with visibility are produced in the intimate sphere, as a woman states, "the mastectomy is something private, but the hair is something very public," producing other ways of dealing with the image.

Finally, we can also recognize other narratives in which the possibilities of re-signifying these dominant ways of seeing take on other forms. Some of our interviewees do not stop wearing wigs, scarves, or turbans; however, the modes of appropriation are different, and so are the alternatives as bodily dispositions.

As we have seen, the processes of visibility for oneself and for others are part of a complex operation that acts coextensively. That is to say, this reflexivity on oneself that inaugurates the gaze cannot be done outside of eyes that are the same eyes from which we also see ourselves.

3. Sexuality, links, and bodily dispositions

We read sexuality as a device of gendered power. Authors such as De Lauretis [18] and Butler [19] provide tributaries and critics of Foucault's [20] reading and read the body as signified in a context of power relations, where sexuality is a historical and specific organization of these relations. It is a politically complex zone in which affective states, pleasures, pains, fantasies are experiences of the body, but as we have already alluded to, it exceeds it. Sexuality in the face of the experience of illness not only alludes to bodily dispositions as ways of being with and toward the other, in which possibilities crossed by this contingency appear, but at the same time leads us to think about how it should be lived, which opens the field to the ethical dimension and to questions about meanings, choices, moralities, possible ways of linking, and the power relations that are established. These are the two aspects that we are interested in focusing on in this section and which are coextensively involved.

The passage through breast cancer, particularly during the course of treatment, produces transformations in women's ways of experiencing sexuality. Given the wide range of aspects from which the object "sexuality" can be approached, we refer here particularly to the dimension of eroticism, which deals with pleasure, in its different forms, enjoyment, and sexual desire without reproductive purposes [21]. We have already mentioned in the previous section that visibility is part of the experience of illness, although we will emphasize its participation in the modes of erotic-affective bonding with their partners.

Depending on the type of treatment, the transition through the disease involves "side effects" for the ways of dealing with sexuality, in which discomfort, pain, and the sensation of discomfort and weakness transform the ways of bonding that had previously remained unquestioned. To this we must add another type of effect, related to weight gain and the surgical interventions themselves, which can lead to a feeling of strangeness toward one's own body, an estrangement from oneself.

Drugs and radiotherapy can produce lesions such as burns, blisters, reduced vaginal elasticity, and genital pain, which is why it is understandable that women during this time find it painful to try to have sexual relations. To this we can add some of the consequences of treatment-induced menopause, which exacerbates the difficulties of "traditional genitalia." The passage through the treatments exposes many women to a new experience as a sexual being, which brings to "consciousness" aspects unnoticed in the incarnated everyday life.

Many women are concerned about a fundamental aspect of this transition in terms of erotic-affective bonds and find themselves faced with the dilemma of "giving in" or suffering from a "painful" sensation, also experienced out of guilt for their own experience of illness, which is inevitably shared by their partner. This aspect is highlighted by other studies, which addresses the guilt experienced by women with breast cancer when they feel unable to respond sexually to their partners [22, 23]. We can read here not only a bodily tension, but also a concern for the other that in most cases ends up disabling pleasure and sexual desire itself. Sexuality is challenged not only with respect to genitality and penetration itself, but also to the encounter itself.

As we mentioned, the moment when the interview was conducted—as a concrete point in the transition of the experience—and the treatments—the "side effects"—are part of the narration about the experience of sexuality. We are now interested in including other aspects that are also significant and that allude, on the one hand, to the type of erotic-affective link they maintain with their partners and, on the other hand, to the treatments, but particularly, to the surgical interventions and to the production of a certain visibility. Some of these women had stable partners who knew and had experienced with them the first signs of what would later become a diagnosis of breast cancer. Faced with the difficulties and the new situation of going through the treatments, a game was established between the order of what was said and what was not said, between assumptions and aspects that they preferred not to be dealt with, and doubts and ambivalent instances where concern for the other prevailed. For this reason, the work of bodily processing is not limited to women, but forms part of a network that is produced in the links with their partners.

In stable couples, despite the difficulties, there was a tacit knowledge not only about the experience of breast cancer, but also about an erotic understanding as a bond. Even at the time of treatment, they possessed an important capital, which allowed them to anticipate. However, it is totally different for women who try or initiate a relationship during the illness, which speaks of greater difficulties and dilemmas for their subjectivities. For those who did not have a stable partner, starting a relationship can be problematic after surgery or mastectomy. For some, this implied an impossibility to establish any kind of erotic-affective links. For other women, undergoing surgery does not make them erotically and sexually inactive, but they do feel obliged to "warn," to anticipate, an aspect that can also be "traumatic."

The modes of sex-affective processing are largely mediated by visibility, where "negotiations" between partners are at stake, determining how the bodily disposition is experienced in relation to the other. For some women, having sex wearing a bra has been one of the ways of dealing with the transformations resulting from the surgeries. In these cases, an internalization of the norm prevails, which also does not allow visibility of the self without the possibility of anguish. The norm here operates by demanding compliance with certain esthetic patterns, as a dominant visual pattern that directs the gaze, even that of the women themselves who experience sexuality as a result of a loss.

In most of the accounts in our research, the types of bonds established by the women speak of loving care and respect for their partners, their decisions and possibilities, as ways of protecting and also being able to propitiate spaces that favor sexual pleasure and sexuality itself, even if traditional genitality is dispensed with. But we should also mention that not all women were able to be contained and accompanied in these moments of transformation and sensitivity. There are harsh accounts that speak of neglect, abuse, and violence, which are linked to the dynamics of the type of relationship they had. For both of them, this experience has affected them to such an extent that they have not been able to return to their relationships with men, extending this experience to all other possible experiences.

In the narratives recovered for this analysis, we can see a predominance of the gaze as an active participant in the modes of production of sexuality. However, it should be noted that for some women the transit of the illness has not been felt only on this level. Sensitivity is a fundamental aspect to be considered after undergoing surgical treatment.

There are mastectomies in which it is possible to preserve the nipple-areola complex, although this does not necessarily mean preserving sensitivity or the "nipple function," that is, sensitivity as an erogenous zone, breastfeeding the baby.

This also invites us to question the role of reconstructive surgery: reconstructive of what? This is the political question that opens up and which participates as a normative regulation of the materiality of bodies and of the ways of experiencing illness.

DOI: http://dx.doi.org/10.5772/intechopen.109502

4. Conclusions

This chapter has dealt with the experience of women with breast cancer by considering the diagnosis as an instance that exceeds a strictly biomedical nomination and that is linked to life itself, to the conditions of being and thinking in the world. This experience is sometimes disruptive insofar as the unexpected interrupts and destabilizes habitualities. There are displacements, transformations in regularities, and also disputes experienced subjectively, but not for this reason, culturally and socially mediated. This operates as a matrix that acts on bodies and participates in ways of living.

In this chapter, we have focused in particular on some bodily transformations, as a figuration of modes of visibility for others and for oneself, but also on the experience of sexuality and the bodily styles that are put into play in the transition to the experience of illness. The generated modes regulate bodily matter [7] on the basis of dynamics of recognition/unrecognition, and these dimensions are settled as spaces of dispute, fully felt by the subjectivities of this study.

Visibility has been an important dimension during the transit of the disease, making the experience of cancer a public experience. The ways of going through bodily transformations have varied, but they are undoubtedly a source of concern for women. Visibility is adjusted on the basis of a work on the self that presupposes a voluntarist corporeality on which a project is based. From a critical reading, we have noticed here the effort that is made by subjectivities, from the use of different artifacts, to reach an invisibility, biased by access to specific resources and often experienced from the discomfort of such devices, which participate as gender technologies, modeling healthy, acceptable, beautiful corporeality, as a signifying chain that operates simultaneously. We could think of a microphysics of the gaze, paraphrasing Foucault [20], which is expressed in the ways of experiencing illness and must be understood in a larger horizon, from cultural regimes that permeate our experiences and ways of seeing. Undoubtedly, there are other possible dimensions of priority analysis, such as the dimension of the place of breasts in the cultural framework and the so-called reconstructive surgeries. This opens up new questions linked to how to approach bodily materiality, although we have decided not to deal with it here and to think about a future development that will give it greater depth.

The other of the questions addressed here dealt with the experience of sexuality, particularly during the course of the treatments. We referred here to the erotic dimension, as a work of bodily processing in the links themselves. What is said and what is not said, the ways of approaching visibility, the type of bond established, the discomfort caused after the passage of treatments linked to pain, the sensation of weakness, and the feeling of heaviness, were, in the narratives studied, some of the aspects that produce discomfort in the bonds.

We can conclude that the transit through the illness, and particularly the interventions and bodily transformations from the passage through the treatments and surgeries, is part of instances of normative regulation, privileged processes from which it was possible to materially explore these dynamics of power. The experience of illness from a significant contiguity with "the feminine" highlights the regimes of cultural intelligibility that mediate and produce bodies, undoubtedly influencing the ways of experiencing illness.

Acknowledgements

The results of this research have been made possible thanks to funding from the National Scientific and Technological Research Council (CONICET).

Conflict of interest

The author declares no conflict of interest.

Notes/thanks/other declarations

My thanks for the trust placed in all the women who have participated in this study. It is their voices, stories, and sensitivities that have allowed this research to take place. It should be noted that all interviews were conducted under the ethical safeguards of confidentiality of those who participated in this study.

Author details

Leila Martina Passerino
Rafaela Research and Transfer Centre (UNRaf-CONICET), Santa Fe, Argentina

*Address all correspondence to: leila.passerino@unraf.edu.ar

References

[1] Bertaux D. The Biographical Approach: Its Methodological Validity and Potentialities. Vol. LXIX. Paris: Traducido por el TCU 0113020 de la Universidad de Costa Rica, de L'approche biographique: Sa validité méthodologique, ses potentialités En Cahiers lnternationaux de Sociologie; 1999. pp. 197-225

[2] Ferrarotti Franco. Life histories as a method. Convergencia, mayo-agosto. 2007;**14**(n° 44):15-40

[3] Arfuch L. The Biographical Space. Dilemmas of Contemporary Subjectivity. Buenos Aires: Fondo de Cultura Económica; 2002

[4] Young IM. [1990] on Female Body Experience. Throwing like a Girl and Other Essays. Oxford: Oxford University Press; 2005

[5] Alcoff Linda. Merleau-Ponty and the feminist theory of experience. Mora. 1999;**N° 5**:122-138

[6] Tajer D. Wounded Hearts. Coronary Vulnerability in Men and Women. Buenos Aires: Paidós; 2009

[7] Butler J. Bodies That Matter: On the Discursive Limits of Sex. New York: Routledge; 1993

[8] Butler J. Gender Trouble: Feminism and the Subversion of Identity. New York: Routledge; 1990

[9] Sheppard LA, Ely S. Breast cancer and sexuality. The Breast Journal. 2008;**14**(2):176-181. DOI: 10.1111/j.1524-4741.2007.00550.x

[10] Miaja M, Platas A, Martinez-Cannon BA. Psychological impact of alterations in sexuality, fertility, and body image in Young breast cancer patients and their partners. Revista de Investigación Clínica. 2017;**69**(4):204-209. DOI: 10.24875/ric.17002279

[11] Hungr C, Sanchez-Varela V, Bober SL. Self-image and sexuality issues among Young women with breast cancer: Practical recommendations. Revista de Investigación Clínica. 2017;**69**(2):114-122. DOI: 10.24875/ric.17002200

[12] Archangelo SCV, Sabino Neto M, Veiga DF, Garcia EB, Ferreira LM. Sexuality, depression and body image after breast reconstruction. Clinics (São Paulo, Brazil). 2019;**74**:e883. DOI: 10.6061/clinics/2019/e883

[13] Den Ouden MEM, Pelgrum-Keurhorst MN, Uitdehaag MJ, De Vocht HM. Intimacy and sexuality in women with breast cancer: Professional guidance needed. Breast Cancer. 2019;**26**(3):326-332. DOI: 10.1007/s12282-018-0927-8

[14] Berger J. Ways of Seeing. London: Penguin; 1977

[15] Nead L. The Female Nude: Art, Obscenity and Sexuality. New York and London: Routledge; 1992

[16] Vigarello G. History of Beauty. The Body and the Art of Beautifying from the Renaissance to the Present Day. Buenos Aires: Nueva Visión; 2005

[17] Labandeira MC. Cinematic Discourse as Semiotics of Subjectivity: A Scene by Fassbinder. IX: AdVersuS; 2012. pp. 84-121

[18] De Lauretis T. Technologies of Gender: Essays on Theory, Film, and

Fiction. Indiana: Indiana University Press; 1987

[19] Butler J. The Psychic Life of Power: Theories in Subjection. Stanford: Stanford University Press; 1997

[20] Foucault M. The history of sexuality. In: An Introduction. Vol. 1. New York: Vintage; 1990

[21] Gamba S. (Coord.) Dictionary of Gender Studies and Feminisms. Buenos Aires: Editorial Biblos; 2007

[22] Langelleir KM, Sullivan CF. Breast talk in breast cancer narratives. Qualitative Health Research. 1998;**8**:76-94

[23] Mathews H, Burke N, Kampriani E, editors. Anthropologies of Cancer in Transnational Worlds. New York: Routledge; 2015

Chapter 6

Breast Cancer in the Elderly

Agnieszka Jagiello-Gruszfeld and Agnieszka Mlodzinska

Abstract

Breast cancer is a serious health problem in the elderly female population. The approach to treating healthy women aged 65–70 years should be similar to treating younger patients with a similar stage and biological subtype of breast cancer. Greater individualization of treatment is necessary in the case of patients with worse parameters of functional efficiency and features of the frail syndrome. It should also be emphasized the need for closer cooperation with geriatricians, especially when defining the management plan and conducting systemic treatment in this group of patients. There is also a great need for research into the proper selection of treatment in elderly breast cancer patients. This is especially important in groups of patients with early and locally advanced breast cancer.

Keywords: breast cancer, elderly, frailty syndrome, comprehensive geriatric assessment

1. Introduction

Cancer is age-related. Increased life expectancy means that cancers in the elderly are becoming ever more common. More than three-quarters of cancer deaths are among those aged 65 years and older, and more than half among those are aged 75 years and older [1].

This poses a challenge, especially for clinical oncologists, when choosing systemic therapy, due to the specificity of this group of patients. Unfortunately, the group of elderly patients is still underrepresented in clinical trials evaluating new cancer therapies. As a result, there is much less evidence-based information to guide proposed medical management.

Many publications emphasize that older patients are less likely to receive the most effective forms of systemic therapies. This can lead to poorer treatment outcomes and negatively affect patients' survival rates [2].

An important problem for the clinical oncologist is the comorbidities, which occur much more frequently in the elderly versus the younger population. Regrettably, comorbidities happen to be treated suboptimally, especially in people with no family support or care, which can cause additional problems complicating decisions about systemic therapy [3].

It should be pointed out that access to systemic therapy in the elderly population can be significantly hampered for social and economic reasons, especially for patients who live a considerable distance from oncological centers and find it difficult to come to regular visits. This factor is less important when it comes to other types of oncological therapies, namely surgery and radiation therapy, as both are not stretched over time and, if necessary, a patient may be hospitalized until the completion of therapy. In the case of systemic therapy, patients need to visit the oncological center regularly (e.g. once a week or once a month), but they usually do not need to stay at the hospital for more than a few hours [4].

The primary risk factor for breast cancer is age. The median age of onset of this type of cancer is about 60 years. Over 40% of women with newly diagnosed breast cancer are 65 years and older. Since the population is clearly aging, the number of breast cancer patients may be expected to increase significantly in the coming years [1].

At present, the screening in most countries does not cover the population of 70 + – year-old women, mostly because this procedure is less cost-effective in comparison with the population of younger women. This is mainly due to the presence of concomitant diseases which reduce life expectancy, as well as the higher cost of treating breast cancer in elderly women. Besides, elder women are much less likely to report regularly for screening mammography. As a consequence, breast cancer detected in women at the age of 70 plus years is often at more advanced stages than in the case of younger women. According to some sources, over 40% of patients aged over 65 years are diagnosed with breast cancer only when distant metastases are already present [5].

Another very important problem in elderly breast cancer patients is systemic perioperative therapy. Although it is not a major problem to assess such patients eligible for endocrine therapy, a decision to assess a patient eligible for chemotherapy in many cases already raises many doubts among oncologists. The problem is even more compounded by the fact that older patients rarely consent to participate in clinical trials or they meet the exclusion criteria. As a result, elderly patients' therapy is suboptimal, usually not intensive enough, or they are sometimes assessed eligible for therapies that are too toxic for them; both options lead to a situation where the ultimate outcomes of treating older patients are worse.

The work published in 2011 by Smith et al. indicates that although the mortality rate from breast cancer in the <75-year-old population in the US declined by 2.5% per year from 1990 to 2007, breast cancer mortality in women aged 75+ years declined by only 1.1% per year [4]. In Europe, breast cancer mortality declined by 13% from 2000 to 2004 compared with the years 1990–1994; however, this decline was much more pronounced among women aged 35–64 years (17%) compared to only 6% for patients aged 65 years and older [5].

2. Factors affecting the choice of a course of action

In most developed countries, 65 is the chronological age assumed to define the elderly. However, there is no doubt that this is a conventional limit, and the chronological age does not coincide with the biological one. Women aged 65 years are frequently individuals with no functional limitations under the conditions of most developed countries; nonetheless, in developing countries, this limit should be perhaps set much lower. The differences between communities can be very clear, e.g. for those born in 2011, the life expectancy is estimated at 48 to 82 years depending on the region of residence [6, 7].

Therefore, when assessing the eligibility for therapeutic management of an elderly breast cancer patient, not only do we need information about the biological features of breast cancer and its progress but also about comorbidities, received medications and most of all, the patient's biological age, as this information should crucially determine further action to be taken. Most geriatric oncologists agree that the key element is to divide the elderly patients into those who are completely stable, with no co-existing medical conditions, i.e. so-called fit patients, and ailing patients with multiple co-existing internal diseases, i.e. frail patients. Thus, the suggested course of action should be based primarily on the patient's biological age.

Generally speaking, advanced age is associated with reduced tolerance to physiological stress, more frequent occurrence of comorbidities, more intense cognitive disorders, and decreased social support. A patient over the age of 70 years can be expected to suffer on average from three comorbidities. It has been shown that most comorbidities such as renal failure, liver failure, and cerebrovascular disease are mostly associated with an increased risk of death from causes other than breast cancer. The occurrence of any serious and chronic comorbidities is assumed to play a major role in determining the predicted survival time in older patients aged 50–79 years and diagnosed with breast cancer.

This is to some extent confirmed by the study results published in 2011 by Schonberg et al. This study evaluates mortality from the cause of death in 66,000 women aged over 67 years after a breast cancer diagnosis compared to a properly selected group of women without breast cancer [8]. Women with ductal carcinoma in situ (DCIS) or stage I invasive breast cancer had a lower risk of death than the controls, and the most common cause of death was cardiovascular disease. Patients with a diagnosed stage II breast cancer had greater mortality than controls but among women aged 80 years and older, cardiovascular disease was still the prevailing cause of death. In contrast, for stage III or IV breast cancer, breast cancer itself was the commonest cause of death, even with the oldest patients.

Undoubtedly, the biggest decision-making problem is the eligibility assessment or the decision to abandon perioperative chemotherapy.

It seems that the most significant factor to take into account when making that decision should be an assessment of the patient's functional status, which is defined as an individual's ability to perform normal daily activities. In their work, Braithwaite et al. studied a cohort of 2200 women with breast cancer who received adjuvant therapy. Functional limitations in this group were associated with older chronological age, lower education level, and obesity. It has been shown that during the median follow-up of 9 years in patients with functional limitations, the risk of death increased from all causes but not from breast cancer (HR 0.90; 95% CI 1.03–1.92) [9].

Ideally, all elderly patients with indications for perioperative chemotherapy according to the generally applicable guidelines should have a comprehensive geriatric assessment (CGA) or at least a functional status assessment, which, unfortunately, is not possible in most cancers, mainly due to lack of time and qualified medical staff [10].

3. Screening procedures

For over 30 years, the main determinants of improved survival rates for cancer patients have been considered early detection of the disease, i.e. the screening tests that make this possible (namely screening mammography) and the introduction of adjuvant therapy. Most randomized studies evaluating the value of mammography screening did not include women aged 75 years or older. Therefore, the epidemiological benefits of screening in this age group are unknown. Observation studies suggest that older women with a life expectancy of 10 years plus should be taken into account in screening tests. The breast cancer mortality is estimated to be reduced by about 0.2% if active mammography screening is extended beyond the age of 70 years. However, in each case, a decision to continue mammography screening in 70 + – year-old women should be made on a case-by-case basis unless other guidelines are developed [11].

4. Breast cancer biology in elderly patients

Most available publications report that breast cancer in older women is less aggressive. In this group, hormone-dependent cancers are diagnosed more frequently, and overexpression of the HER2 receptor, grade 3 cancers, and high Ki67 values are less common.

The odds of developing triple-negative cancer in women aged <40 years are 1.53 times higher than in patients aged over 60 years, but 15–18% of older patients are diagnosed with this breast cancer subtype, which confers a poor prognosis [12].

Age does not significantly affect the cancer's histological subtype, but lobular, mucinous, and papillary carcinomas are slightly more common in older patients. For example, mucinous carcinomas account for 4–6% of cancers diagnosed over the age of 75 years, whereas only 1% of premenopausal women are diagnosed with this type of cancer [12, 13].

5. Distinctions in the management of systemic therapy in elderly patients

When conducting oncological systemic therapy in the geriatric population, various side effects may be observed that are directly related to the type of therapy. Depending on the formation mechanism, they may occur with similar or greater frequency than in younger age groups.

However, when treating the elderly, we also encounter problems that are not at all or very rarely described in younger patients. They mainly concern the aging physiology as well as the psychological and sociological levels [14, 15].

The biology of some cancers and their response to therapy changes as the patient ages. In addition, physiological changes associated with aging can affect the tolerance of the drugs. The lower renal and hepatic performance, as well as low bone marrow reserve, which arises from the physiological changes in the aging body, can fundamentally affect the pharmacokinetics and pharmacodynamics of the drugs.

Comorbidities, mainly cardiovascular and nervous ones, are also much more common in elderly patients. Some of those patients may be malnourished and experience geriatric syndromes such as incontinence, tendency to fall, balance disorders, frailty syndrome, and dementia. In addition, in this group of patients, we often deal with polypragmasy [3, 12, 14].

All of these factors can significantly complicate or even prevent optimal systemic therapy. Furthermore, if patients face other types of medical problems, these can significantly define their life expectancy and considerably impair their quality of life [16]. What is of particular importance is the detection of frailty syndrome. Literature data indicate that over half of elderly oncological patients exhibit some or all features of frailty syndrome. This group of patients specifically is often at increased risk of mortality, postoperative complications, and serious side effects associated with systemic therapy, especially chemotherapy [15, 17].

Psychosocial factors have been described as having a significant impact on therapeutic decisions and the course of treatment. Elderly patients living alone or with a person of a similar age are less likely to accept possible problems that may arise during treatment.

Similar difficulties may arise for people having difficult access to transportation and those residing in nursing homes. In many countries, governmental or nongovernmental initiatives are emerging to reduce barriers to access oncological treatment among the elderly and disabled. These may involve medical staff visiting the patient at their home to inject or infuse drugs, blood draws for laboratory tests, etc., as well as telephone monitoring of the patient's condition to detect possible adverse symptoms in advance.

Patients with dementia pose a significant problem for oncologists. In most clinical situations, people with minor dementia can understand the rules of the suggested therapy and make proper decisions on their own, if given enough time to explain them properly. In the case of people with more advanced dementia, the caregiver must participate in the decision-making process concerning the therapy and further care provided to the patient.

It should also be pointed out that older patients may prefer therapies that have the potential to improve their quality of life, whereas longer survival may be of lower importance for them. The Silvestri study, for example, assessed the preferences for chemotherapy in patients with advanced lung cancer. Only 22% of patients chose chemotherapy for 3 months' improvement in survival, but the majority (68%) would choose chemotherapy if it substantially reduced symptoms without prolonging life [18].

6. Individual approach to systemic therapy in elderly patients

As the dependencies between genetic and environmental factors in the aging process are quite complex, the aging process for each person is slightly different. Therefore, the chronological age alone does not reflect a patient's condition, nor can it be considered a predictor of response to treatment and the occurrence of side effects or other therapy-related problems. To be able to make optimal decisions about systemic therapy in elderly patients, you need to characterize the functional reserve, both from the physical and mental point of view, as well as assess the number and severity of comorbidities and evaluate the patient's social capabilities [17, 19].

It is also important to make certain modifications, if any, to the treatment of comorbidities, that includes consultations with other specialists, especially in the field of geriatrics, but also rehabilitation, nutrition, etc.

During systemic therapy, it is important to implement any methods that can reduce side effects.

The most important element that is fundamentally responsible for the success of systemic therapy in a group of geriatric patients seems to be the individual assessment of the patient's condition before deciding on their eligibility for therapy. This assessment should be done as early as the initial visit to the clinical oncologist [20, 21].

At present, we have several tools that can help us assess the risk of serious complications arising during systemic therapy. The most commonly recommended tools are the CRASH score and CARG score.

Extermann developed the CRASH score calculator (https://moffitt.org/eforms/crashscoreform), which can be used to assess the risk of serious chemotherapy complications among elderly patients based on information about the planned therapy and patient characteristics. The main elements indicating the risk of hematologic toxicities are the instrumental activities of daily living score (IADL), blood lactate dehydrogenase level, diastolic blood pressure value, and estimated toxicity of the chemotherapy regimen. In contrast, the incidence of serious non-hematological complications is supported by the patient's ECOG score, cognitive status using the mini-mental state examination (MMSE) score, nutritional status using the mini-nutritional assessment (MNA) score, and the toxicity of the therapy regimen [22].

Huria was the author of a similar tool, namely the CARG score calculator (https://www.mycarg.org/?page_id=934 or https://www.evidencio.com/models/show/520), which can be used to assess the risk of serious complications of systemic therapy based on such information as the patient's condition (age, the number of falls they have had within the past 6 months, limited social activity, and need for assistance with medications), laboratory test results (creatinine and hemoglobin levels), and the proposed therapy regimen. In addition, Huria emphasized that the Karnofsky Performance Status (KPS) commonly used by oncologists to assess the performance status of the elderly is not useful at all [23].

Recently, we have observed some opinions that point out the importance of optimizing psychosocial and physical health before starting systemic therapy in older patients. This involves the identification of patient's needs in this regard. The International Society of Geriatric Oncology (SIOG), an organization dedicated to addressing oncology issues in the elderly, recommends conducting a comprehensive geriatric assessment (CGA) before undertaking any planned surgical intervention or systemic therapy in elderly oncological patients. The value of this assessment lies not only in determining the risk of possible complications but primarily in seeing it as a possibility of optimization and individualization of treatment [3, 19].

Kalsi published the results of a randomized trial involving 135 cancer patients over the age of 70 years who were eligible for chemotherapy. The observational control group (70 patients) received standard oncological therapy, while the intervention group (65 patients) underwent risk stratification using a patient-completed screening questionnaire; subjects were assigned to appropriate groups, depending on the risk of complications. Those at high risk of complications had a comprehensive geriatric assessment performed and, based on the results, were given plans for appropriate multidisciplinary interventions. It turned out that patients in the intervention group were more likely to follow the expected treatment plan and were less likely to require any modification of therapy [10, 24].

Thus, there seems to be a need to change the approach to oncological therapy of elderly patients taking into account the need to implement measures currently referred to as prehabilitation [25].

7. Surgery and radiotherapy for breast cancer

Unquestionably, unless there are very significant contraindications to anesthesia, stage II, post-neoadjuvant therapy breast cancer patients (and in selected cases stage III patients that have not received neoadjuvant therapy) should be offered surgical therapy, which may involve breast-conserving surgery or mastectomy.

In selected cases, i.e. in patients with a predicted survival time shorter than 5 years, axillary procedures as well as any surgical treatment in general may be abandoned when the preinvasive form of breast cancer has been diagnosed.

However, studies have shown that surgical treatment is often abandoned in elderly patients for various reasons. The study of Bastiaannet et al., which involved more than 120,000 women, showed that older age was associated with a lower percentage of surgeries. Whereas more than 93% of women under 80 years of age underwent surgery, the percentages of radical breast cancer surgery performed in the 80–84, 85–89, and over 90 years of age groups totaled, 83%, 65%, and 41%, respectively. Also, it has been shown that older patients were less often eligible for radiation therapy after breast-conserving surgeries. In that group, in women under the age of 75 years, radiotherapy was used in more than 90% of cases, while in the age groups of 75–79, 80–84, 85–89, and 90+ years, it totaled 86%, 71%, 36%, and 15%, respectively. However, this study does not report on how the decision of radiotherapy was dependent on cancer recurrence risk factors. The same paper claims that the eligibility for hormone therapy (without surgical treatment) rate increased with age. It ranged from <1% in patients below the age of 65 years up to 47% in patients aged 90 years and older [26].

Another study attempted to answer the question of whether the lower number of surgeries performed arose from the functional status or biological age of patients with stage I, II, or III breast cancer. Multivariate analysis showed that women aged 85 years and older were significantly less likely to undergo breast cancer surgery having taken into account the patient's possible negative attitude toward the procedure and their functional status (the odds ratio [OR]: 0.18, 95% CI 0.07–0.44). These data suggest that objective considerations are not always decisive when assessing older patients' eligibility for surgery [27].

Most patients without functional status limitations should be eligible for adjuvant radiotherapy following breast-conservative surgery. However, it should be noted that even during the visit to discuss surgical treatment options with the patient, they should be informed of the radiation therapy options, as some patients may decide not to have radiation therapy for the fear of its consequences or for social reasons [28].

8. Systemic perioperative therapy

Older patients with early forms of breast cancer and perfect or very good functional status may be offered adjuvant therapy per standard treatment guidelines for younger patients. In the case of patients with multiple internal concomitant diseases, cognitive disorders, and functional status limitations, the suggested therapy should mainly depend on the feasibility and expediency of surgical therapy. If surgery had been performed, in most patients with an estimated survival time of up to 5 years, systemic therapy and radiotherapy may be abandoned. On the other hand, those patients that do not agree to surgery or who cannot have surgery due to medical contraindications should receive hormone therapy (in case of hormone-sensitive cancers) or remain under the supervision of an oncologist or a general practitioner (GP).

It is believed at present, that breast cancer patients aged 65–70 years should be initially evaluated in terms of their general condition and internal diseases by an oncologist, and only the preselected patients should undergo geriatric screening tests (mainly to evaluate their functional status). To this end, it is recommended to use the G8, VES-13, TRST 1+ scales, or Groningen Frailty Index. This evaluation should be also performed for all older patients. In the case of some patients, the next necessary step before making any decisions about the therapy may be a comprehensive geriatric evaluation and geriatric consultation [29–31].

This will help to select a group of older patients who should be eligible for or totally excluded from chemotherapy. Additionally, the International Society of Geriatric Oncology (SIOG) guidelines suggest the need for serial evaluation of functional status during adjuvant therapy to identify deterioration of the patient's health and undertake necessary intervention as early as possible [24, 32].

8.1 Fit patients

The treatment management of fit older breast cancer patients is identical to that of younger women and depends primarily on the evaluation of the recurrence risk factors. As a general rule, some patients should be offered neoadjuvant therapy.

The preferred cytostatic agents for perioperative treatment in this group of patients are anthracyclines and taxanes. However, you should remember the risk of myocardial damage after anthracyclines; therefore, women with significant cardiac comorbidities should be excluded from therapy with this group of cytostatic agents.

The study conducted by Pinder et al., which included 44,338 women aged 66–80 years with stage I–III breast cancer with no history of heart failure, showed that with a follow-up median of 56 months, evidence of heart failure after 5 and 10 years after the end of treatment in the group of patients who received anthracyclines (4000 patients) totaled 19% and 38%, whereas in the case of patients that did not receive anthracyclines, they totaled 18% and 33%, respectively. In the case of patients who did not receive any chemotherapy, it totaled 15% and 29%. Heart failure symptoms were observed more frequently in Black patients, as well as in patients with hypertension, diabetes, and coronary artery disease [33].

Other options involving slightly less cardiotoxicity are epirubicin or liposomal anthracyclines.

In patients who cannot receive anthracyclines, a TC (docetaxel with cyclophosphamide) regimen can be used. In a randomized phase III clinical trial published in 2009, four cycles of TC were shown to produce superior median progression-free survival and median overall survival compared with four cycles of AC, in patients with stage I–III cancer aged 65 years and older [34].

Another option is a CMF regimen (cyclophosphamide, methotrexate, 5-fluorouracil), but this is not the preferred option due to the high risk of hematological complications in elderly patients [35].

Where we are dealing with patients with lower performance status or significant internal comorbidities, a reasonable option may be paclitaxel administered weekly for 12 weeks at a dose of 60–80 mg/m2 [36].

Single-agent capecitabine is not recommended as adjuvant therapy in elderly patients. A randomized phase III trial involving 633 patients aged 65 years and older with early-stage breast cancer, which was published in 2009, showed that capecitabine produced worse therapy results. During the follow-up (a follow-up median of 2.4 years), a progression-free survival rate totaled 68% versus 85%, whereas an overall survival rate was 85% versus 91% after a follow-up median of 3 years [37].

Adjuvant therapy combined with trastuzumab and taxanes is recommended for breast cancer patients with overexpression of HER2. Sequencing of anthracyclines is usually not recommended due to the increased risk of heart failure.

Data on the use of docetaxel and carboplatin in combination with trastuzumab, as well as with trastuzumab and pertuzumab, are very limited in women aged 70 years and older. Rather, a TC (docetaxel with cyclophosphamide) regimen should be considered in selected cases in patients with no functional status limitations and higher-stage cancers.

Also, in the case of HER2-positive cancer patients, chemotherapy can be often limited to paclitaxel administered weekly for 12 weeks. In contrast, for patients diagnosed with stage I and II hormone-sensitive, HER2-positive cancer, hormone therapy in combination with trastuzumab may be a sufficient treatment option [37, 38].

For patients with cardiovascular comorbidities, consideration may be given to shortening the length of trastuzumab therapy, as trastuzumab-induced cardiotoxicity is linked to the length of exposure [38, 39].

Until now, there are no guidelines pertaining to the group of older patients regarding prolonged anti-HER2 cancer therapy with neratinib, nor the use of trastuzumab emtansine for the minimal residual disease after the completion of neoadjuvant therapy.

Preoperative hormone therapy is recommended for patients with hormone-sensitive cancers at a locally advanced stage, or for those interested in conserving therapy but whose anatomical conditions prevent it at the time of breast cancer diagnosis. The recommended group of drugs in this case is aromatase inhibitors. They should be administered for 6–9 months and, of course, should be continued after the surgery, as long as the response to therapy is observed [40].

Adjuvant hormonal treatment should be offered to all patients with hormone-sensitive breast cancer, regardless of age. Aromatase inhibitors are preferred in older women due to the greater benefit of such treatment in this patient group versus tamoxifen and a more favorable safety profile. However, for patients at high risk of cardiovascular complications and with advanced osteoporosis or aromatase inhibitor intolerance, tamoxifen is also a reasonable option.

The optimal duration of adjuvant hormone therapy is not fully established. The minimum therapy duration should be 5 years, but in selected patients, it may be recommended to extend the therapy up to 10 years [41, 42].

8.2 Patients with evidence of frailty syndrome

Patients with evidence of a frailty syndrome, short life expectancy, and those wishing to avoid any therapy-related toxicities should be treated on a case-to-case basis [43, 44].

In some patients, systemic therapy can simply be abandoned (except for hormone therapy in hormone-sensitive cancer patients).

Also, in this group, aromatase inhibitors as hormonal therapy are preferred, but there are no results of prospective studies in this patient population comparing the efficacy and safety of tamoxifen versus aromatase inhibitors.

Similarly, no results of randomized trials comparing more aggressive treatments with hormone therapy, or hormone therapy only, have been published.

8.3 Metastatic breast cancer

Metastatic breast cancer remains incurable regardless of the patient's age, and any available therapy is palliative. Only about 20% of metastatic patients survive 5 years.

However, even in older patients with metastases, there is a high risk of death from causes other than breast cancer [8, 12].

The goal of therapy in metastatic patients is to maintain the highest quality of life for as long as possible.

8.4 Triple-negative cancer

The general approach to treating older patients with metastatic triple-negative breast cancer is similar to that followed in younger patients; it consists of using single agents sequentially, except for patients with rapidly progressive symptomatic metastases [45].

Radiation therapy should be considered for older patients with symptomatic brain and bone metastases.

Older age has been proven to be a risk factor for early death in those who present with de novo metastatic triple-negative breast cancer.

In a group of older patients, several single agents are recommended as preferred single agents. These include capecitabine, weekly paclitaxel, nab-paclitaxel, eribulin (as second- and third-line treatment), liposomal doxorubicin, vinorelbine, and gemcitabine [34, 45, 46].

The choice of drug should be based on the toxicity profile. As first-line therapy, response rates vary greatly according to patient characteristics, and average about 30–50%, while progression-free survival time averages about 3 to 6 months. Second- and third-line therapies are less effective.

In comparison with younger age groups, the use of chemotherapy in patients aged 80 years and older has been shown to be associated with a significantly higher rate of hospitalizations (32%), red blood cell concentrates transfusions (18%), and reduced doses of cytostatic drugs, skipping and/or delaying subsequent doses (68%) [47, 48].

Other drugs that can be considered for the treatment of elderly patients include olaparib (poly(ADP-ribose) polymerase inhibitor). However, as with most trials of newer agents, the registration study of that drug in breast cancer patients involved only 15 patients aged 65 years and older [34, 49].

Modulating the immune system using checkpoint inhibitors also shows promise, but almost no data are available from randomized clinical trials in older breast cancer patients [50].

8.5 Hormone-dependent cancer

The primary treatment option for generalized hormone-dependent breast cancer is hormone therapy. Preferred options for first-line therapy are aromatase inhibitors or fulvestrant. In most cases, hormone therapy may be combined with cyclin-dependent kinase 4/6 inhibitors. A particular agent from this group should be selected depending on the expected side effects. Most authors suggest that palbociclib may be the agent best tolerated by elderly patients [51, 52].

The second-line therapy should include a hormonal drug that has not been used yet in combination with a CDK 4/6 inhibitor (provided it has not been used before). The combination of hormone therapy with alpelisib is also recommended in older patients with PIK3CA mutations [53].

In the case of patients with hormone resistance, chemotherapy is also an option, according to standard guidelines for patients with triple-negative cancers.

8.6 Cancer with overexpression of the HER2 receptor

For older patients with HER2-positive cancers, pertuzumab, trastuzumab, and a taxane are recommended as first-line therapy options, similarly to younger age groups, whereas paclitaxel is the preferred option in this case [37, 49].

Patients with poorer functional status may be considered for pertuzumab and trastuzumab in combination with cyclophosphamide administered orally at a dose of 50 mg/day [54].

The combination of dual anti-HER2 blockade with an aromatase inhibitor is also a recommended option in patients with HER2-positive hormone-sensitive cancers.

In the next line of therapy, trastuzumab emtansine (T-DM1) is recommended due to the good safety profile of this drug in the elderly patient population.

For patients with good functional status, other drugs that act on the HER2 receptor may be considered, but information on the safety of these drugs in the group of patients older than 65 years is very limited [47, 49].

8.7 Patients with evidence of frailty syndrome

Patients with generalized breast cancer and evidence of frailty syndrome, significant cognitive disorders, or multiple co-existing internal diseases should be treated on a case-to-case basis. It should be noted that the proposed treatment must not cause more problems for the patient and her family than the cancer itself. Therefore, sometimes the best option may be to use symptomatic therapy only in hospice-palliative care [55].

9. Conclusion

Breast cancer is a serious health problem in the elderly female population. The approach to treating healthy women aged 65–70 years should be similar to treating younger patients with a similar stage and biological subtype of breast cancer.

Greater individualization of treatment is necessary for patients with worse functional status and evidence of frailty syndrome. The need for closer cooperation with geriatricians should be also pointed out, especially when determining the management plan and conducting systemic therapy in this group of patients.

There is also a great need for research on the appropriate choice of therapy for elderly breast cancer patients. This is of particular importance in early and locally advanced breast cancer patients.

Author details

Agnieszka Jagiello-Gruszfeld* and Agnieszka Mlodzinska
Breast Cancer and Reconstructive Surgery Department, Maria Sklodowska-Curie National Research Institute of Oncology, Warsaw, Poland

*Address all correspondence to: agnieszka.jagiellogruszfeld@gmail.com; agnieszka.jagiello-gruszfeld@pib-nio.pl

References

[1] National Cancer Institute Surveillance. Epidemiology and end results: Breast cancer incidence and mortality. http://seer.cancer.gov/statfacts/html/breast.html

[2] Ries LA, Eisner MP, Kosary CL. SEER Cancer Statistics Review 1973-1999. Bethesda, MD, USA: National Cancer Institute; 2009

[3] Biganzoli L, Wildiers H, Oakman C, et al. Management of elderly patients with breast cancer: Updated recommendations of the International Society of Geriatric Oncology (SIOG) and European Society of Breast Cancer Specialists (EUSOMA). The Lancet Oncology. 2012;**13**(4):e148-e160

[4] Smith BD, Jiang J, McLaughlin SS, et al. Improvement in breast cancer outcomes over time: Are older women missing out? Journal of Clinical Oncology. 2011;**29**(35):4647-4653

[5] Berry DA, Cronin KA, Plevritis SK, et al. Effect of screening and adjuvant therapy on mortality from breast cancer. The New England Journal of Medicine. 2005;**353**(17):1784-1792

[6] La Vecchia C, Bosetti C, Lucchini F, et al. Cancer mortality in Europe, 2000-2004, and an overview of trends since 1975. Annals of Oncology. 2010;**21**(6):1323-1360

[7] Kalben BB. Why men die younger: Causes of mortality differences by sex. North American Actuarial Journal. 2000;**4**(4):83-111

[8] Schonberg MA, Marcantonio ER, Ngo L, Li D, Silliman RA, McCarthy EP. Causes of death and relative survival of older women after a breast cancer diagnosis. Journal of Clinical Oncology. 2011;**29**(12):1570-1577

[9] Braithwaite D, Satariano WA, Sternfeld B, et al. Long-term prognostic role of functional limitations among women with breast cancer. Journal of the National Cancer Institute. 2010;**102**(19):1468-1477

[10] Hamaker ME, Jonker JM, de Rooij SE, Vos AG, Smorenburg CH, vanMunster BC. Frailty screening methods for predicting outcome of a comprehensive geriatric assessment in elderly patients with cancer: A systematic review. The Lancet Oncology. 2012;**13**(10):E437-E444

[11] Nelson HD, Tyne K, Naik A, Bougatsos C, Chan BK, Humphrey L. Screening for breast cancer: An update for the U.S. Preventive Services Task Force. Annals of Internal Medicine. 2009;**151**(10):727-737

[12] Tesarova P. Specific aspects of breast cancer therapy of elderly women. Biomedical Research International. 2016;**2016**:1381695. DOI: 10.1155/2016/1381695

[13] Ogunbiyi SO, Lee S, Mathew J, Cheung KL. Primary breast cancer in the elderly: A systematic literature review on histological type and clinical outcome. Future Oncology. 2015;**11**(2):259-265

[14] Shachar SS, Hurria A, Muss HB. Breast cancer in women older than 80 years. Journal of Oncology Practice. 2016;**12**(2):123-132

[15] Chen H, Cantor A, Meyer J, et al. Can older cancer patients tolerate chemotherapy? A prospective pilot study. Cancer. 2003;**97**(4):1107-1114

[16] Di Maio M, Perrone F. Quality of life in elderly patients with cancer. Health and Quality of Life Outcomes. 2003;**1**:44 http://www.ncbi.nlm.nih.gov/pubmed/14525617

[17] Handforth C, Clegg A, Young C, et al. The prevalence and outcomes of frailty in older cancer patients: A systematic review. Annals of Oncology. 2015;**26**(6):1091-1101 http://www.ncbi.nlm.nih.gov/pubmed/25403592

[18] Silvestri G, Pritchard R, Welch HG. Preferences for chemotherapy in patients with advanced non-small cell lung cancer: Descriptive study based on scripted interviews. BMJ. 1998;**317**(7161):771-775. http://www.ncbi.nlm.nih.gov/pubmed/9740561

[19] Turner N, Zafarana E, Becheri D, Mottino G, Biganzoli L. Breast cancer in the elderly: Which lessons have we learned? Future Oncology. 2013;**9**(12):1871-1881

[20] Valero S, Migeot V, Bouche G, et al. Who needs a comprehensive geriatric assessment? A French Onco-geriatric screening tool. Journal of Geriatric Oncology. 2011;**2**(2):130-136

[21] Parry JL, Hall PS, Young J. New horizons in systemic anti-cancer therapy in older people. Age and Ageing. 2018;**47**(3):340-348. DOI: 10.1093/ageing/afy024

[22] Extermann M, Boler I. Reich RR et al Predicting the Risk of Chemotherapy Toxicity in Older Patients: The Chemotherapy Risk Assessment Scale for High-Age Patients (CRASH) Score

[23] Hurria A, Togawa K, Mohile SG, et al. Predicting chemotherapy toxicity in older adults with cancer: A prospective multicenter study. Journal of Clinical Oncology. 2011;**29**(25):3457-3465

[24] Kalsi T, Babic-Illman G, Ross PJ, et al. The impact of comprehensive geriatric assessment interventions on tolerance to chemotherapy in older people. British Journal of Cancer. 2015;**112**(9):1435-1444

[25] Silver JK, Baima J. Cancer prehabilitation. American Journal of Physical Medicine & Rehabilitation. 2013;**92**(8):715-727 http://www.ncbi.nlm.nih.gov/pubmed/23756434

[26] Bastiaannet E, Liefers GJ, de Craen AJM, et al. Breast cancer in elderly compared to younger patients in the Netherlands: Stage diagnosis, treatment and survival in 127,805 unselected patients. Breast Cancer Research and Treatment. 2010;**124**(3):801-807

[27] Lavelle K, Sowerbutts AM, Bundred N, et al. Is lack of surgery for older breast cancer patients in the UK explained by patient choice or poor health? A prospective cohort study. Journal of Cancer. 2014;**110**(3):573-583

[28] Audisio RA, Bozzetti F, Gennari R, et al. The surgical management of elderly cancer patients: Recommendations of the SIOG surgical task force. European Journal of Cancer. 2004;**40**(7):926-938

[29] Land LH, Dalton SO, Jensen M-B, Ewertz M. Influence of comorbidity on the effect of adjuvant treatment and age in patients with early-stage breast cancer. British Journal of Cancer. 2012;**107**(11):1901-1907

[30] Patnaik JL, Byers T, Diguiseppi C, Denberg TD, Dabelea D. The influence of comorbidities on overall survival among older women diagnosed with breast cancer. Journal of the National Cancer Institute. 2011;**103**(14):1101-1111

[31] Extermann M, Balducci L, Lyman GH. What threshold for adjuvant

therapy in older breast cancer patients? Journal of Clinical Oncology. 2000;**18**(8):1709-1717

[32] Hurria A, Levit LA, Dale W, et al. Improving the evidence base for treating older adults with cancer: American Society of Clinical Oncology Statement. Journal of Clinical Oncology. 2015;**33**(32):3826-3833 http://jco.ascopubs.org/cgi/doi/10.1200/JCO.2015.63.0319

[33] Pinder MC, Duan Z, Goodwin JS, Hortobagyi GN, Giordano SH. Congestive heart failure in older women treated with adjuvant anthracycline chemotherapy for breast cancer. Journal of Clinical Oncology. 2007;**25**(25):3808-3815

[34] Yoon J, Knapp G, Quan ML, Bouchard-Fortier A. Cancer-specific outcomes in the elderly with triple-negative breast cancer: A systematic review. Current Oncology. 2021;**28**(4):2337-2345. DOI: 10.3390/curroncol28040215

[35] De Maio E, Gravina A, Pacilio C, et al. Compliance and toxicity of adjuvant CMF in elderly breast cancer patients: A single-center experience. BMC Cancer. 2005;**5**:article 30

[36] Muss HB, Berry DA, Cirrincione CT, et al. Adjuvant chemotherapy in older women with early-stage breast cancer. The New England Journal of Medicine. 2009;**360**(20):2055-2065

[37] Pallis AG, Fortpied C, Wedding U, et al. EORTC elderly task force position paper: Approach to the older cancer patient. European Journal of Cancer. 2010;**46**(9):1502-1513

[38] Freedman RA, Vaz-Luis I, Barry WT, et al. Patterns of chemotherapy, toxicity, and short-term outcomes for older women receiving adjuvant trastuzumab-based therapy. Breast Cancer Research and Treatment. 2014;**145**(2):491-501

[39] Vaz-Luis NL, Keating NU, Lin H, Lii EP, Freedman RA. Duration and toxicity of adjuvant trastuzumab in older patients with early-stage breast cancer: A population-based study. Journal of Clinical Oncology. 2014;**32**(9):927-934

[40] Martí C, Sánchez-Méndez JI. The present and future of Neoadjuvant endocrine therapy for breast cancer treatment. Cancers (Basel). 2021;**13**(11):2538. DOI: 10.3390/cancers13112538. PMID: 34064183; PMCID: PMC8196711

[41] Dowsett M, Cuzick J, Ingle J, et al. Meta-analysis of breast cancer outcomes in adjuvant trials of aromatase inhibitors versus tamoxifen. Journal of Clinical Oncology. 2010;**28**(3):509-518

[42] Ferrigni E, Bergom C, Yin Z, Szabo A, Kong AL. Breast cancer in women aged 80 years or older: An analysis of treatment patterns and disease outcomes. Clinical Breast Cancer. 2019;**19**(3):157-164. DOI: 10.1016/j.clbc.2019.01.007

[43] Yancik R, Wesley MN, Ries LAG, Havlik RJ, Edwards BK, Yates JW. Effect of age and comorbidity in postmenopausal breast cancer patients aged 55 years and older. The Journal of the American Medical Association. 2001;**285**(7):885-892

[44] Luciani A, Jacobsen PB, Extermann M, et al. Fatigue and functional dependence in older cancer patients. American Journal of Clinical Oncology. 2008;**31**(5):424-430 http://content.wkhealth.com/linkback/openurl?sid=WKPTLP:landingpage&an=00000421-200810000-00004

[45] Kumar P, Aggarwal R. An overview of triple-negative breast cancer. Archives of Gynecology and Obstetrics. 2016;**293**:247-269

[46] Begg CB, Carbone PP. Clinical trials and drug toxicity in the elderly. The experience of the eastern cooperative oncology group. Cancer. 1983;**52**(11):1986-1992 http://www.ncbi.nlm.nih.gov/pubmed/6354419

[47] Sud S, Lai P, Zhang T, et al. Chemotherapy in the oldest old: The feasibility of delivering cytotoxic therapy to patients 80 years old and older. Journal of Geriatric Oncology. 2015;**6**:395-400

[48] Ring A, Harari D, Kalsi T, Mansi J, Selby P. Problem Solving in Older Cancer Patients: A Case-Study Based Reference and Learning Resource. Oxford, UK: Clinical Publishing; 2016. p. 272

[49] Pondé N, Wildiers H, Awada A, de Azambuja E, Deliens C, Lago LD. Targeted therapy for breast cancer in older patients. Journal of Geriatric Oncology. 2020;**11**(3):380-388. DOI: 10.1016/j.jgo.2019.05.012

[50] Hutchins LF, Unger JM, Crowley JJ, Coltman CA, Albain KS. Underrepresentation of patients 65 years of age or older in cancer-treatment trials. The New England Journal of Medicine. 1999;**341**(27):2061-2067 http://www.ncbi.nlm.nih.gov/pubmed/10615079

[51] Lee SY, Seo JH. Current strategies of endocrine therapy in elderly patients with breast cancer. BioMed Research International. 2018;**2018**:6074808. DOI: 10.1155/2018/6074808

[52] Battisti NML, De Glas N, Sedrak MS, Loh KP, Liposits G, Soto-Perez-de-Celis E, et al. Use of cyclin-dependent kinase 4/6 (CDK4/6) inhibitors in older patients with ER-positive HER2-negative breast cancer: Young International Society of Geriatric Oncology review paper. Therapeutic Advanced Medicine Oncology. 2018 Nov;**20**(10):175. DOI: 10.1177/1758835918809610

[53] Almodallal Y, Le-Rademacher JG, Cook KD, Yadav S, Singh AB, Lee M, et al. Observations with alpelisib in older patients (≥65 years of age) with breast cancer in a non-clinical trial setting. Breast Cancer Research and Treatment. 2021;**188**(1):15-20. DOI: 10.1007/s10549-021-06277-6

[54] Wildiers H, Tryfonidis K, Dal Lago L, Vuylsteke P, Curigliano G, Waters S, et al. Pertuzumab and trastuzumab with or without metronomic chemotherapy for older patients with HER2-positive metastatic breast cancer (EORTC 75111-10114): An open-label, randomised, phase 2 trial from the Elderly Task Force/Breast Cancer Group. The Lancet Oncology. 2018;**19**(3):323-336. DOI: 10.1016/S1470-2045(18)30083-4

[55] Gironés Sarrió R, Antonio Rebollo M, Molina Garrido MJ, Guillén-Ponce C, Blanco R, Gonzalez Flores E, et al. General recommendations paper on the management of older patients with cancer: The SEOM geriatric oncology task force's position statement. Clinical & Translational Oncology. 2018;**20**(10):1246-1251. DOI: 10.1007/s12094-018-1856-x

Chapter 7

Management of the Triple Negative Locally Advanced Breast Cancer

Amir Iqbal Memon, Ikram Din Ujjan and Aisha Masroor Bhatti

Abstract

One out of eight women is suffering from the breast cancer. 2.3 million New cases is predicted by 2023 worldwide. Triple negative breast cancer (TNBC) is having 10–15% incidence. As categorized with the lack of estrogen, progesterone and human epidermal growth factor receptor 2 neu receptor expression. Though it presents with narrow management opportunities that makes it to be the poor prognostic as well as survival rate. The management of the TNBC includes: neoadjuvant treatment then surgery and the adjuvant treatment or the surgery as the first step and then the adjuvant treatment options accordingly. The discussion are still going on to set a management protocol for the triple negative breast cancers with positive outcome and the good disease free survival. Neoadjuvant or adjuvant chemotherapy decreases the estradiol levels and thus improves the survival. The immune check points and immune modulators are under the research and the trials are still going on to treat the TNBC with the improved outcomes. It has been concluded that the management of the TNBC, still wanting the guidelines as tumor-specific targeted therapies is in trials.

Keywords: triple negative breast cancer (TNBC), locally advanced breast cancer (LABC), modified radical mastectomy (MRM), chemotherapy and immunotherapy

1. Introduction

Breast cancer is the leading cancer globally [1] and when it presents as TNBC, it carries the worst prognosis [2]. As the commonly diagnosed malignancy with the second cause of mortality among women with cancer [3]. Incidence of the breast cancer has been increasing from the western word to the east. It has increased the mental burden to the patients and the families of the affected individual's younger women.

TNBC is described as the lack of the hormone receptor status. As estradiol heights among TNBC patients were considered as favorable outcome [4]. Fortunately the incidence of TNBC is only 15–20% of invasive breast cancers [5], its hostile behavior, comprising prior recurrence with high proliferation and metastasis [6, 7]. International Breast Cancer Conference delivered a novel description of breast cancer molecular subtypes that are: luminal A (ER/PR^+, $HER2^-$, $Ki67^+ < 20\%$), luminal B ($ER/PR^+ < 20\%$, $HER2^-$, $Ki67^+ \geq 20\%$); $HER2^+$ B2 (ER/PR^+, HER2 overexpression), HER2 overexpression (ER^-, PR^-, $HER2^+$) and basal-like TNBC (triple negative) [1]. TNBC is so hostile that it leads to poor survival of the diagnosed cases and makes it

IntechOpen

shorter. As the short disease free survival with the death ratio in the initial years of identification. Half of the TNBC patients usually presents with the metastatic disease.

Though molecular phenotype, of the TNBC presents without the receptors expression, proving it most difficult to manage. To control the local disease we have surgical options like modified radical mastectomy (MRM) and lumpectomy or wide local excision (WLE) in breast conserving surgery (BCS) and for the systemic disease add neo-adjuvant or adjuvant chemotherapy. As chemotherapy to these patients can be an option to regress the tumor size and the stage and make it an operable in case of locally advanced disease stage and make the survival considerably good [8].

TNBC has narrow management opportunities that makes it vulnerable. While it is usually known that TNBC that diagnosed timely in its initial stages is responding well to the chemotherapy instead of indistinct management plan. Specifically the inoperable and locally advanced TNBC has a good outcome with the Neoadjuvant therapy.

The residual TNBC lesions ultimately prone to the relapse of the disease. The metastatic disease will get benefit from the neoadjuvant course with platinum-based therapy, combination therapy of paclitaxel per week as adjuvant course will be used [9].

TNBC patients recently receiving FDA-approved regimen of chemotherapy plus immunotherapy [10]. TNBC has the specific features that leads it towards the immunotherapy [11]. As the TNBC tumor has additional tumor-infiltrating lymphocytes (TILs), which correlate to the improved responses to immune check point inhibitors (ICIs), and the high levels of tumor-infiltrating lymphocytes in TNBC proves with better-quality prognosis in initial phase of the TNBC. TNBC also has better PD-L1 expression and making it more useful for the future targeted therapies for ICIs and anti–PD-1 therapies. TNBC has an overexpression of no synonymous mutations, that provide tumor-specific neoantigens for specific T cells to support the targeted behavior towards the tumor reinforced by ICIs [6]. The trials of the immunotherapy with or without the chemotherapy is ongoing to conclude the treatment regimen for the TNBC patients. The blend of ICIs and chemotherapeutic agents has also established the primarily control towards the TNBC. Metastatic progress is more in the favor of liver, chest and brain [12].

Metastatic TNBC has an effect by the Platinum compounds that work by DNA crosslinking and are of better efficiency towards the gBRCA1/2 transformation carriers, while combination therapy with PARP inhibition with veliparib provides the better-quality survival as well [13].

2. Risk factors and pathogenesis

Genetic mutations and the hereditary factors have been the key element for the aggressive behavior of this Cancer with the association of BARCA1 25% BARCA2 75% [5]. Germ line BRCA1 is the most frequently associated with the TNBC but still the debate is going on as there is the variation of the genetics and the ethnicity along with the caner presentation and the prognosis.

The other risk factors are:

- Reproductive history (nulliparity)
- Age
- Dense breasts

- Having cancer or certain benign breast neoplasms
- Breast cancer running in the family
- Contact to radiation
- History for the diethylstilbestrol (DES).

3. Management

TNBC presents with the restricted management options that leads it to the recurrence and metastasis with an unfortunate diagnosis. As it lack the hormone receptors status that target the disease and improves the survival. Chemotherapy looks to be the central approach towards the systemic management of TNBC with the surgery is to control the local disease.

3.1 Chemotherapy

It is the main treatment modality in the TNBC. It can be used as neo-adjuvant as well as the adjuvant setting depending upon the tumor staging.

After the local disease cure by the operative options followed by the adjuvant management by the chemotherapy, the disease free survival (DFS) will be observed. DFS is correlated with the pathological complete response (pCR). Neoadjuvant therapy have more chances to get a high pCR in patients with TNBC and reflected as substitute consequence of the outcome of the disease [12].

3.2 Taxane

Taxel act as the antitumor agent through the macrophages by initiating the apoptosis. The guidelines by national comprehensive cancer network endorse the sandwich of the regimens consists of taxane, anthracycline, cyclophosphamide, Cisplatin, & fluorouracil. Currently, Taxel/Docetaxel + Adriamycin + cyclophosphamide (TAC), Docetaxel + cyclophosphamide (TC), Adriamycin + cyclophosphamide (AC), cyclophosphamide + methotrexate + fluorouracil (CMF), cyclophosphamide + Adriamycin + fluorouracil (CAF), and cyclophosphamide + Epirubicin + fluorouracil + paclitaxel/Docetaxel (CEF-T) are among favored adjuvant therapeutic regimens designed for TNBC. Suitable chemotherapy medications and its optimization for the patients with favorable outcome [1].

3.3 Anthracycline

Anthracycline and anthracycline antibiotics are a group of chemotherapy medications derived from *Streptomyces peucetius* var. *caesius*, having more power to treat the variety of the cancers in comparison to the other regimens. Ongoing clinical educations and studies proved the ideal plans of anthracycline adjuvant to treatment TNBC with dosage of doxorubicin is 60 mg/m^2 and that of Epirubicin is 100 mg/m^2. Anthracyclines that are FEC-100 (100 mg/m^2 Epirubicin), decreases 25–30% danger of relapse as well as mortality. Data currently suggesting that subsequently chemotherapy with anthracycline for the 6 months improves the mortality rate by 38% in patients of 50 years and below age at the time of diagnosis, whereas the mortality rate in patients with 50 to 69 years at the time of identification, reduced by 20%.

The CREATE-X experimental trial indicated that 6–8 cycles of adjuvant capecitabine (1250 mg/m^2 from days 1 to 14, every 21 days) with better-quality DFS and OS in the TNBC cohort. The significance of aiming adjuvant capecitabine among patients had residual disease was presently emphasized with outcomes of the phase 3 GEICAM/CIBOMA trial. Phase 3 trial of 876 participants diagnosed with initial stage TNBC and accomplished average adjuvant or neoadjuvant chemotherapy was planned towards evaluation the impact of capecitabine (1000 mg/m^2 from days 1 to 14, every 21 days) as an adjuvant therapy irrespective of their pCR status. Though the major transformation was not significant among 5-year DFS and OS between the treatment groups, emphasizing that still there is necessity to select a resistant groups. Outcome among CREATE-X trial currently strength the oncologist and surgeons for management of initial stage TNBC through neoadjuvant chemotherapy and comprehend the group, who ought to have capecitabine. Capecitabine must be considered, ongoing trials are assessing novel agents for the management of the TNBC with residual disease after neoadjuvant treatment [12].

Enhanced markers required to update improved-quality range and managing by the checkpoint inhibitors. Advanced prognosis is observed with checkpoint inhibitors when they are combined with chemotherapeutic agents as an initial therapy. The behavior of malignant tumor is categorizing the possible molecular targets and future researches are also valuing novel small molecule agents for the management of the TNBC with AKT inhibition and numerous others. The management model with chemotherapy agents as "one size fits all" methodology is fluctuating constructed on the behavior and have to be polished more to cover the multiple subtypes [14].

Studies showed that Anthracycline as a single drug up-to-date the pCR rates of 14 to 47%, however consecutive anthracycline and taxane combination therapies had reported pCR of 17 to 39%. Although the research studies are still in the way to express the peak rates of pCR with the chemotherapeutic regimens [12].

3.4 Surgical management

Multiple surgical options are available from the minimal invasive BCS to the MRM and the immediate reconstruction of the breast [5]. Breast and the axilla are the two different entities to treat. Axillary staging and the nodal involvement and the dissection will be done accordingly. As the presentation is usually in advanced stage and the BCS is not A primary treatment for aggressive and advance tumor, so the better option is to start the neo-adjuvant chemotherapy and assess the tumor response to the chemotherapy, again stage the disease and plan the surgery accordingly if possible then the BCS is the best option to the MRM.

Patients with stages I and II TNBC, will be benefited by BCS plus radiotherapy (BCS + RT), mastectomy only (MRM) or MRM plus radiotherapy (MRM + RT), still there is no single point surgical management has been concluded for the TNBC [15]. Disease free survival study revealed that BCS along with the simultaneous RT had considerable predictive effect than MRM and MRM + RT in the early management of the diagnosis. The axilla will be treated as a separate entity with the sentinel lymph node biopsy in case of clinically and radiological impalpable nodes was defined as removal of at least four lymph nodes and axillary node dissection was defined as removal of ≥10 nodes at least up to level-II clearance that is required for the specific staging of the disease [10].

Recent National Comprehensive Cancer Network (NCCN) Guidelines recommend breast surgery (breast conservation surgery or mastectomy) and axillary staging for all TNBC patients diagnosed with the early disease. Study presented that the BCS + RT had better predictive effect than MRM and MRM with RT in the cohort of early staged diagnosed TNBC cases in terms of overall survival. Cox proportional model revealed MRM and MRM along with the RT remained to have unfavorable outcome to the prognosis as related with BCS + RT survival P value is 0.006 [15].

3.5 Immunotherapy

It acts on the immune check points.

3.5.1 Immune check point monotherapy

As the outcome results to ICIs are higher in cases with TNBC, but the monotherapy effectiveness is still low and under the research control.

PD-1 inhibitor pembrolizumab, avelumab and atezolizumab established a hopeful (ORR) of 18.5% among 32 cases among PD-L1 + ve TNBC. Though, successive bigger phase II KEYNOTE-086 study (NCT02447003) establish an ORR of 5.3% among 170 participants PD-L1 unselected pretreated cancers. Remarkably, 84 treatment-naïve participants included, ORR observed 21.4%, signifying ICIs had better efficiency with 1st line metastatic malignancy. By the favor of that impression, the phase III KEYNOTE-119 trial (NCT02555657) with cases had metastatic TNBC, not revealed any progress among ORR, PFS, or OS by monotherapy pembrolizumab vs. chemotherapy (monotherapy), while participants had peak PD-L1 impression experienced the tendency for better advantage by pembrolizumab [6].

Two research studies by chemotherapy with or without atezolizumab, presently increasing. The IMpassion131 trial (NCT03125902) have to explore the significances of first line atezolizumab along with paclitaxel compared with paclitaxel only in terms of overall improvement, while IMpassion132 study describe atezolizumab as first line joined by chemotherapeutic agents may progress consequences linked through chemotherapeutic only among participants presenting with recurrence of the disease within the year of adjuvant therapy. Several enduring early-stage disease trials will additional explain the effectiveness of ICIs in TNBC cases as neoadjuvant and adjuvant therapies.

Biomarkers assume advantage to immunotherapy in TNBC are required to sort out the cases with more advantage of ICIs monotherapy, progress blended treatments that overwhelmed the resistance of ICI. Individual with two authenticated biomarkers presently occur, mismatch repair deficiency and manifestation of PD-L1 on immune cells. Nonetheless, mismatch repair deficiency ensues hardly among carcinoma breast and usually among initial stage presentation, those with diagnosed as metastatic TNBC with PD-L1 -ve presently accepted SP-142 assay.

3.5.2 Management of metastatic TNBC by immunotherapy

The II KEYNOTE-086 Cohort A, had appraised Pembrolizumab (inhibitor of PD-1) as it was single arm research, among diagnosed cases of triple negative metastatic breast carcinoma. They had assessed pembrolizumab effectiveness among 170 patients who were kept in this research trial, irrespective of expression of PD-L1. 62% patients enrolled in study had expression of PD-L1 + ve cancers (n = 105).

The response rate 4.7%, seems to be not significant, only one case achieving a complete response and 7 cases with limited response. The overall survival was 8.9 months among all the participants and 8.3 vs. 10 months in the PD-L1 + ve and -ve cohorts separately.

Cohort B of KEYNOTE-086 appraised pembrolizumab as the first line treatment of patients diagnosed by PD-L1 + ve triple negative breast carcinoma. Around 84 participants included in the study, out of that 73 (87%), experienced traditional neo-adjuvant or adjuvant chemotherapeutic medications. ORR were 23.1%, three patients achieving a CR and 16 had PR. 12 participants, presently were at data limit. Median PFS 2.1 months and median OS 16.1 months.

Pembrolizumab evaluated by phase III KEYNOTE-119 (NCT02555657) trial. 622 participant diagnosed as TNBC, randomized 1:1 to have pembrolizumab compared with monotherapy chemotherapy (capecitabine, eribulin, gemcitabine, or vinorelbine) as second- or third-line therapy. But the results are pending and expected to be presented at an future meeting [14].

Impassion130 (NCT02425891), phase III randomized research trial assessing nab-paclitaxel with PD-L1 inhibitor (atezolizumab) vs. nab-paclitaxel with placebo among diagnosed participants as first line management for metastatic or inoperable locally advanced triple –ve breast carcinoma. Neoadjuvant or adjuvant treatment may be permissible if more than 1 year from end of therapy. Participants with PD-L1 + ve when >1% staining is present within immune cells. Co-primary endpoints were PFS and OS in ITT and PD-L1+ participants [14].

4. Follow-up

TNBC progression has exceptional behaviors that leads it towards metastasis and prone to recurrence. As its violent behavior presents it as metastatic cancer even in its primary progress of the disease. The close evaluation is compulsory, at least the first 3-years after controlling the primary disease to control it and make it to be a better disease free survival.

5. Conclusion

The management of the TNBC is the interesting among all cases with breast carcinoma. As TNBC has higher chances of disease relapse, metastasis, and limited survival. The documentation of markers in near future will support the management guidelines in TNBC remains a clinically indolent. Immunotherapy acts in ICIs, promises the pronounced outcomes by immunotherapy agent (ATEZOLIZUMAB). As with unlimited hope and confidence that future ongoing research studies will add more understanding of the progression of the TNBC and will enhance the options for the management that leads towards the better survival.

Novel management options have offered the hope for the improved survival with better outcome by the upcoming period.

Conflict of interest

"The authors declare no conflict of interest."

Acronyms and abbreviations

LABC	Locally Advanced Breast Cancer
TNBC	Triple Negative Breast Cancer
ER	Estrogen receptor
PR	Progesterone receptor
HER2 NEU	Human epidermal growth factor receptor 2 neu
MRM	Modified radical mastectomy
RT	Radiotherapy
BL1	Basal-like 1
BL2	Basal-like 2
M	Mesenchymal
MSL	Mesenchymal stem-like
IM	Immunomodulatory
LAR	Luminal androgen receptor
BCS	Breast conserving surgery
WLE	Wide local excision
NCCN	Current National Comprehensive Cancer Network
ICIs	Immune check point inhibitors
pCR	Pathological complete response
DFS	Disease-free survival
ORR	Overall response rate
TMB	Tumor mutational burden
CR	Complete response
PR	Partial response

Author details

Amir Iqbal Memon*, Ikram Din Ujjan and Aisha Masroor Bhatti
Lumhs Jamshoro, Pakistan

*Address all correspondence to: dramiriqbalmemon@gmail.com

References

[1] Yin L, Duan J-J, Bian X-W, Yu S-c. Triple-negative breast cancer molecular subtyping and treatment progress. Breast Cancer Research. 2020;**22**(1):1-13

[2] Zagami P, Carey LA. Triple negative breast cancer: Pitfalls and progress. NPJ Breast Cancer. 2022;**8**(1):1-10

[3] Garrido-Castro AC, Lin NU, Polyak K. Insights into molecular classifications of triple-negative breast cancer: Improving patient selection for treatment heterogeneity of triple-negative breast cancer. Cancer Discovery. 2019;**9**(2):176-198

[4] Septiani RV, Soewoto W, Budhi IB. Chemotherapy effect on estradiol levels in patients with triple-negative breast cancer: A clinical prospective study from Indonesia. Open Access Macedonian Journal of Medical Sciences. 2022;**10**(B):477-481

[5] Amro A, Newman LA. Surgical management of triple-negative breast cancer. Triple-Negative Breast Cancer. 2018:55-69

[6] Keenan TE, Tolaney SM. Role of immunotherapy in triple-negative breast cancer. Journal of the National Comprehensive Cancer Network. 2020;**18**(4):479-489

[7] Gianni L, Huang C-S, Egle D, Bermejo B, Zamagni C, Thill M, et al. Abstract GS3-04: Pathologic complete response (pCR) to neoadjuvant treatment with or without atezolizumab in triple negative, early high-risk and locally advanced breast cancer. NeoTRIPaPDL1 Michelangelo randomized study. Cancer Research. 2020;**80**(4_Supplement):GS3-04-GS3

[8] Sharma RK, Gogia A, Deo SVS, Sharma D, Mathur S, Sagiraju HKR. Does pathological complete remission after neoadjuvant chemotherapy translate to longer relapse-free survival in patients with triple-negative breast cancer in the Indian population. Journal of Clinical Oncology. 2021;**39**(15_suppl):e12618

[9] Lebert J, Lester R, Powell E, Seal M, McCarthy J. Advances in the systemic treatment of triple-negative breast cancer. Current Oncology. 2018;**25**(s1):142-150

[10] Obeng-Gyasi S, Asad S, Fisher JL, Rahurkar S, Stover DG. Socioeconomic and surgical disparities are associated with rapid relapse in patients with triple-negative breast cancer. Annals of Surgical Oncology. 2021;**28**(11):6500-6509

[11] Zhu Y, Zhu X, Tang C, Guan X, Zhang W. Progress and challenges of immunotherapy in triple-negative breast cancer. Biochimica et Biophysica Acta (BBA)-Reviews on Cancer. 2021;**1876**(2):188593

[12] Bergin AR, Loi S. Triple-negative breast cancer: Recent treatment advances. F1000Research. 2019:8

[13] Eikesdal HP, Yndestad S, Elzawahry A, Llop-Guevara A, Gilje B, Blix ES, et al. Olaparib monotherapy as primary treatment in unselected triple negative breast cancer. Annals of Oncology. 2021;**32**(2):240-249

[14] Lyons TG. Targeted therapies for triple-negative breast cancer. Current Treatment Options in Oncology. 2019;**20**(11):1-13

[15] Wang S, Sun Y, Zhao S, Wei F, Yang G. Breast conserving surgery (BCS)

with adjuvant radiation therapy showed improved prognosis compared with mastectomy for early staged triple negative breast cancer patients: Running title: BCS had better prognosis than mastectomy for early TNBC patients. Mathematical Biosciences and Engineering. 2020;**17**(1):92-105

Chapter 8

Inter-Relationship of Ki-67 and Triple-Negative Breast Cancer

Ankit Jain, Vijayakumar Chellappa and Kadambari Dharanipragada

Abstract

Triple-negative breast cancer (TNBC) is a heterogeneous group characterized by an early onset, aggressive course of the disease, a higher tendency of visceral metastases, and a poorer prognosis. It is also associated with basal-like phenotype and germline mutations for BRCA genes in 10–20% and somatic mutations in 3–5% of cases. Based on gene expression profiling, TNBC is divided into four tumor-specific subtypes (Basal-like 1, Basal-like 2, Mesenchymal, and Luminal androgen receptor) with different clinical, prognostic, and therapeutic implications. The Ki-67 antigen, a non-histone nuclear protein, is a surrogate marker to assess tumor proliferation. As TNBCs are expected to be highly proliferating tumors, a higher baseline Ki-67 level has been seen. Although a higher Ki-67 level is associated with a higher pathological complete response rate, the best cutoff point of this marker as a prognostic and predictive factor in TNBC remains unclear.

Keywords: triple negative, breast cancer, Ki 67 expression, chemotherapy response, prognosis, predictive marker, survival, quality of life

1. Introduction

According to GLOBOCAN 2020, female breast cancer surpassed lung cancer as the leading cause of cancer globally in 2020, with 2.3 million new cases worldwide [1]. Breast cancer is a heterogeneous disease encompassing different entities with distinct morphological features and clinical behaviors. The St. Gallen guidelines, the American Society of Clinical Oncology, and the College of American Pathology have defined triple-negative breast cancer (TNBC) as breast cancer with:

1. Less than 1% of tumor cells expressing ER and PR via IHC [2].

2. Her-2-neu negative: Immunohistochemistry (IHC) staining of 0 or 1 +, a Fluorescent in-situ hybridization (FISH) result of less than 4.0 HER2 gene copies per nucleus, or FISH ratio of less than 1.8 (FISH to be done in case IHC is 2+, equivocal) [3].

2. TNBC vs. Basal

TNBC is labeled based on IHC negativity of ER/PR/Her-2neu on tumor cells. However, based on gene expression profiles established through the 50-gene Prediction Analysis of Microarray (PAM50) assay, four "intrinsic subtypes" are defined: Luminal A, Luminal B, Basal-like, and Her-2-neu enriched. TNBC represents approximately 15–20% of all patients with breast cancer and shares various similarities with basal-like cancer [4]:

i. TNBC occurs in premenopausal young women under 40 years old

ii. More aggressive disease course with a peak in recurrence between 1 and 3 years after diagnosis. Survival time is also shorter, and the mortality rate is 40% within the first 5 years after diagnosis

iii. Approximately 46% of TNBC patients will have distant metastasis at presentation

iv. The metastasis often involves the brain and visceral organs rather than the lungs or bones.

v. Due to the lack of targeted therapies, chemotherapy and surgery are the mainstays in treatment for TNBC

The basal-like subtype of breast cancer is characterized by a gene expression profile similar to that of the basal-myoepithelial layer of the normal breast; cytokeratins (5/6, 14, and 17), P-cadherin, EGFR17, and EGFR gene amplification (rarely) [5]. TP53 gene mutations are observed in up to 85% of cases [5, 6]. However, basal-like breast cancers, unlike "basal"/myoepithelial cells of normal breast, uniformly express cytokeratins 8 and/or 18 [5]. This questions microarray-based taxonomy of breast cancers that suggested that basal-like cancers would arise from basal/myoepithelial cells. This has been answered in a recent study with the possibility that a subgroup of basal-like breast cancers may originate from luminal progenitors rather than basal myoepithelial cells of the breast [7].

Although TNBC and basal-like share many similarities and the terms are very often used interchangeably, they are different. Not all basal-like cancers lack ER, PR, and HER2, and not all TNBCs show a basal-like phenotype by expression array analysis (25% discordance) (**Figure 1**) [8].

Reasons for this discordance can be:

1. False positivity/false negativity of the IHC-based assays for determining the HR or HER2 status (inter-laboratory and inter-method discordance rates of 20%) [8]

2. Intra-tumor Heterogeneity: It is difficult that two different subtypes coexist in same tumor [8]

3. Some TNBCs do not express basal markers and are classified as normal breast-like. (Probably an artifact of gene expression profiling due to samples with disproportionately high content of stromal and normal breast epithelial cells) [5]

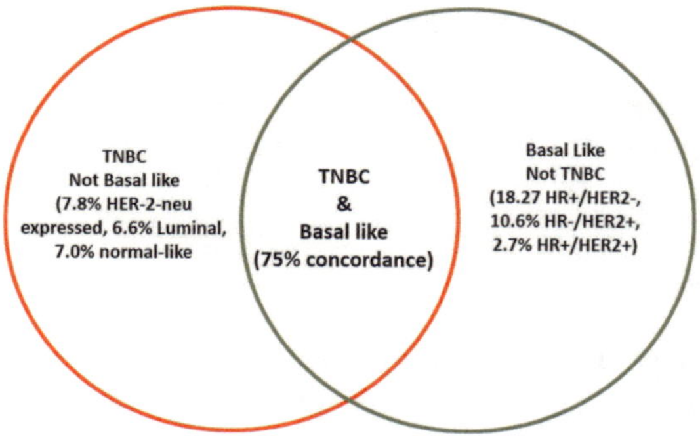

Figure 1.
Concordance between TNBC (IHC BASED) AND BASAL LIKE (genetic array analysis.

4. Multigene expression data using hundreds of genes better capture the accurate biological profile compared with three or four individual surrogate biomarkers used to label TNBC [6]

2.1 BRCA1-Associated TNBC

Basal-like tumors show similar molecular genetic profiles to tumors arising in BRCA1 carriers. Both sporadic basal-like tumors and tumors with BRCA 1 mutations express basal keratins, and both groups cluster together in gene expression profiling [9]. Germline mutations for BRCA genes occur in 10–20% of TNBC patients, and somatic mutations are seen in 3–5% [10]. Apart from somatic mutation in BRCA1 gene: [5, 6]

1. BRCA1 hypermethylation and/or loss of heterozygosity may give rise to a BRCA1-like molecular profile in wild-type TNBC

2. Sporadic invasive ductal carcinomas with basal-like phenotype express ID4, a negative regulator of BRCA15

3. Frequent loss of several other genes involved in BRCA1-dependent homologous recombination (HR) repair has been demonstrated in basal-like/triple-negative cancer [9]

BRCA1-like features are characterized by: [5]

1. Basal-like phenotype (associated with the BRCA1 phenotype but not with the BRCA2 phenotype)

2. Present as interval tumor

3. ER-negativity, EGFR expression, c-MYC amplification

4. TP53 mutations (85%) [5], loss of RAD51 focus formation

    a. Extreme genomic instability and sensitivity to DNA-crosslinking agents

5. Predominantly hematogenous spread over axillary nodes and bones

6. Sensitive to DNA-damaging agents such as platinum compounds, or poly (ADP-ribose) polymerase (PARP) inhibitors or their combination

2.2 TNBC subtypes

In 2011, Lehmann et al. performed gene expression profiling of tumor samples from 587 TNBC patients and divided TNBC into six subtypes: [9, 11]

1. Basal-like-1 (BL-1):

    a. Abnormal expression of cell cycle regulating and DNA repair-related genes (high amplification of MYC, PIK3CA, CDK6, AKT2, KRAS, IGF1R, and CDKN2A/B)

    b. High frequency of heterozygous or homozygous deletion of DNA repair-related genes such as BRCA2, PTEN, MDM2, RB1, and TP53

    c. A high Ki-67 mRNA expression is observed on nuclear Ki-67 staining (>70%).

    d. Nearly all of the cell lines with BRCA1 and BRCA2 mutations have gene expression patterns that correlate with this subtype [12]

2. Basal-like-2 (BL-2): Abnormal activation of growth factor signaling pathways such as the EGFR, MET, NGF, Wnt/β-catenin, and IGF-1R pathways

3. Mesenchymal-like subtype (M): Also called metaplastic breast cancer

    a. Highly activated cell migration-related signaling pathways, extracellular matrix-receptor interaction pathways, and differentiation pathways (Wnt pathway, anaplastic lymphoma kinase pathway, transforming growth factor (TGF)-β signaling)

    b. The M subtype has sarcoma-like or squamous epithelial cell-like tissue characteristics

    c. Prone to develop resistance to chemotherapeutic drugs

4. Mesenchymal stem-like subtype (MSL): Low levels of cell proliferation-related genes and high levels of stem cell-related genes

5. Immuno-modulatory subtype (IM):

    a. Characterized by increased expression of immune cell-associated genes and pathways such as the Th1/Th2 pathway, NK cell pathway, B cell receptor signaling pathway, dendritic cell (DC) pathway, T cell receptor signaling, interleukin (IL)-12 pathway, and IL-7 pathway.

b. Substantially overlap with a gene signature for medullary breast cancer, high-grade histology with a favorable prognosis.

c. This subtype has the best prognosis [9]

6. Luminal Androgen Receptor (LAR):

a. Although the LAR subtype does not express ER receptors, it does have highly activated hormonal-related signaling pathways (including steroid synthesis, porphyrin metabolism, and androgen/estrogen metabolism).

b. ESR1 (the gene encoding ERα) and other estrogen-regulated genes (PGR, FOXA, XBP1, GATA3) are present on micro-array profiling. Thus, there is molecular evidence of ER activation. However, they may be classified as "ER-negative" because <1% of these tumor cells express low levels of ER protein on IHC analysis

c. Androgen receptor (AR) is highly expressed (mRNA level is nine times) as well as high expression of AR on IHC (10 times)

This classification was validated by Masuda et al. [13]. They further compared the TNBC subtypes between the PAM50 basal-like subtype and non-basal-like subtypes (other subtypes grouped). All tumors in the BL1 and BL2 subtypes belonged to the basal-like PAM50 subtype, and most tumors in the LAR subtype belonged to the non-basal-like PAM50 group. In the non-basal-like group, there were only three TNBC subtypes, LAR, MSL, and M; most of these tumors were the LAR subtype (59%). They further found that even though BL-1 and BL-2 are highly proliferative tumors, the BL-1 subtype had the highest pathological complete response (pCR) rate, and the BL2 subtype had the lowest pCR rate. Similarly, consistent with LAR's low pCR rate, the luminal A and B intrinsic subtypes, hormonally regulated tumors, showed less response to chemotherapy. Therefore, the LAR group had delayed recurrences compared with the other groups and did not have the lowest OS rate despite having a low pCR rate.

Burstein et al. distinguished TNBC subtypes into four types only: luminal-AR (LAR), mesenchymal (MES), basal-like immune-suppressed (BLIS), and basal-like immune-activated (BLIA) [14]. However, in an updated analysis, Lehman et al. reported that transcripts in the previously described IM and MSL subtypes were contributed from infiltrating lymphocytes and tumor-associated stromal cells, respectively [15]. Therefore, in their new refined classification, TNBC molecular subtypes were reduced from six (TNBCtype-6) to four (TNBCtype-4) tumor-specific subtypes (BL1, BL2, M, and LAR) (**Table 1**). PAM50 subtype "calls" distribution among the TNBC subtypes showed that most BL1, BL2, and M were basal-like, while LAR was enriched in HER2 and luminal subtypes.

2.3 Benefits of sub-classifying TNBC

A. All the subtypes of TNBC have different clinic-pathological features, affecting their prognosis.

1. Age: Non-basal TNBC was reported in older patients than basal TNBC. LAR subtype was diagnosed in women of older age than all other subtypes.

TNBC subtypes Lehman et al. [11]	TNBC subtypes Burstein et al. [14]	TNBC subtype-4 Lehman et al. [15]
Basal-like 1 (BL1)	Basal-like Immune suppressed (BLIS)	Basal-like 1 (BL1)
Basal-like 2 (BL2)	—	Basal-like 2 (BL2)
Immunomodulatory (IM)	Basal-like Immune-activated (BLIA)	—
Mesenchymal (M)	Mesenchymal (MES)	Mesenchymal (M)
Mesenchymal Stem-like (MSL)	—	—
Luminal androgen receptor (LAR)	Luminal androgen receptor (LAR)	Luminal androgen receptor (LAR)

Table 1.
Different classification of subtypes of TNBC.

2. Grade: Basal TNBC tumors are more likely to be of a higher grade than non-basal TNBC. BL1 tumors are higher grade, and LAR tumors are lower grade. In contrast to lower histological grade, non-basal TNBC presents significantly more advanced clinical disease and a higher stage than basal TNBC

3. Histopathology: BL1 tumors were mainly ductal carcinomas without notable atypical histology. In contrast, infiltrating lobular carcinomas were nearly exclusive to the LAR subtype. Medullary breast cancer histological types were present in BL1, BL2 and, LAR and absent in the M subtype.

4. Regional nodes: Regional spread to lymph nodes was similar in basal (29%) and non-basal (31%). Approximately half (47%) of LAR TNBC patients have regional spread, whereas the node involvement was lower for the M TNBC subtype (21%).

5. Distant Metastasis: The M subtype is prone to a higher frequency of lung metastasis (46%) than all other subtypes (25%). Whereas bone metastasis was significantly higher for the LAR subtype (46%) than all other subtypes (16%).

6. pCR: pCR rates were similar in basal and non-basal subtypes. The BL-1 subtype had the highest pCR rate, and the BL2 and LAR subtypes had the lowest pCR rate. Moreover, BL1 patients had significantly higher pCR than all other subtypes (49% vs. 31%).

7. Overall survival (OS): BL1 patients had significantly better OS than all other TNBCtype-4 subtypes combined. Moreover, BL1 patients displayed better relapse-free survival, with nearly 60% survival even at 10 years. The IM subtype displayed the best overall and relapse-free survival. The LAR subtypes had better survival despite a decreased response to neoadjuvant chemotherapy. The decreased response of AR-positive TNBC tumors to neoadjuvant chemotherapy has recently been validated with the report of significantly lower pCR [16].

8. Distant relapse-free survival (DRFS): Despite having better pCR to neoadjuvant chemotherapy (34% vs. 11%), TNBC patients had significantly worse DRFS survival than non-TNBC [15]. However, TNBC patients that achieved a pCR on chemotherapy had a far better DRFS than those patients that did not. BL2 patients have the worst outcome, with a median survival of 2.4 years. In contrast, the BL1 subtype had the best long-term DRFS, with 72% of patients relapse-free at a 7-year follow-up.

B. Treatment Options (**Table 2**)

1. Basal Like: Cells have a complex DNA damage response and repair mechanisms to maintain genomic integrity. The most deleterious lesion, double-strand breaks are repaired by either HR (homologous recombination) or non-homologous end joining. Patients with mutations in the breast cancer susceptibility proteins BRCA1 and BRCA2A have cancers due to deficiency in HR repair. Moreover, these are dependent on other DNA repair mechanisms, the most prominent of which is the peroxisome proliferator-activated receptor (PARP)-based. Therefore, PARP inhibitors have significant antitumor effects on BRCA1/2-deficient tumors, and the inhibition effect on BRCA1-mutant tumors is 100–1000 times higher than

Molecular subtypes	Cellular pathways	Therapeutic target
Basal-like 1 (BL1)	Cell cycle	PARP inhibitors
	DNA repair	Platinum agents
	Proliferation	Conventional chemotherapy
Basal-like 2 (BL2)	Growth factor pathways	mTOR inhibitors
	Metabolic pathways (glycolysis and gluconeogenesis)	Growth-factor inhibitors
Immunomodulatory (IM)	Immune cell processes	Immune-checkpoint inhibitors
Mesenchymal (M)	Cell motility, differentiation, and growth factor signaling	mTOR inhibitors
		EMT-targeted therapy
		CSC-targeted therapy
		AXL inhibitor
Mesenchymal Stem-like (MSL)	Low proliferation	PI3K inhibitors
	Angiogenesis	Antiangiogenic therapy
		SRC antagonist
Luminal androgen receptor (LAR)	Androgen receptor	Antiandrogen blockade
	Luminal gene expression	CDK4/6 inhibitors
	Molecular apocrine subtype	Immune-checkpoint inhibitors

Source: Silva D et al. [10] licensed under CC BY-NC 4.0.

Table 2.
Molecular pathways in TNBC subtypes as therapeutic targets.

in tumors without such mutations [4]. The basal-like subgroup has increased expression of proliferation-related genes and DNA repair genes; therefore, they may be sensitive to anti-mitotic drugs such as taxanes and platinum and PARP inhibitors such as olaparib and veliparib.

2. Immune Check Point Regulators: Tumor cells can evade recognition and destruction by the host immune system through the immune checkpoint system. Under normal circumstances, the immune system reacts to foreign antigens that accumulate in the lymph nodes or spleen and promotes antigen-specific T-cell proliferation. Programmed cell death protein 1 (PD-1) binds to PD-L1 and can transmit signals to inhibit T cell proliferation and promote T cell depletion [17]. PD-L1 expression in tumor cells or its presence in the tumor microenvironment has been positively associated with triple-negative status in breast cancer [17]. Moreover, high PD-L1 levels have also been correlated with pCR after neoadjuvant chemotherapy and improved clinical outcomes in TNBC [17]. Pembrolizumab, a monoclonal anti PD-1, and Atezolizumab anti-PD-L1 antibody are under trials for their role in TNBC.

3. LAR subtypes: The LAR subtype is characterized by high AR and an activating mutation in the kinase domain of PIK3CA. Antiandrogens, such as combination of bicalutamide with a PI3K inhibitor or enzalutamide, are being explored to target LAR subtypes.

4. Epidermal growth factor receptor (EGFR): EGFR is expressed in 45–70% of TNBC and is associated with poor prognosis [10]. EGFR inhibitors are being evaluated in metastatic settings with not-so-promising results [18]. It has been seen that the EGFR downstream signaling pathways were still activated in most patients after EGFR-targeted treatment, suggesting that there might be other pathways involved in a bypass activation [4]. As a result, EGFR-targeted treatment alone cannot achieve significant efficacy. Use of growth factor inhibitors in BL-2, M, and MSL subtypes combined with other downstream signal transduction inhibitors might achieve better results [4].

2.4 Ki-67

The Ki-67 antigen, a nonhistone nuclear protein, was identified by Scholzer and Gerdes in 1983 in a Hodgkin lymphoma cell line [19]. The Ki-67 antigen encodes two protein isoforms with 345 and 395 kDa molecular weights [20]. This protein is expressed in the G1, S, G2, and M phase of the cell cycle but is absent in resting cells (G0) [20, 21]. Therefore, the nuclear expression of Ki-67 can be evaluated to assess tumor proliferation by IHC. The Ki-67 protein has a half-life of only 1–1.5 hours. Therefore, the quantity of Ki-67 present at any time during the cell cycle is regulated by a precise balance between synthesis and degradation [20].

2.5 Is Ki-67 a prognostic or a predictive marker?

A prognostic biomarker indicates the likely course of the disease in an untreated individual, and a predictive biomarker identifies subpopulations of patients most likely to respond to a given therapy. An increased Ki-67 is linked to a worse prognosis and an increased response to neoadjuvant chemotherapy. As Ki-67 represents proliferating tumor, a high level will translate to an increased response. However, same is not true for prognoses. Increased Ki-67 is an adverse prognostic factor in HR-positive tumors, and patients with low Ki-67 tumors have the best prognosis [21]. Whereas, in HR-negative tumors, low proliferating tumors have the worst prognosis. This phenomenon is also reported by Cortazar et al. in their meta-analysis, which shows that increased pCR rates are linked to better survival in the HR-negative subgroup [22]. At the same time, chemotherapy response does not affect the prognosis in HR-positive tumor. Based on this, Denkert et al. reported the biological plausibility of three different groups of tumors [21]:

1. Low proliferating tumors are not responding to chemotherapy but have a good prognosis (low Ki-67 linked to a good outcome)

2. High proliferating tumors are chemotherapy-sensitive, high Ki-67 is linked to an increased chance of pCR and improved survival (high Ki-67 linked to a good outcome)

3. High proliferating tumors are chemotherapy-resistant, increased Ki-67 is linked to reduced survival (high Ki-67 linked to a poor outcome)

2.6 Problems in Ki-67 assessment

1. Ki-67 cutoff as a measure of cell proliferation should be considered in the tumor's histological type context: [6, 21] For example, a Ki-67 rate of 16% would indicate very high proliferation in a classic invasive lobular cancer; however, the same Ki-67 rate would indicate just about average proliferation in an Invasive Ductal Carcinoma [6]. Similarly, baseline Ki-67 values for TNBC are much higher than those for luminal tumors [23, 24]

2. Intratumoral heterogeneity [6, 21]:

    a. Spatial heterogeneity: the number of cells needed to be counted for consistent results might be much lower in tumors with low proliferation and high in tumors with high proliferation

    b. Temporal heterogeneity: This is commonly observed as a result of therapy. Several studies have shown that the short-term reduction of Ki-67 after 2 weeks of therapy is predictive of the outcome of endocrine therapy [5, 6, 21]

3. Inter-observer variability based on different evaluation approaches for different pathologists

2.7 Cutoff for TNBC

In the 2011 St. Gallen recommendations, a cutoff of 14% for the separation of luminal A and B tumors is suggested [25]. In 2013, the cutoff was revised to 20%, signifying 20% as the cutoff level for differentiating low proliferating Luminal A from high proliferating Luminal B [26]. However, the best cutoff point of this marker as a prognostic and predictive factor in TNBC remains unclear.

1. According to Zhu et al., the optimal cutoff value of Ki-67 for TNBC is 30% [27]. At a cutoff point of 30%, worse DFS and OS were observed in the Ki-67 high group.

2. Aleskandarany et al. reported the baseline mean Ki-67 value of Luminal cancer as 22 compared with 64.5 for TNBC tumors [23]. Therefore, 10% was the optimal cutoff in the luminal class separating low from moderate/high proliferative subgroups. In contrast, the cutoff for TNBC was found to be 70%. Moreover, there was no association of Ki-67 with survival compared to the luminal subtype.

3. In the study by Arafah et al., the median result of the KI-67 expression was 70%, with a range of 20–95% [24]. Moreover, High Ki-67 (>30%) was significantly associated with positive sentinel lymph node status, higher nuclear grade, diagnosis of an invasive tumor, advanced clinical stage, and adverse survival outcome.

4. Epithelial-mesenchymal transition (EMT) [24]: TNBC has also recently been linked to this phenomenon, which is characterized by the loss of the epithelial characteristics of the cells while they acquire a mesenchymal phenotype. This is a plausible explanation for distant metastases in breast cancer, skipping regional nodes. The high expression of KI-67 was correlated with an increased expression of Vimentin, a marker for EMT.

5. In the study by Keam et al., high Ki-67 (>10%) was associated with poor survival [28].

6. According to Wang et al., a high Ki-67 (>40%) level is associated with young age, higher grade, poor overall and recurrence-free survival [29].

7. A meta-analysis by Wu et al. reported the heterogeneity in cutoff value for Ki-67 for different studies, ranging from 10 to 50% [30]. Also, high Ki-67 is associated with worse overall and recurrence-free survival.

2.8 pCR

1. Arafah et al. reported a statistically significant association of high Ki-67 with the inability to achieve pCR [24].

2. Nishimura et al. reported that high Ki-67 levels and TNBC status were associated with higher pCR [31]. Moreover, no pathological responder in cases with Ki-67 < 25%

3. In the study by Keam et al., TNBC with high Ki-67 showed a higher pCR rate (18.2%) to neoadjuvant chemotherapy than TNBC with low Ki-67 (0.0%) [28].

2.9 Is there a triple-negative paradox?

Higher Ki-67 predicts a higher response to chemotherapy and a higher pCR rate, which generally means a good prognosis [21]. However, high Ki-67in TNBC is associated with poor recurrence-free or overall survival. This was termed as a "triple negative paradox." However, this paradox can be explained by a higher likelihood of relapse in patients whose pCR was not achieved. In a study by Keam et al., only 18.2% of TNBC patients achieved pCR, and patients with high Ki-67 residual disease had statistically significant poor prognoses than patients with residual disease and low Ki-67 or patients with pCR with high Ki-67 [28]. Similarly, in a study by Carey et al., only 27% of patients with basal subtype achieved pCR [32]. Therefore, in patients with TNBC, the higher number of non-pCR patients tilt the results toward poor prognoses resulting in the so-called "triple negative paradox."

Only 20–30% of patients with TNBC achieved pCR on neoadjuvant chemotherapy [21, 32], and pCR was strongly associated with prolonged overall survival [15, 33, 34]. Moreover, patients with TNBC who achieve pCR have the same prognosis as patients with non-TNBC [33]. However, among patients who did not achieve pCR, patients with TNBC have a significantly poorer outcome than patients with non-TNBC [33].

3. Conclusions

Although marred by intratumoral heterogeneity and inter-observer variability, true to the highly proliferative nature of TNBCs, higher baseline Ki-67 levels are seen as compared to luminal tumors. A higher Ki-67 is associated with a higher pCR rate in TNBC. However, the best cutoff point of this marker as a prognostic and predictive factor in TNBC remains to be seen even after many researchers have explored this idea. Moreover, the "triple negative paradox" concept is more of a myth arising from more non-pCR patients in the TNBC group.

Acknowledgements

Thanks to Dr. Biswajit Dubashi , Professor, Department of Medical Oncology, Jawaharlal Institute of Postgraduate Medical Education and Research (JIPMER), Puducherry, India, for reviewing the manuscript and suggesting improvements.

Conflict of interest

The authors declare no conflict of interest.

Acronyms and abbreviations

AXL	tyrosine-protein kinase receptor
BL	basal-like
CDK	cyclin-dependent kinase
CSC	cancer stem cells
DNA	deoxyribonucleic acid
EGFR	epidermal growth factor receptor
EMT	epithelial-mesenchymal transition
FGFR	fibroblast growth factor receptors
IGF-1R	insulin-like growth factor receptor

IL	interleukin
IM	immunomodulatory
LAR	luminal androgen receptor
MET	hepatocyte growth factor
MSL	mesenchymal stem like
mTOR	mammalian target of rapamycin
PARP	poly ADP-ribose polymerase
PD1	programmed cell death 1
PDGFR	platelet-derived growth factor receptors
PD-L1	programmed death-ligand 1
PI3K	phosphatidylinositol 3-kinase
SRC	Proto-oncogene tyrosine-protein kinase Src
TGFβ	transforming growth factor beta
TNBC	triple-negative breast cancer

Author details

Ankit Jain, Vijayakumar Chellappa* and Kadambari Dharanipragada
Department of Surgery, Jawaharlal Institute of Postgraduate Medical Education and Research (JIPMER), Puducherry, India

*Address all correspondence to: vijaymmc01@gmail.com

References

[1] Sung H, Ferlay J, Siegel RL, et al. Global cancer statistics 2020: GLOBOCAN estimates of incidence and mortality worldwide for 36 cancers in 185 countries. CA: A Cancer Journal for Clinicians. 2021;**71**:209-249. DOI: 10.3322/caac.21660

[2] Hammond ME, Hayes DF, Dowsett M, et al. American Society of Clinical Oncology/College of American Pathologists guideline recommendations for immunohistochemical testing of estrogen and progesterone receptors in breast cancer. Journal of Clinical Oncology. 2010;**28**:2784-2795. DOI: 10.1200/JCO.2009.25.6529

[3] Wolff AC, Hammond ME, Schwartz JN, et al. American Society of Clinical Oncology/College of American Pathologists. American Society of Clinical Oncology/College of American Pathologists guideline recommendations for human epidermal growth factor receptor 2 testing in breast cancer. Archives of Pathology & Laboratory Medicine. 2007;**13**:18-43. DOI: 10.5858/2007-131-18-ASOCCO

[4] Yin L, Duan JJ, Bian XW, Yu SC. Triple-negative breast cancer molecular subtyping and treatment progress. Breast Cancer Research. 2020;**22**:61. DOI: 10.1186/s13058-020-01296-5

[5] Badve S, Dabbs DJ, Schnitt SJ, et al. Basal-like and triple-negative breast cancers: A critical review with an emphasis on the implications for pathologists and oncologists. Modern Pathology. 2011;**24**:157-167. DOI: 10.1038/modpathol.2010.200

[6] Sahin A, Zhang H. Invasive Breast Carcinoma: In Pathobiology of Human Disease: A Dynamic Encyclopedia of Disease Mechanisms. Elsevier Inc.; 2014. pp. 934-951. DOI: 10.1016/B978-0-12-386456-7.03204-4

[7] Lim E, Vaillant F, Wu D, et al. Aberrant luminal progenitors as the candidate target population for basal tumor development in BRCA1 mutation carriers. Nature Medicine. 2009;**15**(8): 907-913. DOI: 10.1038/nm.2000

[8] Prat A, Adamo B, Cheang MC, Anders CK, Carey LA, Perou CM. Molecular characterization of basal-like and non-basal-like triple-negative breast cancer. The Oncologist. 2013;**18**:123-133. DOI: 10.1634/theoncologist.2012-0397

[9] Hubalek M, Czech T, Müller H. Biological subtypes of triple-negative breast cancer. Breast Care (Basel). 2017; **12**:8-14. DOI: 10.1159/000455820

[10] Silva D, Mesquita A. Evolving evidence for the optimization of neoadjuvant therapy in triple-negative breast cancer. Breast Cancer (Auckl.). 2022;**16**:1178. DOI: 10.1177/11782234221107580

[11] Lehmann BD, Bauer JA, Chen X, et al. Identification of human triple-negative breast cancer subtypes and preclinical models for selection of targeted therapies. The Journal of Clinical Investigation. 2011;**121**: 2750-2767. DOI: 10.1172/JCI45014

[12] Stefansson OA, Jonasson JG, Johannsson OT, et al. Genomic profiling of breast tumours in relation to BRCA abnormalities and phenotypes. Breast Cancer Research. 2009;**11**:R47. DOI: 10.1186/bcr2334

[13] Masuda H, Baggerly KA, Wang Y, et al. Differential response to neoadjuvant chemotherapy among 7 triple-negative breast cancer molecular

subtypes. Clinical Cancer Research. 2013;**19**:5533-5540. DOI: 10.1158/1078-0432.CCR-13-0799

[14] Burstein MD, Tsimelzon A, Poage GM, et al. Comprehensive genomic analysis identifies novel subtypes and targets of triple-negative breast cancer. Clinical Cancer Research. 2015;**21**:1688-1698. DOI: 10.1158/1078-0432.CCR-14-0432

[15] Lehmann BD, Jovanović B, Chen X, et al. Refinement of triple-negative breast cancer molecular subtypes: Implications for neoadjuvant chemotherapy selection. PLoS One. 2016;**11**:e0157368. DOI: 10.1371/journal.pone.0157368

[16] Asano Y, Kashiwagi S, Onoda N, et al. Clinical verification of sensitivity to preoperative chemotherapy in cases of androgen receptor-expressing positive breast cancer. British Journal of Cancer. 2016;**114**:14-20. DOI: 10.1038/bjc.2015.434

[17] Pardoll DM. The blockade of immune checkpoints in cancer immunotherapy. Nature Reviews. Cancer. 2012;**12**:252-264. DOI: 10.1038/nrc3239

[18] Carey LA, Rugo HS, Marcom PK, et al. TBCRC 001: Randomized phase II study of cetuximab in combination with carboplatin in stage IV triple-negative breast cancer. Journal of Clinical Oncology. 2012;**30**:2615-2623. DOI: 10.1200/JCO.2010.34.5579

[19] Scholzen T, Gerdes J. The Ki-67 protein: From the known and the unknown. Journal of Cellular Physiology. 2000;**182**:311-322. DOI: 10.1002/(SICI)1097-4652(200003)182:3<311::AID-JCP1>3.0.CO;2-9

[20] Li LT, Jiang G, Chen Q, Zheng JN. Ki67 is a promising molecular target in the diagnosis of cancer (review). Molecular Medicine Reports. 2015;**11**:1566-1572. DOI: 10.3892/mmr.2014.2914

[21] Denkert C, Budczies J, von Minckwitz G, Wienert S, Loibl S, Klauschen F. Strategies for developing Ki67 as a useful biomarker in breast cancer. Breast. 2015;**24**:S67-S72. DOI: 10.1016/j.breast.2015.07.017

[22] Cortazar P, Zhang L, Untch M, et al. Pathological complete response and long-term clinical benefit in breast cancer: The CTNeoBC pooled analysis. Lancet. 2014;**384**(9938):164-172. DOI: 10.1016/S0140-6736(13)62422-8

[23] Aleskandarany MA, Green AR, Benhasouna AA, et al. Prognostic value of proliferation assay in the luminal, HER2-positive, and triple-negative biologic classes of breast cancer. Breast Cancer Research. 2012;**14**:R3. DOI: 10.1186/bcr3084

[24] Arafah MA, Ouban A, Ameer OZ, Quek KJ. KI-67 LI expression in triple-negative breast cancer patients and its significance. Breast Cancer (Auckl.). 2021;**15**:1178. DOI: 10.1177/11782234211016977

[25] Gnant M, Harbeck N, Thomssen C. Summary of the consensus discussion. Breast Care (Basel). 2011;**2011**(6):136-141. DOI: 10.1159/000328054

[26] Untch M, Gerber B, Harbeck N, et al. 13th St. Gallen International Breast Cancer Conference 2013: Primary Therapy of Early Breast Cancer Evidence, Controversies, Consensus—Opinion of a German Team of Experts (Zurich 2013). Breast Care. 2013;**8**:221-229. DOI: 10.1159/000351692

[27] Zhu X, Chen L, Huang B, et al. The prognostic and predictive potential of Ki-67 in triple-negative breast cancer.

Scientific Reports. 2020;**10**:225. DOI: 10.1038/s41598-019-57094-3

[28] Keam B, Im SA, Lee KH, et al. Ki-67 can be used for further classification of triple negative breast cancer into two subtypes with different response and prognosis. Breast Cancer Research. 2011; **13**:R22. DOI: 10.1186/bcr2834

[29] Wang W, Wu J, Zhang P, et al. Prognostic and predictive value of Ki-67 in triple-negative breast cancer. Oncotarget. 2016;7:31079-31087. DOI: 10.18632/oncotarget.9075

[30] Wu Q, Ma G, Deng Y, et al. Prognostic value of Ki-67 in patients with resected triple-negative breast cancer: A meta-analysis. Frontiers in Oncology. 2019;**9**:1068. DOI: 10.3389/fonc.2019.01068

[31] Nishimura R, Osako T, Okumura Y, Hayashi M, Arima N. Clinical significance of Ki-67 in neoadjuvant chemotherapy for primary breast cancer as a predictor for chemosensitivity and for prognosis. Breast Cancer. 2010;**17**: 269-275. DOI: 10.1007/s12282-009-0161-5

[32] Carey LA, Dees EC, Sawyer L, et al. The triple negative paradox: Primary tumour chemosensitivity of breast cancer subtypes. Clinical Cancer Research. 2007;**13**:2329-2334. DOI: 10.1158/1078-0432.CCR-06-1109

[33] Liedtke C, Mazouni C, Hess KR, et al. Response to neoadjuvant therapy and long-term survival in patients with triple-negative breast cancer. Journal of Clinical Oncology. 2008;**26**:1275-1281. DOI: 10.1200/JCO.2007.14.4147

[34] von Minckwitz G, Untch M, Blohmer JU, et al. Definition and impact of pathologic complete response on prognosis after neoadjuvant chemotherapy in various intrinsic breast cancer subtypes. Journal of Clinical Oncology. 2012;**30**:1796-1804. DOI: 10.1200/JCO.2011.38.8595

Chapter 9

Bcl-2 Immunoexpression in Invasive Ductal Carcinoma and Its Evaluative Correlation with Molecular Sub-Types and BR-Grade and TNM Stage

Poornima Pandey and Arvind Bhake

Abstract

Invasive Ductal carcinoma is the most common histological type of breast cancer. It constitutes about 80 percent of all breast cancer diagnoses. The molecular pathogenesis of breast cancer involves multiple gene types. Bcl-2 is one of them. Bcl-2, is an anti-apoptotic protein which is up regulated by oestrogen in breast cancer patients. The immunoexpression of Bcl-2 detection is being carried out by immunohistochemical methods as described in many published studies. Bcl-2 as is known acts through transcriptional induction in pathogenesis of breast cancer. The present chapter describes the role of Bcl-2 in pathogenesis, significance and its relationship with BR Grade and TNM stage. The present chapter specifically describes its observation of Bcl-2 immunoexpression and relationship with molecular subtypes of breast carcinoma.

Keywords: Bcl-2, breast cancer, BR grade, TNM stage, molecular sub-types

1. Introduction

The Breast cancer has become great concern for global health scenario and health providers [1]. The incidence of it has surpassed the cervical cancers in Indian female [2]. The world over laboratory physicians across the world are engaged in assessing new and novel prognostic and predictive markers that would bring about best possible outcome at breast cancer treatment. The modern day practice of onco-pathology revolves more around predictive prognostic markers that would enable the appropriate adjuvant therapies and management of cancer. The challenges in breast cancer management is to predict its prognostic outcome, benefits of adjuvant therapy, surgical management and immunotherapy.The another challenge in breast cancer treatment is to understand molecular defect and thereby assessment of prognosis, and corrective therapies that would involute the primary tumour as well as metastasis [1, 2].

The conventional pathological prognostic factors in breast cancers which were until relied heavily were lymph node status, tumour size, tumour stage, tumour grade, Nottingham prognostic index and many others [2, 3].

With advent in understanding of pathogenesis of breast cancer many cell surface molecules, cytoplasmic signalling pathways, the nuclear transcriptional activities and many others have come under scanner which relates with breast cancer prognosis and treatment outcomes, especially with chemotherapeutic interventions and monoclonal antibody therapies [4].

Among many such families of the genes, Bcl-2 has been studied extensively for its commonality at participation in the pathogenesis of solid tumours especially the cancers of breast, prostate, lung, colo-rectum and ovaries [5, 6].

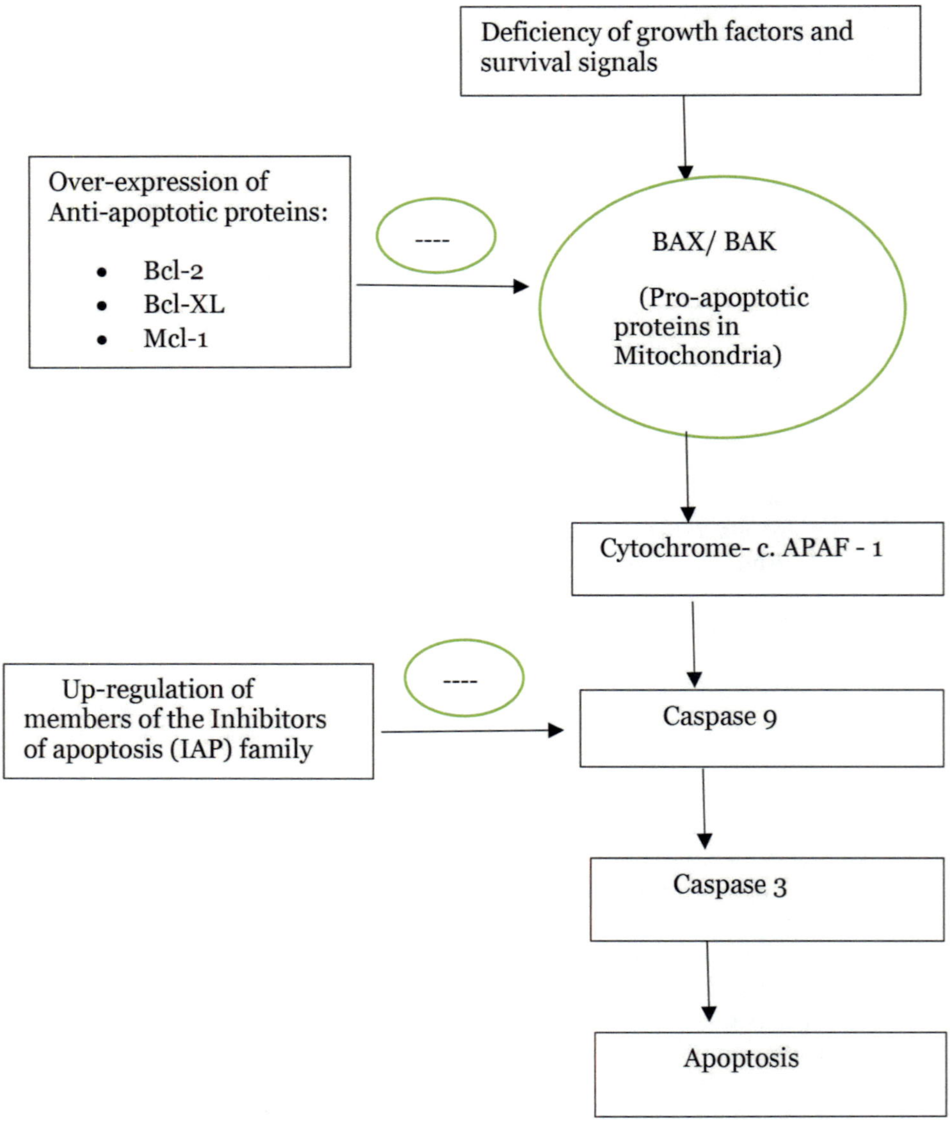

Figure 1.
Flowchart – Evasion of cell death.

Bcl-2 is an anti-apoptotic protein normally expressed in mammary tissue and is up-regulated by oestrogen in breast cancer through direct consequence of transcriptional induction.

Bcl-2 is a principle member of anti-apoptotic proteins along with Bcl-XL and MCL-1. The release of pro-apoptotic proteins in the cells such as cytochrome-c is through the integrity of the mitochondrial outer membrane. This is tightly controlled by Bcl-2 family of proteins. Bcl-2 is overexpressed due to chromosomal translocations and certain mutational changes. Bcl-2 protein also resides in the cytosol and ER membranes. Impermeability by Bcl2 protein prevents the leakage of cytochrome and thereby limits the process of apoptosis. The one way, Bcl-2 genes and their proteins plays an important role in intrinsic pathway of apoptosis [7]. Therefore Bcl-2 genes is one of the genes which is at the centre stage in the pathogenesis of the breast cancer (**Figure 1**).

A few studies in published literature did correlation between Bcl-2 immunoexpression and clinico-pathological variables, disease free survival, prognostic factors, Nottingham prognostic index, TNM stage and treatment outcome [8, 9]. A few studies have proposed that Bcl-2 expression be considered as a molecular subtype of invasive ductal carcinoma because of clinical implications [10, 11].

The search for publications over this topic originating in India was found to be marginal which correlated clinicopathological variables, molecular subtypes of breast cancer and BR-grades [12, 13].

The Bcl-2 expression as published in the western literature have shown its predictive utility and therefore its inclusion in the reporting of histopathology is considered as an essential component [14, 15]. Detecting Bcl-2 immunoexpression in the tumour cell therefore create a frame for appropriate treatment and management of invasive ductal carcinoma.

2. Methodology

The chapter includes the observation on Bcl-2 immunoexpression in invasive ductal carcinoma and its evaluative correlation with BR grade, TNM stage and molecular subtypes as gathered from published literature. Most of the published literature detected Bcl-2 immunoexpression by immunohistochemistry performed on paraffin sections of breast lumps diagnosed as invasive ductal carcinoma.

The authors of the present chapter adopted the methodology for performing the immunohistochemistry in demonstration of Bcl-2, ER, PR and Her 2 on paraffin tissue section as described in the previous studies [6].

The present study included 50 cases whose complete demographic details, clinical examination of the breast lumps, relevant clinical examination, mastectomy details, gross examination finding of specimen, subsequent tissue diagnosis, BR grading, and TNM staging was carried out. The work included only those cases of invasive ductal carcinoma whose complete clinical records and follow up of at least 6 months were available.

The studies whose results are a part of the present chapter performed immunohistochemistry by standard methods meant for it, in detection of ER, PR, Her 2 nu and Bcl-2. The results and interpretation of positivity and score of immunohistochemistry for Bcl-2 and ER, PR, Her 2 were aligned.

The statistical tests used for comparison of the results contained in the present chapter were similar as performed by the authors of other studies.

3. Short review, results and discussion

The chapter contributor's work in this field over the 50 cases of invasive ductal carcinoma is depicted in a tabular forms below.

The Bcl-2 immunoexpression was seen in 33 of 50 cases (66%). There were 30 (60%) women who were below age of 51 and 20 (40%) were 51 and above years. The age versus Bcl-2 immunoexpression is charted in **Table 1**.

Of the 30 women who were below age of 51 showed Bcl-2 immunoexpression on 21 instances (70%) while 12 of 20 (60%) showed Bcl-2 immunoexpression in women more than 50 years of age. The youngest patient of invasive ductal carcinoma was 26 years while oldest one was 84 years. The immunoexpression of Bcl-2 was observed to be 100% in women of invasive ductal carcinoma in between the age of 31 to 40 years.

The distribution of Bcl-2 immunoexpression across BR grade is shown in **Table 2**.

It was observed that Bcl-2 immunoexpression is independent of BR grade.

TNM stage and immunoexpression in 50 cases of invasive ductal carcinoma is shown in **Table 3**.

The TNM stage of invasive ductal carcinoma when plotted against Bcl-2 immuno-expression revealed 15 Bcl-2 immunoexpressions in 20 cases of stage II disease and 7

Age Range	No. of cases/ Percentage	Bcl-2 Immuno-expression				Total No. Cases showing Positive Bcl-2 Expression/ Percentage
		Negative	1(+)	2(++)	3(+++)	
21–30 years	03(06%)	01	01	—	01	02(66.6%)
31–40 years	07(14%)	—	01	03	03	07(100%)
41–50 years	20(40%)	08	04	05	03	012(60%)
51–60 years	11(22%)	03	04	02	02	08(72.7%)
61–70 years	05(10%)	02	01	01	01	03(60%)
71–80 years	03(06%)	02	01	—	—	01(33.3%)
81–90 years	01(02%)	01	—	—	—	00(0%)
Total (21–90) years	50 (100%)	17	12	11	10	33(66%)

Table 1.
Bcl-2 Immuno-expression and age range of invasive ductal carcinoma.

BR-Grade	No. of cases/ Percentage	Bcl-2 Immuno-expression				Total No. Cases showing Positive Bcl-2 Expression/ Percentage
		Negative	1(+)	2(++)	3(+++)	
Grade I	12(24%)	05	—	05	03	08(66.6%)
Grade II	29(58%)	08	07	06	07	20(68.9%)
Grade III	09(18%)	04	05	—	—	05(55.5%)
Total	50(100%)	17	12	11	10	33(66%)

Table 2.
Bcl-2 Immuno-expression and BR-grade.

TNM Stage	No. of cases/ Percentage	Bcl-2 Immuno-expression				Total No. Cases showing Positive Bcl-2 Expression/ Percentage
		Negative	1(+)	2(++)	3(+++)	
Stage I	17(34%)	07	01	04	05	10(58.82%)
Stage II	20(40%)	05	06	06	03	15(75%)
Stage III	09(18%)	02	04	01	02	07(77.7%)
Stage IV	04(08%)	03	01	—	—	01(25%)
Total	50(100%)	17	12	11	10	33(66%)

Table 3.
Bcl-2 Immuno-expression and TNM stage.

Molecular Sub-type	No. of cases/ Percentage	Bcl-2 Immuno-expression				Total No. Cases showing Positive Bcl-2 Expression/Percentage
		Negative	1(+)	2(++)	3(+++)	
Luminal A	18(36%)	05	04	07	02	13(72.2%)
Luminal B	11(22%)	03	03	01	04	08(72.7%)
Triple negative breast cancer (TNBC)	13(26%)	07	02	01	03	06(46.15%)
Her- 2 enriched	08(16%)	02	02	02	01	05(62.5%)
Total	50(100%)	17	12	11	10	33(66%)

(TNBC, Triple negative breast cancer).

Table 4.
Bcl-2 Immuno-expression and molecular sub-type.

of the 9 stage III disease thus the comparisons of Bcl-2 immunoexpression in between TNM stages was found to be non-specific.

The molecular subtype of invasive ductal carcinoma and its relationship with Bcl-2 is shown in **Table 4**.

It was observed that Bcl-2 immuno-expression by percentage was more in Luminal A molecular subtype of invasive ductal carcinoma followed by Luminal B and Her2 enriched (**Figure 2**).

The higher frequency of correlation between the Bcl-2 immunoexpression with molecular subtype Luminal A of breast cancer as observed in present study is attributed to oestrogen up regulating of Bcl-2 imuunoexpression. The higher frequency of immunoexpression of Bcl-2 with molecular subtype of Luminal A of breast cancer too has been observed in the other studies.

The p-value distribution of the various studies for relationship between molecular subtype of invasive ductal carcinoma and Bcl-2 immunoexpression is shown in **Table 5**.

The studies depicted in **Table 5** concluded of evidences of Bcl2 immuno-expression correlates well with molecular subtype of Luminal A of invasive ductal carcinoma to which the contributors of present chapter agree.

The included studies for their observations are cited below paragraphically explaining about Bcl-2 immuno-expression and its evaluative correlation with BR Grade, TNM stage and molecular subtypes of invasive ductal carcinoma including comparisons.

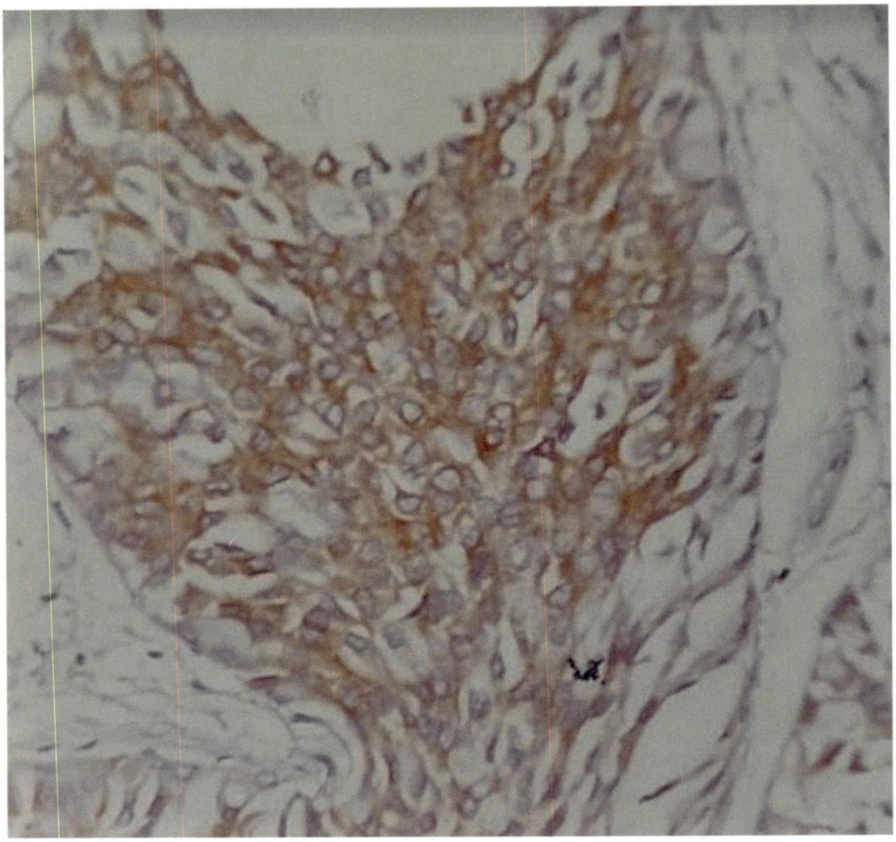

Figure 2.
IHC Bcl-2, invasive ductal carcinoma (luminal a molecular subtype, 40×).

Sharmila, Praba [2] have studied 30 cases of invasive ductal carcinoma for expression of Bcl-2 in immunohistochemistry (IHC). The immunohistochemistry was carried out by standard methods. The objective of study was to analyse Bcl-2 expression and its relationships with ER, PR, HER-2 status, histological grade and Nottingham prognostic index. The study observed that 7 cases of the Invasive Ductal Carcinoma showed intense Bcl-2 staining while 23 cases showed no expression. The Grade I tumour showed 45.5% positive immuno-expression followed by Grade II at 14.3%. The correlation of Bcl-2 expression with ER status showed that 7 out of 12 ER positive cases expressed Bcl-2 with statistically significant values. The study concluded that BCl2 expression in invasive ductal carcinoma, directly related with lower histological grade, small tumour, size, ER and PR positive status. It is inversely related to HER-2 nu status.

Cecka, et al. [3] did study on expression of Bcl-2 in 57 females suffering from primary breast cancer who were treated with neo-adjuvant chemotherapy. The immunohistochemistry for BCl2 were performed either on the surgical specimens or core cut biopsies with Streptavidin and Biotin method with peroxidise detection system. The results of immunohistochemistry when correlated with the findings of Bcl-2 have shown the following p-values with individual variables.

Tumour size (0.56), grading (0.53), ER (0.003), PR (0.36), Ki-67 score (0.07), Her-2 nu (0.24) and p53 (0.88). Hence the study concluded that there exists no significant association of Bcl-2 expression with clinical variable except ER status.

DOI: http://dx.doi.org/10.5772/intechopen.109297

S.No.	Studies	Year	Number of cases in study	Country of Source	Bcl-2 Immuno-expression		p -value	
					Number/ Percentage	Molecular subtype	Total	Molecular subtype
1.	Sharmila,Praba [2]	2020	30	India	44.4% 25.6%	Luminal A and Normal breast like tumours Luminal B, Her2 nu enriched, Triple Negative	$p < 0.05$ $p = 0.236$	Luminal A and Normal breast like tumours Luminal B, Her2 nu enriched, Triple Negative
2.	Cecka et al. [3]	2008	57	Russia	52.8% 23.2%	Luminal A Luminal B, Her2 nu enriched, Triple Negative	$p = 0.003$ $p = 0.561$	Luminal A Luminal B, Her2 nu enriched, Triple Negative
3.	Callagy et al. [4]	2006	930	United Kingdom	57.4%	Luminal A and Normal breast like tumours	$p < 0.001$	Luminal A and Normal breast like tumours
4.	Kamaruzman et al. [5]	2019	53	Malaysia	22.4%	Luminal A and Normal breast like tumours	$p < 0.005$	Luminal A and Normal breast like tumours
5.	Adams, Cory [6]	2007	45	Australia	19.3%	Luminal A and Normal breast like tumours	$p < 0.003$	Luminal A and Normal breast like tumours
6.	Eom et al. [8]	2016	1356	Korea	40.9% 37.1% 9.6% 12.4%	Luminal A Luminal B Her2 enriched Triple Negative	$p < 0.001$ $p < 0.001$ $p < 0.001$ $p < 0.001$	Luminal A Luminal B Her2 enriched Triple Negative
7.	Dawson et al. [9]	2010	11,212	United kingdom	62.3%	Luminal A, Luminal B and Her2 enriched	$p < 0.001$	Luminal A, Luminal B and Her2 enriched
8.	Lehmann et al. [10]	2011	3247	Tennessee(USA)	43.1%	Triple Negative	$p = 0.451$	Triple Negative
9.	Hwang et al. [11]	2012	7230	Seoul (Republic of Korea)	51.2%	Luminal A	$p < 0.001$	Luminal A
10.	Min et al. [12]	2016	203	Seoul (Republic of Korea)	34.2%	Luminal A and Normal breast like tumours	$p < 0.005$	Luminal A and Normal breast like tumours
11.	Wijesinghe et al. [13]	2018	208	Srilanka	33.1%	Her2 nu enriched	$p = 0.001$	Her2 nu enriched

S.No.	Studies	Year	Number of cases in study	Country of Source	Bcl-2 Immuno-expression		p -value	
					Number/ Percentage	Molecular subtype	Total	Molecular subtype
12.	Bayoudh et al. [14]	2010	84	Tunisia (North Africa)	42.1%	Triple Negative	p = 0.002	Triple Negative
13.	Rashid, AL-Sakkal [15]	2015	100	Iraq	61%	Luminal A and Luminal B	p = 0.030	Luminal A and Luminal B
14.	Present Study	2022	50	India	72.2% 72.7% 46.15% 62.5%	Luminal A Luminal B TNBC Her 2 enriched	p = 0.04(S) p = 0.78(NS) p = 0.95(NS) p = 0.68(NS) p = 0.36(NS)	Luminal A Luminal B TNBC Her 2 enriched Overall

Table 5.
Study and results (p-value) distribution.

Callagy et al. [4] did study to evaluate that in first 5 years after diagnosis, Bcl-2 is predictor of breast cancer outcome independently, and serves as a useful tool as prognostic marker besides Nottingham prognostic index. A total of 13 markers expression was evaluated in 930 breast cancer patients on a tissue microarray. Out of all the markers Bcl-2 was the best marker. Through this study it's also evaluated that whether a single marker or a series of markers could improve prognostic potential of Nottingham prognostic index.

Kamaruzman, et al. [5] published study related to nanotherapeutics in breast cancer wherein they observed that the expression of Bcl-2 was observed in 22.4% of molecular subtype of Luminal a of invasive breast cancer.

Adams, Cory [6] did a new study which was innovative as it encouraged to ponder us upon that most of cytotoxic stresses imposed on a cell lead to activation of BH3 only proteins as important signal of stress. These BH3 proteins belong to Bcl-2 family which help us to understand their role in cancer development, and through this search for important class of anticancer drugs can be done.

Eom et al. [8] did study to evaluate the relation between the prognostic outcomes and Bcl-2 expression among the molecular sub-types. A study was conducted taking into account 1356 patients who were newly diagnosed with breast cancer between November 2006 and November 2011. Mainly Immunohistochemistry (IHC) was used to measure status of - ER, progesterone receptor, human epidermal growth factor receptor 2, and Bcl-2 expression. In this study breast cancer was classified into five molecular sub-types namely, luminal A, luminal B with positive status, luminal B with negative status, human epidermal growth factor receptor 2 expression, and triple negative sub-types. The clinico-pathological variables were analysed which assessed the correlation between Bcl-2 expression and clinical outcomes such as relapse free survival and disease- specific survival according to the five molecular sub-types.

Dawson et al. [9] have established the rationale of performing Bcl-2 immunohistochemistry in prognostic stratification of invasive ductal carcinoma. Their work included the conglomeration of 5 studies wherein the relationship between Bcl-2 and molecular subtypes of breast carcinoma was followed. The study observed the significant p-value ($p < 0.01$) in ER positive breast cancer (Luminal A subtype).

Lehmann et al. [10] observed 43.1% of their cases showing Bcl-2 immunoexpression. However, the study observed no relationship between Bcl-2 immuno-expression and molecular subtype of breast cancer. A similar observation of discordant relationship in between molecular subtype of luminal A and Bcl-2 immuno-expression by Wijesinghe et al. [13] and Bayoudh et al. [14]

The study of Hwang et al. [11] observed the Bcl-2 immunoexpression in 51.2% cases and luminal A subtype held its association with significant p-value ($p < 0.01$).

Min et al. [12] observed 34.2% of the breast cancer expressing Bcl-2 and its significant correlation with luminal A subtype of breast cancer ($p < 0.05$).

Rashid, AL-Sakkal [15] studied 61 cases of primary breast cancer in which 71% of ER positive cases and 59% of PR positive cases depicted positive Bcl-2 oncoprotein expression, having p-values ($p = 0.030$) and ($p = 0.001$) respectively.

4. Conclusion

Bcl-2 is an independent prognostic marker for breast cancer although its expression frequency may differ but it plays definite prognostic role in breast cancer. It is observed that Luminal A molecular subtype of invasive ductal carcinoma has a frequent association with Bcl-2 immuno-expression. There are some limitations to use of immunohistochemistry staining method as the results may be affected by intra-tumoral heterogeneity.

Author details

Poornima Pandey* and Arvind Bhake
Department of Pathology, Jawaharlal Nehru Medical College, Datta Meghe Institute of Higher Education and Research, Wardha, Maharashtra, India

*Address all correspondence to: poornima.pan22@gmail.com

References

[1] Sung H, Ferlay J, Siegel RL, Laversanne M, Soerjomataram I, Jemal A, et al. Global cancer statistics 2020: GLOBOCAN estimates of incidence and mortality worldwide for 36 cancers in 185 countries. CA: a Cancer Journal for Clinicians. 2021;**71**(3):209-249. DOI: 10.3322/caac.21660

[2] Sharmila G, Praba V. BCL2 expression in ductal carcinoma of breast and its association with other clinicopathologic variables. IP Achieves of Cytology and Histopathology Research. 2020;**5**(1):75-80. DOI: 10.18231/j.achr.2020.015

[3] Čečka F, Hornychová H, Melichar B, Ryška A, Jandík P, Mergancová J, et al. Expression of Bcl-2 in breast cancer: Correlation with Clinicopathological characteristics and survival. Acta Medica International (Hradec Kralove, Czech Repub). 2008;**51**(2):107-112. DOI: 10.14712/18059694.2017.11

[4] Callagy GM, Pharoah PD, Pinder SE, Hsu FD, Nielsen TO, Ragaz J, et al. Bcl-2 is a prognostic marker in breast cancer independently of the Nottingham prognostic index. Clinical Cancer Research. 2006;**12**(8):2468-2475. DOI: 10.1158/1078-0432.CCR-05-2719

[5] Kamaruzman NI, Aziz NA, Poh CL, Chowdhury EH. Oncogenic signaling in tumorigenesis and applications of siRNA Nanotherapeutics in breast cancer. Cancers. 2019;**11**(5):632. DOI: 10.3390/cancers11050632

[6] Adams JM, Cory S. The Bcl-2 apoptotic switch in cancer development and therapy. Oncogene. 2007;**26**(9):1324-1337. DOI: 10.1038/sj.onc.1210220

[7] Kumar V, Abbas AK, Aster JC. Robbins Basic Pathology. 10th ed. Philadelphia, USA: Elsevier - Health Sciences Division; Book printed in Canada. 2017

[8] Eom YH, Kim HS, Lee A, Song BJ, Chae BJ. BCL2 as a subtype-specific prognostic marker for breast cancer. Journal of Breast Cancer. 2016;**19**(3):252. DOI: 10.4048/jbc.2016.19.3.252

[9] Dawson S-J, Makretsov N, Blows FM, Driver KE, Provenzano E, Quesne JL, et al. BCL2 in breast cancer: A favourable prognostic marker across molecular subtypes and independent of adjuvant therapy received. British Journal of Cancer. 2010;**103**(5):668-675. DOI: 10.1038/sj.bjc.6605736

[10] Lehmann BD, Bauer JA, Chen X, Sanders ME, Chakravarthy AB, Shyr Y, et al. Identification of human triple-negative breast cancer subtypes and preclinical models for selection of targeted therapies. The Journal of Clinical Investigation. 2011;**121**(7):2750-2767. DOI: 10.1172/JCI45014

[11] Hwang K-T, Woo JW, Shin HC, Kim HS, Ahn SK, Moon HG, et al. Prognostic influence of BCL2 expression in breast cancer. International Journal of Cancer. 2012;**131**(7):E1109-E1119. DOI: 10.4048/jbc.2017.20.1.54

[12] Min K-W, Kim D-H, Do S-I, Pyo J-S, Chae SW, Sohn JH, et al. High Ki67/BCL2 index is associated with worse outcome in early stage breast cancer. Postgraduate Medical Journal. 2016;**92**(1094):707-714. DOI: 10.1136/postgradmedj-2015-133531

[13] Wijesinghe HD, Thuvarakan P, Samarasekera A, S. Lokuhetty MD. Prognostic indices predictive of short-term disease-free survival of breast carcinoma patients receiving primary surgical treatment in Sri Lanka. Indian

Journal of Pathology & Microbiology. 2018;**61**(4):505-509. DOI: 10.4103/IJPM. IJPM_321_17

[14] Kallel-Bayoudh I, Hassen HB, Khabir A, Boujelbene N, Daoud J, Frikha M, et al. Bcl-2 expression and triple negative profile in breast carcinoma. Medical Oncology. 2011;**28**(S1):55-61. DOI: 10.1007/s12032-010-9694-x

[15] Rashid PA, AL-Sakkal NS. Immunoexpression of Bcl2 in breast carcinoma: Association with clinicopathological parameters. Journal of Kurdistan Board of medical specialities. April 2015;**1**(1):119-127

Chapter 10

Correlation between Ultrasound Findings and Molecular Subtypes of Breast Cancer

Eman Soliman Metwally, Rahma Mohammed Abed Alghazal and Ah Haggaa Ali

Abstract

Breast cancer is the most common malignant tumor and the major cause of death among women worldwide. Molecular subtyping of breast cancer is important to individualize its management, to understand prognosis of disease and avoid overtreatment. The current study aimed at correlating the breast cancer subtypes with their different ultrasound criteria. The ultrasound findings might have an important role in predicting different groups. The current study is a retrospective study. Which was conducted on 40 females patients with breast cancer; during the period from November 2020 till March 2021.The age were 45–65 years old. They were presented to the Radiology Department, ·Ain-Shams University, Faculty of Medicine. The selected cases had been afforded from: the Breast-unit of General Surgery Hospital, El Demerdash University Hospital, Clinical Oncology & Nuclear Medicine Department. When analyzing the main four breast cancer subtypes in the current work we found that the rates of Luminal A was 34%, Luminal B was 40%, HER2 was 15%, and TNBC was 11%. LA subtype was strongly associated with hypoechoic lesions showing irregular shape, speculated margin surrounded by desmoplastic reaction with posterior shadowing. LB subtype was associated with irregular shape and speculated margin with absence of desmoplastic reaction. Human Epidermal Growth Factor (HER2) subtype in the current study was found to be associated with irregular shape, lobulated margin, absent desmoplastic reaction with posterior acoustic mixed shadowing and enhancement. This could be related to suspicious microcalcifications. Triple Negative Breast Cancer (TNBC) lesions in the present work were predominantly oval in shape with• circumscribed margin; the benign looking malignant lesions which carry the worst prognosis. Based on the latter finding, the good radiologist should be aware about ultround features of different molecular subtype in order not to under diagnose a malignant breast lesion. The sonographic features as margin, shape, posterior acoustic features were significantly associated with molecular subtypes. The histopathological grade and hormone receptor status. Being able to predict the molecular subtype. The current study recommend that the radiologist should be aware about different imaging features of different molecular subtypes especially the triple negative breast cancer which had the most benign looking criteria aiming for better lesion characterization and to allow the patient to benefit from earlier non-invasive, cheap diagnosis and the curable on time treatment.

IntechOpen

Keywords: breast cancer, ultrasound features, molecular subtypes

1. Introduction

Cancer Breast is a heterogeneous and complex disease with different morphologic, biologic, and molecular features. The histopathological characteristics of tumors had been used to determine the management of breast cancer. However They do not provide sufficient information due to tumor heterogeneity [1–3].

Distinct molecular subtypes of breast cancer had been defined based on gene expression. Molecular subtyping of breast cancer is essential to individualize its management, to understand prognosis of disease and avoid overtreatment [4].

Ultrasonographic imaging features of breast cancer, including the tumor shape, margin, boundaries, posterior features, multiplicity, orientation, and calcification, are significant predictive sonographic signs of different molecular subtypes [5].

Previous literatures had indicated an excellent improvement in U/S technologies. It would be possible to have highly sensitive machines be able to differentiate malignant solid breast masses from benign ones based on their different U/S criteria [6].

Many studies correlated the ultrasonography features of malignant lesions with their grade, while limited studies discussed the correlation with molecular subtypes of breast cancer. Overlap of benign and malignant ultrasound morphology descriptors still represents a challenge to breast imaging radiologists. Knowing the descriptors of the different molecular subtypes may help radiologists to decrease both false positive and false negative diagnosis [3–6].

2. Aim of the work

The present study aimed at detecting the correlation between ultrasound morphological features and different molecular subtypes of breast cancer which could increase the diagnostic ultrasound accuracy.

3. Patients and methods

The current study is a retrospective study. Which was conducted on females patients with breast cancer. They were presented to the Radiology Department, Ain-Shams University, Faculty of Medicine. The selected cases had been afforded from: The Breast-unit of General Surgery Hospital, El Demerdash University Hospital, Clinical Oncology & Nuclear Medicine Department.

- Number of patients: 40 female patients had breast cancer.
- Time: during the period from November 2020 till March 2021.
- Age: 45–65 years old ±10.58.

An informed consent explaining the procedure details was obtained from all patients prior to inclusion in this study. The study was conducted according to the stipulations of the ASU ethical and scientific committee. The privacy of participants and confidentiality of data were guaranteed during the various phases of the study. The inclusion criteria were: Female patients with breast cancer, only. The exclusion Criteria were: a) History of neoadjuvant therapy; b) Ductal carcinoma in situ; c) Patients had started any local or systemic therapy.

3.1 Study methods

Forty female patients had breast cancers were selected for the present study the inpatient wards as well as outpatient clinic were admitted for bilateral Sonomammographic examination. An U/S device; GE (Pristima), Siemens (Mammomat 1000) & Samsung (Accuvix XG) machines in Ain Shams University Medical Hospital. A linear probe of 9–15 MHz was used.

The technique was done after exposure of the breast with the patient lying supine and her ipsilateral hand raised above the head the UIS probe was oriented perpendicular to the chest wall. Radial scanning technique, in a clockwise fashion wising the nipple as a center point wall followed. Scanning of each breast quadrant in the sagittal and transverse planers were performed. Scanning axially lymph nodes.

The examination time took about 20 minutes. All the real-time scanning was performed by a radiologist with at least 5 years of experience in breast U/S. More experienced radiologist with at least 7–10 years' experience rechecked the findings. As a way of a double-blind analysis. The final interpretation and diagnosis were obtained.

3.2 Histopathologic diagnosis, image analysis and interpretation of conventional ultrasound

U/S guided biopsy was scheduled for patients with suspicious breast lesions. The procedure was performed by at least 7–10 years experienced radiologist. Biopsy was taken under complete aseptic condition. Sterilization of the area of interest with betadine was done; the latter was followed by sterilization the U/S probe. The radiologist used sterile gloves and injected a local anesthesia followed by introduction of the Tru-cut needle. The needle under ultrasound guidance targeted the lesion. At least four core biopsies were taken.

Tissues biopsied were sent to the Pathology Department. The tissues were formalin fixed, paraffin embedded and subsequently used for IHC staining with appropriate antibodies to detect the hormonal status of the lesions (ER, PR, HER2 gene expression and Ki-67). The cutoff point for ER positive, PR-positive expression was 10%. HER-2 status was graded as 0, 1+, 2+ and 3+. The HER-2 status of 3+ was deemed to be positive, while statuses of O and 1+ were deemed to be negative. Fluorescence in situ hybridization (FISH) was performed on all grade 2 samples. Samples with a > 2-frold-change in expression were regarded as negative. Samples with a < 2-fold increase were regarded as positive for gene amplification. Ki67 was visually scored for the percentage of tumor cell nuclei with positive immunostaining above background. Over **Histopathologic diagnosis** by following and receiving the pathology report from the patient.

3.3 Statistical analysis

Recorded data were analyzed using the statistical package for social sciences, version 20.0 (SPSS Inc., Chicago, Illinois, USA). Quantitative data were expressed as mean ± standard deviation (SD). Qualitative data were expressed as frequency and percentage.

The following tests were done: Chi-square (x^2) test of significance was used in order to compare proportions between qualitative parameters. The confidence interval was set to 95% and the margin of error accepted was set to 5%. So, the p-value was considered significant as the· following: - Probability (P-value). P-value ≤ 0.05 was considered significant. P-value ≤ 0.001 was considered as highly significant. P-value >0.05 was considered insignificant.

4. Results

The current study comprised 40 female patients with cancer breast. The resulting analysis of the main four breast cancer subtypes of the current work among the patients showed the following figures:

- LA: 34% i.e. 14 patients.
- LB: 40% i.e. 16 patients.
- TNBC: 11% i.e. 4 patients.
- HER2: 15% i.e. 6 patients (**Tables 1–5**).

		n	Row%	Column %	P value
Age groups	<=50 yrs	8	33.3%	55.9%	
	>50 yrs	6	34.9%	44.1%	0.429
Density	Fatty	8	33.9%	55.9%	
	Fibroglandular	6	34.1%	44.1%	0.832
Shape	Oval	2	15.4%	11.8%	
	Irregular	12	40.5%	88.2%	<0.001
Margin	Circumscribed	2	13.3%	5.9%	
	Lobulated	4	20.0%	17.6%	
	Speculated	8	47.3%	76.5%	
Echogenicity	Hyper				
	Iso	2	27.8%	14.7%	
	Hypo	12	35.4%	85.3%	0.713
E	Enhancement	2	18.2%	11.8%	
S	Shadowing	10	51.1%	70.6%	
M	Mixed	2	19.4%	17.6%	
Number of	Single	10	33.8%	64.7%	
Lesion	Multiple	4	34.3%	35.3%	0.219
Calcification	No	8	30.6%	55.9%	
	Yes	6	39.5%	44.1%	0.025

		n	Row%	Column %	P value
Size grouped	<2	10	38.3%	52.9%	
	> = 2	4	30.2%	47.1%	0.036
Surrounding	No	10	32.4%	67.6%	
Parenchyma	Yes	4	37.9%	32.4%	0.613
Desmoplastic reaction	No	5	22.1%	44.1%	
	Yes	9	59.4%	55.9%	<0.001

Table 1.
Showing age, U/S criteria of LA subtype.

		N	Row %	Column %	P value
Age groups	<=50 yrs	10	40.4%	60.5%	
	>50 yrs	6	34.9%	39.5%	0.429
Density	Fatty	10	41.1%	60.5%	
	Fibroglandular	6	34.1%	39.5%	0.832
Shape	Oval	5	34.6%	23.7%	
	Irregular	11	39.2%	76.3%	<0.001
Margin	Circumscribed	2	40.0%	15.8%	
	Lobulated	4	33.3%	26.3%	
	Speculated	10	40.0%	57.9%	
Echogenicity	Hyper				
	Iso	2	33.3%	15.8%	
	Hypo	14	39.0%	84.2%	0.713
E	Enhancement	2	36.4%	21.1%	
S	Shadowing	10	34.0%	42.1%	
M	Mixed	4	45.2%	36.8%	
Number of	Single	14	38.5%	65.8%	
Lesion	Multiple	2	37.1%	34.2%	0.219
Calcification	No	11	46.8%	76.3%	
	Yes	5	23.7%	23.7%	0.025
Size grouped	<2	8	40.4%	50.0%	
	> = 2	8	35.8%	50.0%	0.036
Surrounding	No	11	40.8%	76.3%	
parenchyma	Yes	5	31.0%	23.7%	0.613
Desmoplastic	No	10	41.2%	73.7%	
Reaction	Yes	6	31.3%	26.3%	<0.001

Table 2.
Showing age, U/S criteria of LB subtype.

		n	Row %	Column %	P value
Age groups	<=50 yrs	1	15.8%	69.2%	
	>50 yrs	3	9.3%	30.8%	0.429
Density	Fatty	2	10.7%	46.2%	
	Fibroglandular	2	15.9%	53.8%	0.832
Shape	Oval	3	34.6%	69.2%	
	Irregular	1	5.4%	30.8%	<0.001
Margin	Circumscribed	3	46.7%	53.8%	
	Lobulated	0	13.3%	30.8%	
	Speculated	1	3.6%	15.4%	
Echogenicity	Hyper				
	Iso	1	16.7%	23.1%	
	Hypo	3	12.2%	76.9%	0.713
E	Enhancement	2	31.8%	53.8%	
S	Shadowing	1	6.4%	23.1%	
M	Mixed	1	9.7%	23.1%	
Number of	Single	4	16.9%	84.6%	
lesion	Multiple	0	5.7%	15.4%	0.219
Calcification	No	3	14.5%	69.2%	
	Yes	1	10.5%	30.8%	0.025
Size grouped	<2	3	17.0%	61.5%	
	>=2	1	9.4%	38.5%	0.036
Surrounding	No	4	14.1%	76.9%	
parenchyma	Yes	0	10.3%	23.1%	0.613
Desmoplastic	No	4	17.6%	92.3%	
reaction	Yes	0	3.1%	7.7%	<0.001

Table 3.
Showing age, U/S criteria of TNBC subtype.

		n	Row %	Column %	P value
Age groups	<=50 yrs		15.8%	69.2%	
	>50 yrs	9	9.3%	30.8%	0.429
Density	Fatty	8	10.7%	46.2%	
	Fibroglandular	7	15.9%	53.8%	0.832
Shape	Oval	4	34.6%	69.2%	
	Irregular	11	5.4%	30.8%	<0.001
Margin	Circumscribed	0	46.7%	53.8%	
	Lobulated	10	13.3%	30.8%	
	speculated	5	3.6%	15.4%	

		n	Row %	Column %	P value
Echogenicity	Hyper				
	Iso	4	16.7%	23.1%	
	Hypo	11	12.2%	76.9%	0.713
E	Enhancement	3	31.8%	53.8%	
S	Shadowing	4	6.4%	23.1%	
M	Mixed	8	9.7%	23.1%	
Number of	Single	7	16.9%	84.6%	
lesion	Multiple	8	5.7%	15.4%	0.219
Calcification	No	5	14.5%	69.2%	
	Yes	10	10.5%	30.8%	0.025
Size grouped	<2	2	17.0%	61.5%	
	>=2	13	9.4%	38.5%	0.036
Surrounding	No	9	14.1%	76.9%	
parenchyma	Yes	6	10.3%	23.1%	0.613
Desmoplastic	No	13	17.6%	92.3%	
reaction	Yes	2	3.1%	7.7%	<0.001

Table 4.
Showing age, U/S criteria of HER2 subtype.

		n	Row%	Column%	P value
LA subtype: For 14 patients					
Pathology	IDC	12	29.9%	76.5%	
	ILC	2	61.5%	23.5%	
Grade	1	12	43.9%	73.5%	
Grouped	2	2	20.9%	26.5%	0.050
		n	**Row%**	**Column%**	**P value**
LB subtype: For 16 patients					
Pathology	IDC	38	39.1%	89.5%	
	ILC	2	30.8%	10.5%	
Grade	1	22	35.1%	52.6%	
Grouped	2	18	41.9%	47.4%	0.050
		n	**Row%**	**Column%**	**P value**
TNBC subtype: For 4 patients					
Pathology	IDC	3	13.8%	92.3%	
	ILC	1	7.7%	7.7%	
Grade	1	1	7.0%	30.8%	
Grouped	2	3	20.9%	69.2%	0.050

		n	Row%	Column %	P value
HER2 subtype: For 6 patients					
Pathology	IDC	6	17.2%	100.0%	
	ILC	0	0.0%	0.0%	
Grade	1	4	14.0%	53.3%	
Grouped	2	2	16.3%	46.7%	0.05

Table 5.
Showing the histopathological results and grade in different molecular subtypes.

4.1 Luminal A breast cancer case presentation

52-year-old female patient presented, symptomless, was imaged for screening.
Family history of breast cancer: positive (**Figure 1**).
Histopathological examination result:
Invasive ductal carcinoma grade II.

Immunohistochemical revealed:
ER: positive
PR: positive
HER2: negative
Ki-67: 2%

4.2 Luminal B HER2 –ve breast cancer case presentation

58-year-old female patient presented with right breast lump. Family history: Negative (**Figure 2**).

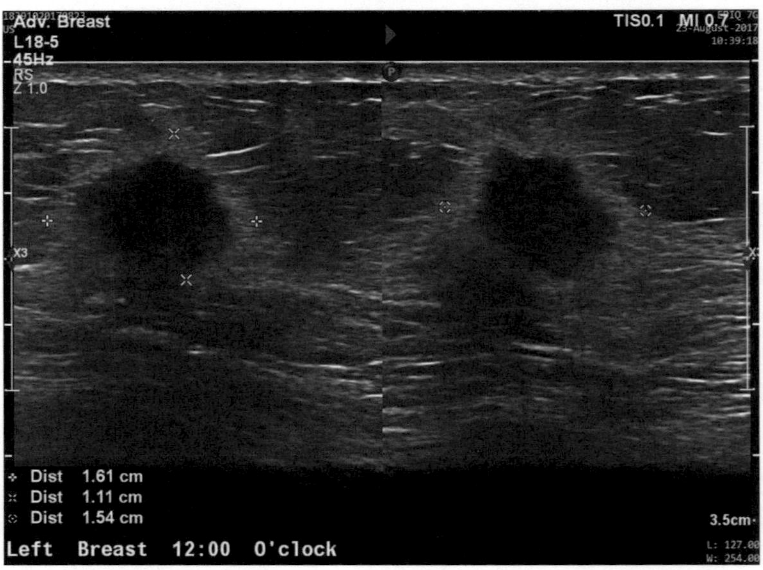

Figure 1.
U/S showing hypoechoic lesion, irregular in shape with spiculated margin, measuring 1.6x1.1 cm in its maximum dimensions surrounded by desmoplastic reaction and showing posterior acoustic shadowing.

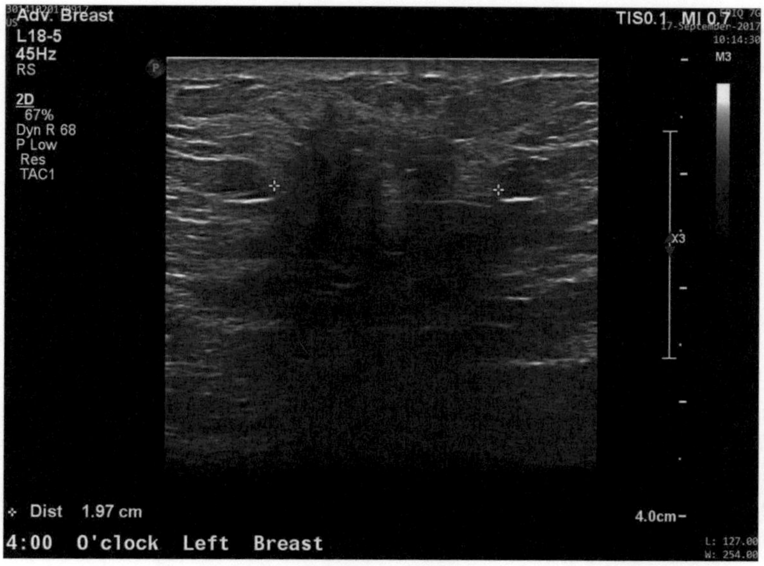

Figure 2.
U/S of fibroglandular breast showing hypoechoic irregular lesion with speculated margin, measuring 2 cm in its maximum dimension not surrounded by desmoplastic reaction with posterior acoustic shadowing. The parenchyma showed mild distortion.

Histopathological examination result:
Invasive ductal carcinoma grade II

Immunohistochemistry revealed:
ER: positive
PR: negative
HER2: negative
Ki-67: 50%

4.3 Luminal B HER2 –ve breast cancer case presentation

65-year-old female patient presented with right breast mass. Family history: Positive (**Figure 3**).

Histopathological examination result:
Invasive duct carcinoma grade II

Immunohistochemistry revealed:
ER: positive
PR: negative
HER2: negative
Ki-67: 50%

4.4 Luminal B HER2 ±ve breast cancer case presentation

60-years-old female patient presented with left breast lump. Family history: Negative (**Figure 4**).

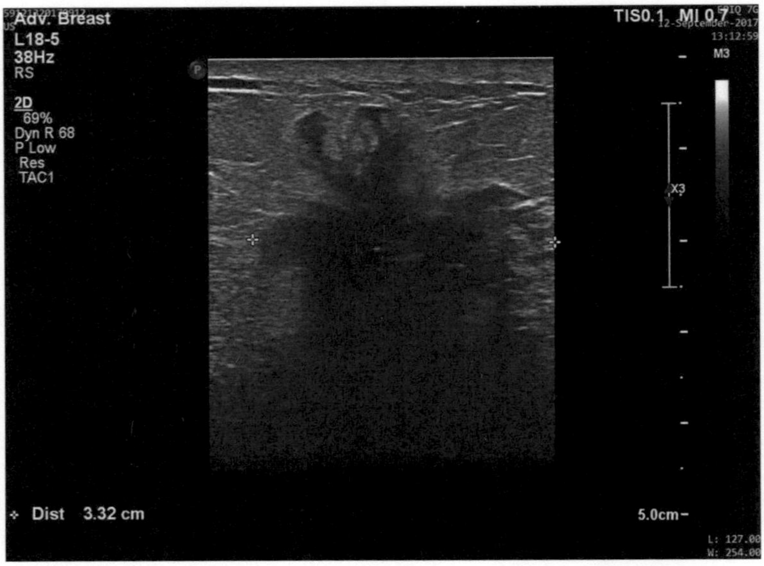

Figure 3.
U/S breast showing irregular shaped lesion with speculated margin measuring 3.3 cm in its maximum dimension showing posterior acoustic shadowing.

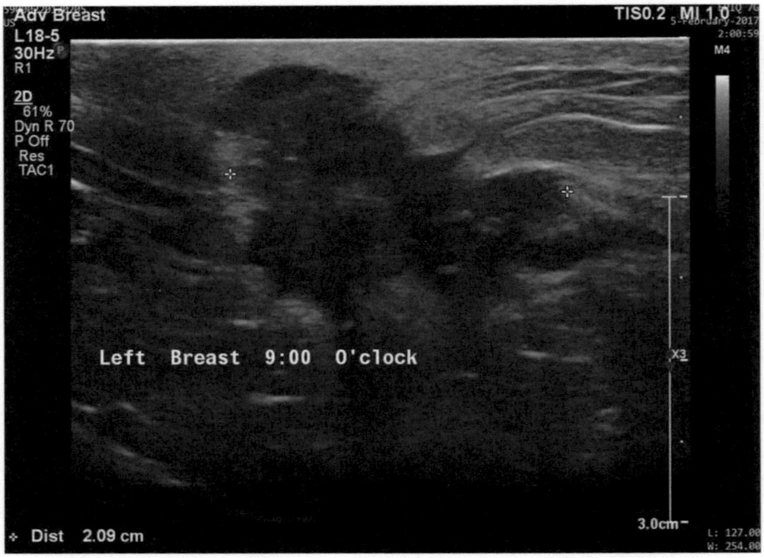

Figure 4.
U/S of fibroglandular breast showing hypoechoic focal lesion, irregular in shape with speculated margin and not surrounded by desmoplastic reaction, mixed posterior acoustic shadowing and enhancement. The parenchyma showed distortion and few calcific foci.

Histopathological examination result:

Invasive duct carcinoma grade III

Immunohistochemical results revealed:

ER: positive
PR: negative

HER2: positive
Ki-67: 30%

4.5 Triple negative breast cancer case presentation

47-years-old female patient presented with left breast mass. Family history: Negative (**Figure 5**).

Histopathological examination result:
Invasive ductal carcinoma grade III.

Immunohistochemistry results:
ER: negative
PR: negative
HER2: negative
Ki-67: 30%

4.6 Triple negative breast cancer case presentation

45-year-old female patient presented with right breast mass. Family history: Negative (**Figure 6**).

Histopathological examination result:
Invasive ductal carcinoma grade III.

Immunohistochemistry results:
ER: negative
PR: negative
HER2: negative
Ki-67: 50%

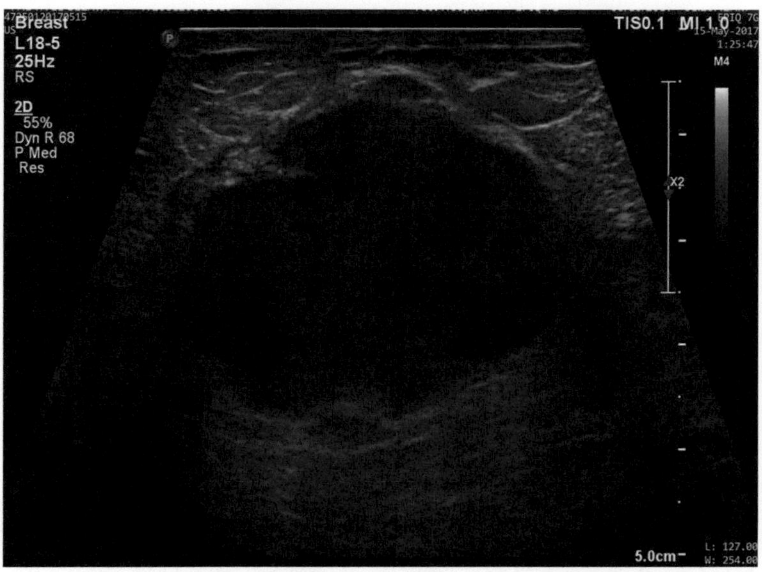

Figure 5.
U/S showed fibroglandular breast with hypoechoic oval shaped lesion with circumscribed margin, measuring 4.3x3.6 cm in its maximum dimensions showing posterior acoustic enhancement with edge attenuation. The lesion is not surrounded by desmoplastic reaction.

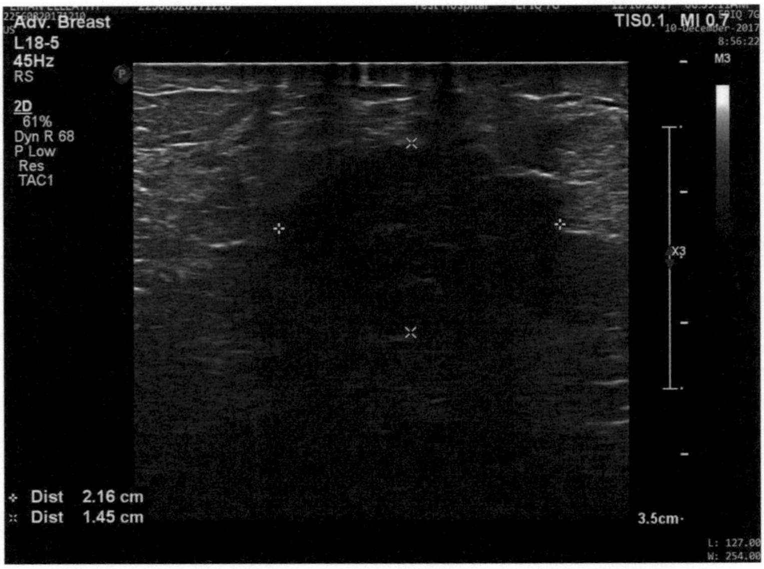

Figure 6.
U/S breast showing hypoechoic oval shaped lesion with circumscribed margin, measuring 2.2x1.5 cm in its maximum dimensions showing mixed posterior acoustic shadowing and enhancement. The lesion is not surrounded by desmoplastic reaction. No associated parenchymal distortion or calcification noted.

4.7 HER2 breast cancer case presentation

52-years-old female patient presented with right breast lump.
Family history: Positive (**Figure 7**).
Histopathological examination result:
Invasive ductal carcinoma grade III.

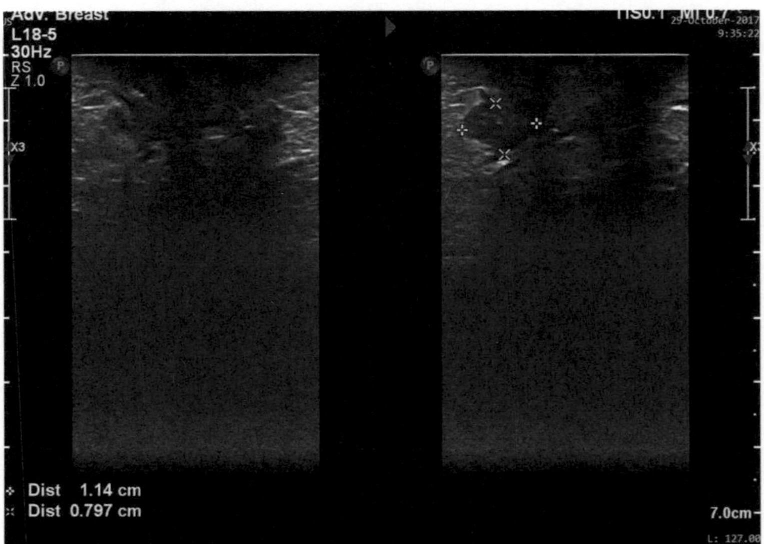

Figure 7.
U/S of breast showing hypoechoic irregular shaped lesion. The lesion was associated with parenchymal distortion and other satellite lesions. The largest measuring 1.2 x 2.1 cm in its maximum dimensions.

Immunohistochemistry revealed:
ER: negative
PR: negative
HER2: positive.

The current study comprised 40 female patients with breast cancer. When analyzing the main four breast cancer subtypes. The present results showed the percentage rates of the subtypes-as: LA 34%. LB 40%, HER2 15%, and TNBC 11%.

The result of the present work showed LB subtype represented 40% and the cases followed by LA subtype 34%. While [6] in their study showed that LA subtype was 37.8°(.o and LB subtype was 36.8%.

The differences between the current work and [6] did not rank to valuable statistical difference.

The mean age of the patients was 50 +/− 10 with a range from 45 to 65:years. Correlation between each subtype.with age and density had been done. The significance of the correlation of subtype of the lesion and density of the breast was related to the age groups.

Since dense fibroglandular breast was associated with younger age group and fatty breast was associated with older age group was described by [7].

In the present study, LA subtype included 14 patients with 8 patients > 50 years and 6 patients <50 years. The result was not consistent with [8] study which had reported that most of LA patients' age was above 50 years.

LB subtype represented 16 patients of the current study with 10 patients> =50 years and 6 patients <50 years. The result was congruent with [8] which showed a higher percentage of the studied LB patients were less than 50 years of age.

HER2 subtype included 15 patients of our study with 6 patients>50 years and 9 patients<50 years. This was consistent with [6]. They found that HER2 breast cancer lesions were significantly associated with advanced age.

TNBC subtype included 4 patients, 3 of them were > 50 years and one patient <50 years. Which indicates that TNBC was more associated with younger age group. The same results had been founded by [6, 9] studies that showed the majority of TNBC lesions were encountered with younger age group.

In the present study, HER2 lesions were more encountered in fatty breast. However the rest of subtypes showed no significant predominance in a certain: breast density. These findings were consistent with [8] findings that showed that HER2 subtype was significantly observed in postmenopausal women; but inconsistent in TNBC subtype. In the present work TNBC showed a strong association with dense fibroglandular breast.

Oval shaped lesions with circumscribed margin were found significantly associated with TNBC lesions (69% of the cases) ($p < 0.001$) and least observed in LA lesions where only 11% of them showed oval circumscribed margin. In contrast–irregular.-shaped lesions were significantly observed in LA subtype (88% of the cases) with a P value < 0.001. In addition 76% of LB cases and 73% of HER2 cases were associated with irregular shape ($P < 0.001$).

Speculated margin was observed in most of LA lesions (76% of the cases), while lobulated margin was more observed in HER2 lesions (66.7%).These findings were congruent with [9–11] findings. They showed tumors with regular shape and circumscribed margins were more often triple negative breast cancer lesions showing hormone negativity while irregular shape and non-circumscribed margins was significantly associated with luminal tumors and hormone receptor positivity.

In the present study posterior shadowing was significantly associated with luminal tumors while posterior enhancement was found to be more observed with TNBC lesions (53%). Mixed enhancement and shadowing were associated with HER2 lesions which was observed in 53.3% of our HER2 cases.

These findings were consistent with [12] had stated that posterior enhancement is an eminent feature characterizing TNBC.

Kin et al. [13] findings were typically consistent with our study regarding the posterior acoustic shadowing feature in luminal subtypes. The current our results were not associated with [14] that showed that HER2 lesions were more associated with posterior enhancement.

Desmoplastic reaction was observed in LA lesions (55.5% of LA cases) with a P value < 0.001. Other subtypes showed no significant correlation with this criterion. Our finding was typically consistent with [6, 9] findings suggesting that desmoplastic reaction could denote slowly growing tumors.

All lesions were found to be more hypoechoic than isoechoic.

Hyperechoic lesions were not found at all in all the examined masses. Hypoechogenieity was significantly associated with TNBC, a result that found to be consistent with the one reported by [13].

Multiplicity of the lesion was more frequently encountered in HER2 subtype lesions and was not significantly observed in other subtype. This _is consistent with [13] that related this finding to the associated intraductal component that is found to be clearly associated with HER2+ receptor.

In the present study calcifications was found to be clearly encountered in ER2, subtyp lesions (,67%) with much less association with other subtype (P = 0.025).

This was found to be in accordance with [15] showing that the expression of HER2 oncogene was strongly correlated with the presence of calcification upon ultrasound. Additionally [12] noticed that the presence of calcification was significantly associated with HER2+ status.

Associated parenchymal distortion was more observed in LA and HER2 subtypes. This was consistent with [15] study that showed that LB subtype was the least associated with architectural distortion. Intraductal extension in HER2 subtype might have a role in architectural distortion as stated by [13].

Tumors larger than 2 cm were frequently associated with HER2+ status. These included HER2 and LB HER2+ subtypes which both together constitute 33% of total number of cases (P = 0.036). Smaller lesions were significantly seen in hormone receptor ER and /or PR positive breast masses. These results were correlated to the findings of [8].

TNBC lesions less than 2 cm were observed in one out of four patients, while the remaining three lesions were more than or equal 2 cm, and these findings were not consistent with [8, 16]. They showed that larger lesions were more associated with TNBC subtype. Invasive ductal carcinoma was the histopathological type the most common of breast cancer in the present study. Invasive lobular breast tumor was encountered in 23% of LA subtype's masses.

5. Conclusion

The sonographic features as margin shape, posterior acoustic features were significantly associated with molecular subtypes. The histopathological grade and hormone receptor status. Being able to predict the molecular subtype. The current study recommend that the radiologist should be aware about different imaging features of different molecular subtypes especially the triple negative breast cancer which had the most benign looking criteria aiming for better lesion characterization and to allow the patient to benefit from earlier non invasive, cheap diagnosis and the curable on time management.

Author details

Eman Soliman Metwally, Rahma Mohammed Abed Alghazal* and Ah Haggaa Ali
Faculty of Medicine, Department of Radiology, Ain Shams University, Egypt

*Address all correspondence to: rahmaalghazal3@gmail.com

References

[1] Irshad A, Leddy R, Pisano E, et al. Assessing the role of ultrasound in predicting the biological behavior of breast cancer. AMR. 2013;**200**:284-290

[2] Sung JS, Stamler S, Brooks J, Kaplan J, Lee CH. Breast cancers detected at screening MR imaging and mammography in patients at high risk: Method of detection reflects tumor histopathological results. Radiology. 2016;**280**(3):716-722

[3] Sood R, Rositch AF, Shakoor D, et al. Ultrasound for breast cancer detection globally: A systemic review and meta analysis. Journal of Global Oncology. 2019;**5**:1-7

[4] Bombonatic A, Sgroi DC. The molecular pathology of breast cancer progression. The Journal of Pathology. 2018;**223**(2):18

[5] Lamiaa M, Rania A. Role of ultrasound in predicting molecular subtypes of invasive breast ductal carcinoma. Egyptian Journal of Radiology and Nuclear Medicine. 2020; **51**:138

[6] Zhang L, Li J, Xiao Y, Cui H, et al. Identifying ultrasound and clinical features of breast Cancer molecular subtypes by ensemble decision. Scientific Reports. 2015;**5**:11085

[7] Willett AM, Michell MJ, Lee MJ Best Practice Diagnostic Guidelines for Patients Presenting with Breast Symptoms, 2010.

[8] Celebi F, Pilanc K, Ordu C, et al. The role of ultrasonographic findings to predict molecular subtype, histologic grade, and hormone receptor status of breast cancer. Diagnostic and lnterventional Radialoy. 2015;**21**:448-453

[9] Fletcher CD. Diagnostic Histopathology of Tumors. Elsevier; 2017

[10] Au-Yong IT, Evans AJ, Taneja S, Rakha EA, Green AR, et al. Sonographic correlations with the new molecular classification of invasive cancer. European Radialogy. 2009;**19**:2342-2348

[11] Larsen MJ, Kruse TA, Tan QH, et al. Classifications within molecular subtypes enables identification of BRCA1/BRCA2 mutation carriers by RNA tumor profiling. PLoS. 2013;**8**: e64268

[12] Whitman GJ, Albarracin CT. Triple negative breast cancer: What the radiologist needs to know. Seminars in Roentgenology. 2018;**46**(1):26-39

[13] Kin J, Yu D, Youngmee K, et al. Genomic characteristics of breast Cancer nominate molecular subtypes that predict chemotherapy response. Molecular Cancer Research. 2020;**19**(3): 1541-1558

[14] Ko ES, Lee BH, Kim HA, Noh WC, Kim MS, Lee SA. Triple-negative breast cancer: Correlation between imaging and pathological findings. European Radialogy. 2015;**20**(5):1111-1117

[15] Kojima Y, Tsunoda H. Mammography and ultrasound features of tripfe-negative breast-cancer. Breast Cancer. 2011;**18**(3):146-151

[16] Evans AJ, Rakha EA, Green AR, Ball G. Ellis I 0: The mammographic correlations of a new immunohistochemical classification of invasive cancer. CLI. 2018;**63**:1228-1223

Chapter 11

A Short Communication: Non-acid Nucleic Blood Multi-Factors Panels for Primary Breast Cancer Detection – A Systematic Review and Network Meta-Analysis

Vahid Raja, Ziba Farajzadegan, Marjan Mansourian, Khojaste Ghasemi, Mohammad Sadegh Aboutalebi, Rasool Nouri and Fariborz Mokarian

Abstract

This study aimed to compare the non-acid nucleic blood multi-factor panels together and with mammography in terms of sensitivity, specificity, and accuracy in primary breast cancer detection (I, II, III, and IV). We systematically reviewed studies assessing non-acid nucleic blood tumor markers panels' diagnostic value in both healthy women and patients (before any anticancer treatment) for the detection of primary breast cancer. Out of the 2358 titles initially identified, 12 studies and 9 panels were included in the network meta-analysis. Panels I (MSA + B2m) and J (GATA3 + E-cadherin) had the highest sensitivity in all stages of primary breast cancer but had no significant difference with mammography. Panels L (MSA + CA15–3) and B (M-CSF- + CA15–3) had the highest specificity in all stages compared to other panels but no remarkable difference with mammography. Panels J (GATA3 + E-cadherin) and I (MSA + B2m) respectively had the highest accuracy in primary breast cancer detection but no considerable difference with mammography in terms of accuracy. Panel J, including GATA3 + E-cadherin, demonstrated a higher diagnostic value for primary breast cancer detection (I, II, III, and IV) than the rest of the panels.

Keywords: primary breast cancer, blood tumor markers, timely diagnosis, sensitivity and specificity, multi-factor panels, network meta-analysis

1. Introduction

Based on our previous study [1], the necessity of a noninvasive, accessible, cost-effective, and reliable method for breast cancer detection based on blood factors was proved. Furthermore, blood multi-factor panels can be the best choice for such a method thanks to improving the sensitivity and specificity of cancer detection considerably compared to the individual state. In that study [1], we had determined the best non-acid nucleic blood multi-factor panels for breast cancer detection in early stages and locoregional breast cancer (I, II, and III). In this brief study, however, we compared the best non-acid nucleic blood multi-factor panels in primary breast cancer detection (I, II, III, and IV) by conducting a network meta-analysis. In fact, this study aimed to offer new insight into the diagnostic value of the best panels of non-acid nucleic blood tumor markers to detect primary breast cancer along all stages not only in early stages. The breast malignancy that emerges and can be diagnosed for the first time is named primary breast cancer, and if it recurs after primary treatment including surgery, chemotherapy, hormone therapy, and radiotherapy individually or collectively, it will be named secondary breast cancer [2]. Primary breast cancer comprises locoregional (I, II, III) and metastatic stages (IV) [3].

2. Materials and method

The systematic reviews of the observational studies were conducted based on PRISMA guidelines (Preferred Reporting Items for Systematic Reviews and Meta-analysis) [4]. Eligibility criteria, search strategy (supplementary material 1 B), databases, study selection, data extraction, and statistical analysis conformed to our former study [1]. The difference is that, in this brief study, we systematically reviewed the studies that have simultaneously assessed several tumor markers in the form of a panel to diagnose and detect breast cancer in all stages of primary breast cancer (I, II, III, and IV).

The included panels were **B**: M-CSF + CA15–3, **C**: VEGF + CA15–3, **D**: VEGF + M-CSF + CA 15–3, **E**: VEGF+ M-CSF, **F**: p16+ c-MYC+ P53, **G**: CA15–3 + CEA, **I**: MSA + B2m, **J**: GATA3 + E-cadherin and **L**: MSA + CA15–3.

All these panels were made based on simultaneous measurement of two or three blood tumor markers in patients and healthy people using a compatible linear combination method [5]. Panels (B, C, D, E, F, G) were assessed in more than one study (multiple studies), and panels (I, J, L) were only assessed in one study (single study). We conducted direct and indirect paired comparisons of the sensitivity, specificity, and accuracy of the included blood tumor markers panels for diagnosing primary breast cancer in all stages. All the investigations were conducted in comparison to mammography (M) as the gold standard [6–8], like our previous study (**Figure 1**) [1].

3. Results and discussion

3.1 Study selection

Study selection conformed to our former study [1]. However, in this brief study, among the 54 studies relevant to our research question which contained 86 unique blood tumor markers panels (supplementary material 2) conforming to our eligibility criteria, only 12 studies and 9 panels presented enough data for estimating sensitivity and specificity in all stages (I, II, III, and IV) of primary breast cancer and could be included in the systematic review and network meta-analysis. These 12 studies were similar in terms of pre-analytical procedures and analytical methods (**Table 1**).

All the included and excluded studies are presented in **Figure 2**.

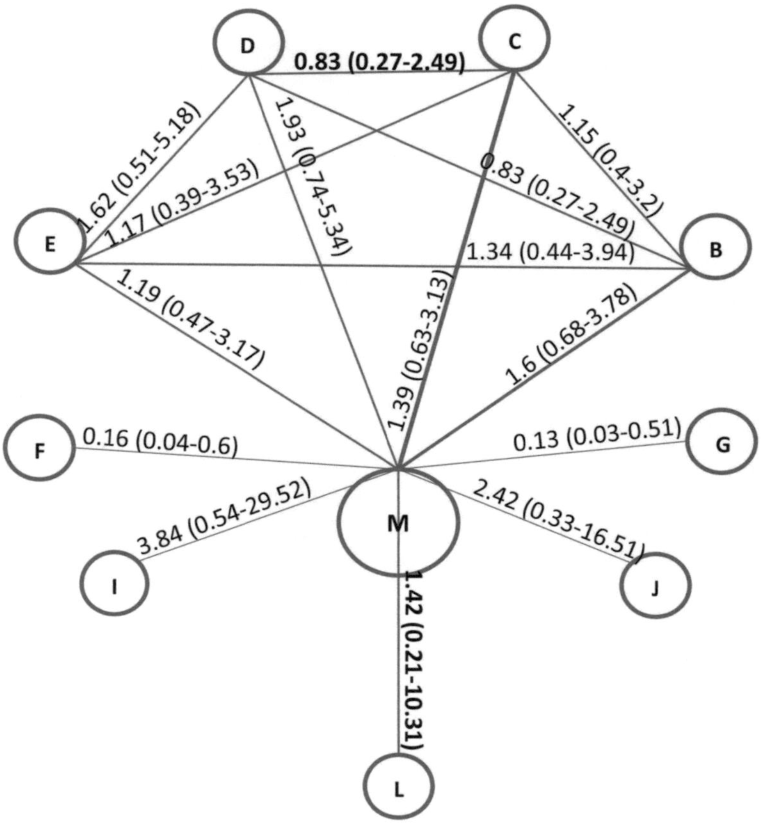

Figure 1.
Multiple comparison of different panels for sensitivity. B: M-CSF + CA15–3, C: VEGF + CA15–3, D: VEGF + M-CSF + CA 15–3, E: VEGF+ M-CSF, F: p16+ c-MYC+ P53, G: CA15–3 + CEA, I: MSA + B2m, J: GATA3 + E-cadherin. L: MSA + CA15–3 M = mammography.

Association between diagnosis of primary breast cancer and blood tumor markers panels:

Panels I (MSA + B2m) and J (GATA3 + E-cadherin) had the highest sensitivity in primary breast cancer but did not have noticeable differences with mammography. Panels G (CA15–3 + CEA) and F (p16+ c-MYC+ P53) had the lowest sensitivity than the rest of the panels and mammography as mammography exhibited a remarkably better function than them, with OR = 0.13 and 95% CL (0.04–0.46) and OR = 0.15 and 95% CL (0.04–0.52) (**Figure 3a**, **Table 2**). In diagnostic tests, sensitivity had a vital role in screening diseases [21]. As a result, we can claim that the panels which had the highest sensitivity can be promising diagnostic tests in primary breast cancer screening, which included panels I and J in all stages of primary breast cancer. Panels L (MSA + CA15–3) and B (M-CSF + CA15–3) had the highest specificity but did not have remarkable differences with mammography. Panels G (CA15–3 + CEA) and D (VEGF + M-CSF + CA 15–3) had the lowest specificity as mammography demonstrated a superior function in specificity, with OR = 0.06 and 95% CL (0.01–0.39) and OR = 0.06 and 95% CL (0.02–0.19) (**Figure 3b**, **Table 3**). Mammography had a better function in specificity than a large number of panels, since it exhibited the highest specificity after panel L with OR = 2.54 and 95% CL (0.1–177.46) in diagnosing

First author and year	Country	Study design	Sample size and population	Clinical stages	Panel	Number of panel components	Sensitivity	Specificity	Accuracy	Method of chemical evaluation	Type of sample	Score
S Zajkowska, M.. 2016 [9]	Poland	Case–control	240 Bc:120 B:60 H:60 Median age (range) 54 (34–72)	I:29 II:30 III:31 IV:30	VEGF + CA 15–3 M-CSF + CA 15–3 VEGF + M-CSF + CA 15–3 VEGF+ M-CSF*	2 2 3 2 VEGF M-CSF CA 15–3	96.25 91.25 96.25 90 76.25 60 83.75	65 67.5 57.5 76 85 90 75	80.6 79.3 76.8 83	ELISA CMIA	plasma	11
Sacks, N. P. 1987 [10]	Australia.	Case–control	131 **Bc:72** **B:13** **H:46**	I/ II:34 III/ IV:38	MSA + CA15–3	2	84	100	89.2	ELISA	serum	11
Liu, Y. 2017 [11]	China	Case–control	248 **Bc102** **H146** **50.88 ± 7.12**	I/ II:57 III/ IV:45	*p16+ c-MYC + TP53	3 p16 c-MYC TP53	30 27.5 11.8 24.5	90 90 90 90	65.3	ELISA	serum	10
Molina, Rafael 1998[12]	Spain	Case–control	292 **Bc186** **B56** **H50**	I/ II:118 III/ IV:68	Ca15.3 + CEA	2 Ca15.3 CEA	29.2 15.6 18.3	90	51.2	ELISA	serum	9.5
Ławicki, Sławomir 2016 [13]	Poland	Case–control	200 **Bc100** **B50** **H50** **48(20–78)**	I/ II/ III:77 IV:23(with metastases)	VEGF +CA15–3	2 VEGF CA 15–3	84 61 65	90 96 96	87	ELISA	plasma	11
Lawicki, S. 2017 [14]	Poland	Case–control	200 **Bc100** **B50** **H50** **48(20–78)**	I/ II/ III:77 IV:23	VEGF+ CA 15–3	2 VEGF CA 15–3	83 60 64	90 95 95	86.5	ELISA	plasma	11.5

DOI: http://dx.doi.org/10.5772/intechopen.108803

First author and year	Country	Study design	Sample size and population	Clinical stages	Panel	Number of panel components	Sensitivity	Specificity	Accuracy	Method of chemical evaluation	Type of sample	Score
Tjandra, JJ 1988 [15]	Australia	Case–control	161 **Bc109** **B31** **H21**	I:32 II:24 III/ IV:53	MSA + B2m	2 MSA B2m	93 88 39	90 95 90	90.3	Radioimmunoassay + ELISA	serum	12
Ławicki, S 2013 [16]	Poland	Case–control	190 **Bc110** **B40** **H40** **44 (30–78)**	I:25 II:35 III:25 IV:25(with metastases)	M-CSF + CA15–3	2 M-CSF CA 15–3	85 60 53	90 95 95	87.1	ELISA	plasma	11
Ławicki, Sławomir 2013 [17]	Poland	Case–control	200 **Bc100** **B50** **H50** **51 (40–70)**	I/ II/ III:75 IV:25(with metastases)	VEGF+ CA 15–3 M-CSF+ CA 15–3 VEGF+ M-CSF VEGF+ M-CSF+ CA 15–3	2 2 2 3 VEGF M-CSF CA 15–3	61 67 63 75 44 53 36	86 86 86 78 92 94 92	73.5 76.5 74.5 76.5	ELISA	plasma	11
Luo, M. 2019 [18]	China	Case–control	200 **Bc120** **H80** **59.88 ± 9.05 (32–70)**	I/ II:47 III/ IV:73	GATA3 + E-cadherin GATA3 E-cadherin	2	90 87.5 82.5	91.7 73.3 87.5	90.6	ELISA	serum	11.5
Looi, Koksun 2006 [19]	China	Case–control	123 **Bc41** **H82** **Multi cancer**		p16 + c-MYC + P53	3	43.9	97.6	79.6	ELISA	serum	8

First author and year	Country	Study design	Sample size and population	Clinical stages	Panel	Number of panel components	Sensitivity	Specificity	Accuracy	Method of chemical evaluation	Type of sample	Score
Guadagni, Fiorella 2001 [20]	Italy	Case–control	2191 **BC 1453 B738 mean age, 57 years (range 25–97 years**	I:392 II:562 III:153 IV:48 Metastatic:240 Local recurrence:58	CEA + CA 15.3	2 CA 15.3 CEA	39 33 16.7	85	54	RIA kit	serum	9.5

B: benign; H: Healthy; ELISA: the enzyme-linked immunosorbent assay; CMIA: luminescent microparticle immunoassay; RIA: radioimmunoassay.
The scoring system based on the CASP checklist (specified for diagnostic studies) was applied to all studies.
The sensitivity, specificity, and accuracy of all studies were evaluated in all stages of primary breast cancer (I, II, III, and IV).
**Based on linear combination (5).*

Table 1.
Characteristics of articled included in network meta-analysis.

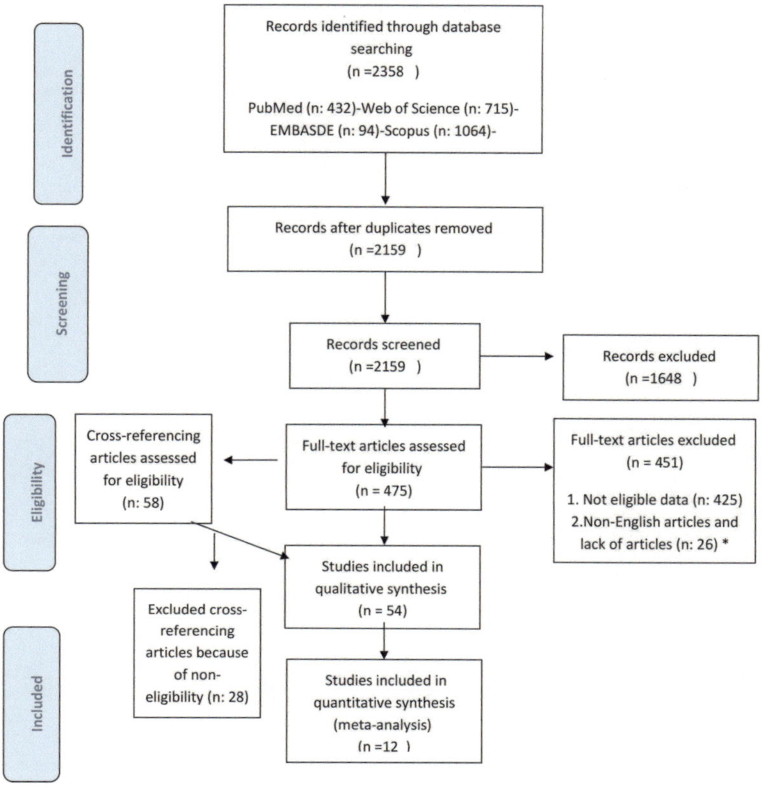

Figure 2.
*Flow diagram of included and excluded articles. *Although we sent emails to articles' authors to get their full texts, we did not receive any answers.*

primary breast cancer. Panels J (GATA3 + E-cadherin) and I (MSA + B2m) possessed the highest accuracy in primary breast cancer but did not show significant differences with mammography. Panel L (MSA + CA15–3) did not demonstrate considerable differences with panel I; therefore, we could consider them approximately similar regarding accuracy. Panels G (CA15–3 + CEA) and F (p16+ c-MYC+ P53) possessed the lowest accuracy in primary breast cancer as mammography exhibited a considerably superior function in accuracy, with OR = 0.15 and 95% CL (0.07–0.3) and OR = 0.37 and 95% CL (0.17–0.74) (**Figure 3c, Table 4**).

The best panels based on total function: **J: GATA3 + E-cadherin, I: MSA + B2m.**

In diagnosing primary breast cancer, panels J and I exhibited the highest accuracy and total function compared to other panels. Overall, we recommend panel J because it had an even better function in accuracy than panel I, despite being minor (**Table 1**) and its study had a larger sample size (200). Panel J was made of GATA3 and E-cadherin. GATA3 is a transcription factor that plays a crucial role in the development and progression of breast cancer and can reverse the epithelial-mesenchymal transition. It also regulates the proliferation, differentiation, and development of cells. E-cadherin is a member of the cadherin family mainly expressed in epithelial cells. E-cadherin mediates the adhesion of allogeneic epithelial cells and plays a key role in epithelial cell aggregation and adhesion. Studies have demonstrated that the expression of cadherin is closely related to the invasion of breast cancer [18].

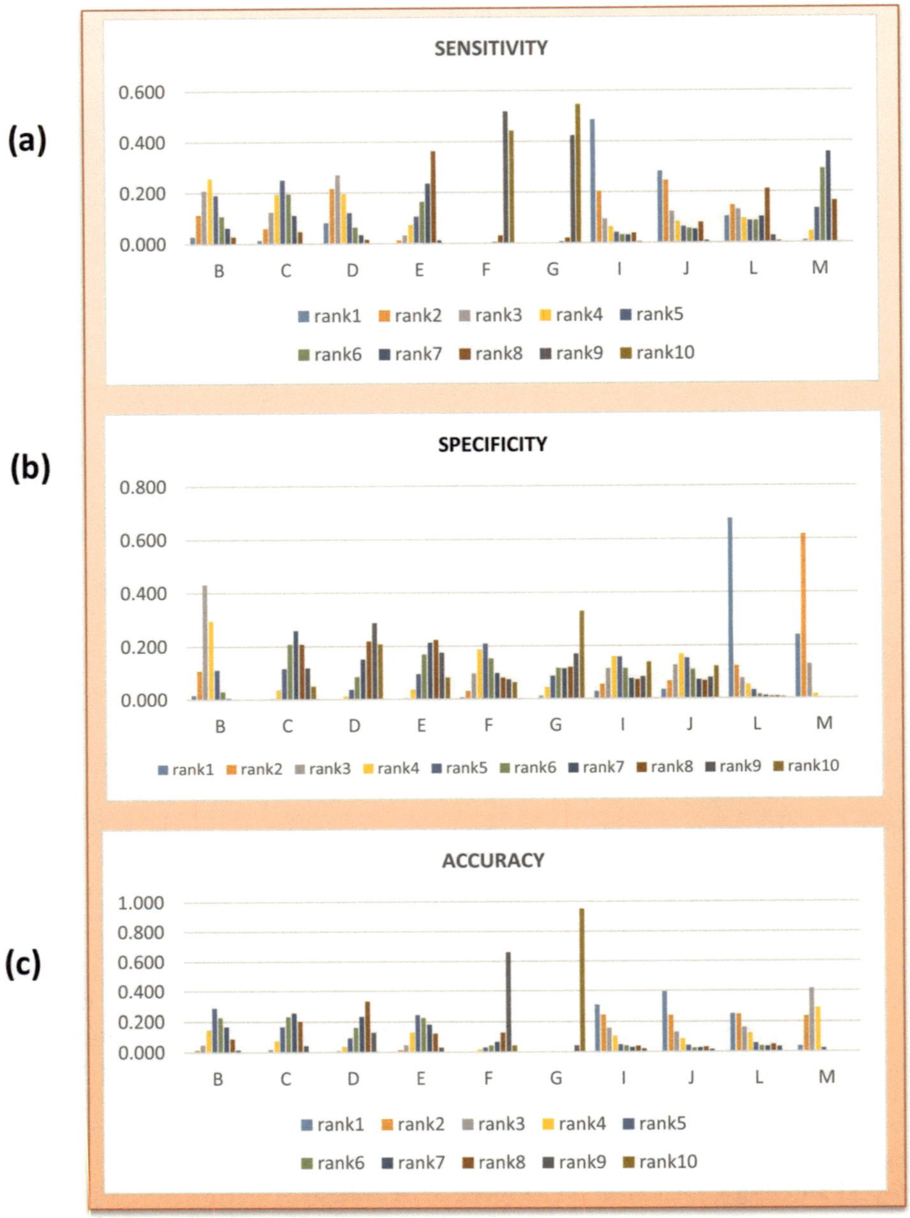

Figure 3.
Estimated rank probability of all panels' sensitivity, specificity, and accuracy. B: M-CSF + CA15–3, C: VEGF + CA15–3, D: VEGF + M-CSF + CA 15–3, E: VEGF+ M-CSF, F: p16+ c-MYC+ P53, G: CA15–3 + CEA, I: MSA + B2m, J: GATA3 + E-cadherin. L: MSA + CA15–3 M = mammography.

4. Conclusion

In conclusion, panel J including GATA3 + E-cadherin with a sensitivity of 90 and specificity of 91.7 demonstrated a higher diagnostic value for primary breast cancer than the rest of the panels as it exhibited higher function in accuracy than mammography, with OR = 1.38 and 95% CL (0.42–4.41), although it was not remarkable. After

DOI: http://dx.doi.org/10.5772/intechopen.108803

	B	C	D	E	F	G	I	J	L	M
B	1									
C	1.18 (0.42–2.96)	1								
D	0.83 (0.28–2.29)	0.71 (0.25–2)	1							
E	1.73 (0.62–4.83)	1.47 (0.56–4.24)	2.09 (0.72–6.32)	1						
F	**10.52 (2.42–46.72)**	**9.01 (2.16–39.41)**	**12.73 (2.85–60.57)**	**6.13 (1.34–27.66)**	1					
G	**11.94 (2.69–56.3)**	**10.21 (2.36–46.39)**	**14.57 (3.07–70.46)**	**6.93 (1.49–32.44)**	1.12 (0.19–6.78)	1				
I	0.44 (0.05–3.44)	0.37 (0.05–2.95)	0.52 (0.06–4.22)	0.25 (0.03–2.01)	**0.04 (0.01–0.4)**	**0.04 (0.01–0.37)**	1			
J	0.64 (0.09–4.78)	0.54 (0.08–4.16)	0.77 (0.1–6.26)	0.37 (0.05–2.95)	**0.06 (0.01–0.57)**	**0.05 (0.01–0.52)**	1.46 (0.11–22.19)	1		
L	1.13 (0.16–7.97)	0.98 (0.14–6.79)	1.37 (0.19–10.07)	0.65 (0.09–4.78)	**0.11 (0.01–1)**	**0.09 (0.01–0.87)**	2.6 (0.18–36.26)	1.79 (0.13–22.86)	1	
M	1.59 (0.69–3.53)	1.35 (0.65–2.94)	1.91 (0.78–4.88)	0.91 (0.38–2.26)	**0.15 (0.04–0.52)**	**0.13 (0.04–0.46)**	3.63 (0.55–25.11)	2.47 (0.37–15.96)	1.4 (0.24–8.3)	1

B: M-CSF + CA15–3, C: VEGF + CA15–3, D: VEGF + M-CSF + CA 15–3, E: VEGF+ M-CSF, F: p16+ c-MYC+ P53, G: CA15–3 + CEA, I: MSA + B2m, J: GATA3 + E-cadherin L: MSA + CA15–3 M = Mammography.

Table 2.
Relative effects and its 95% credible interval of all pairwise panels for sensitivity based on Bayesian network meta-analysis method.

	B	C	D	E	F	G	I	J	L	M
B	1									
C	**4.75 (1.41–16.11)**	1								
D	**6.86 (1.97–25.88)**	1.46 (0.42–5.27)	1							
E	**5.19 (1.42–18.95)**	1.08 (0.31–3.99)	0.75 (0.2–2.74)	1						
F	2.8 (0.33–24.19)	0.58 (0.07–4.87)	0.4 (0.04–3.57)	0.53 (0.06–4.86)	1					

	B	C	D	E	F	G	I	J	L	M
G	6.82 (0.76–63.76)	1.43 (0.16–12.82)	1 (0.11–9.29)	1.33 (0.14–12.7)	2.62 (0.17–35.24)	1				
I	2.74 (0.16–61.57)	0.57 (0.03–12.81)	0.39 (0.02–8.77)	0.53 (0.03–12.6)	1 (0.04–30.25)	0.39 (0.02–13.06)	1			
J	2.4 (0.14–48.49)	0.51 (0.03–9.19)	0.34 (0.02–6.66)	0.46 (0.03–9.64)	0.85 (0.03–22.94)	0.34 (0.01–9.86)	0.87 (0.02–42.75)	1		
L	0.16 (0.01–4.92)	0.03 (0.01–1.04)	**0.02 (0.01–0.72)**	**0.03 (0.01–0.89)**	0.06 (0.01–2.68)	**0.02 (0.01–0.96)**	0.06 (0.01–3.68)	0.07 (0.01–4.26)	1	
M	0.42 (0.14–1.2)	**0.09 (0.03–0.24)**	**0.06 (0.02–0.19)**	**0.08 (0.02–0.25)**	**0.15 (0.02–0.96)**	**0.06 (0.01–0.39)**	0.16 (0.01–2.05)	0.18 (0.01–2.3)	2.54 (0.1–177.46)	1

B: M-CSF + CA15–3, C: VEGF + CA15–3, D: VEGF + M-CSF + CA 15–3, E: VEGF+ M-CSF, F: p16+ c-MYC+ P53, G: CA15–3 + CEA, I: MSA + B2m, J: GATA3 + E-cadherin L: MSA + CA15–3 M = Mammography.

Table 3.
Relative effects and its 95% credible interval of all pairwise panels for specificity based on Bayesian network meta-analysis method.

	B	C	D	E	F	G	I	J	L	M
B	1									
C	1.11 (0.65–1.9)	1								
D	1.24 (0.7–2.18)	1.11 (0.65–1.97)	1							
E	1.03 (0.59–1.81)	0.92 (0.54–1.64)	0.83 (0.46–1.46)	1						
F	1.8 (0.77–4.42)	1.61 (0.7–4)	1.45 (0.61–3.77)	1.78 (0.73–4.23)	1					
G	**4.42 (1.92–10.23)**	**3.98 (1.74–9.25)**	**3.58 (1.44–8.49)**	**4.32 (1.79–10.29)**	2.45 (0.85–6.76)	1				
I	0.54 (0.15–1.81)	0.48 (0.14–1.62)	0.44 (0.12–1.48)	0.53 (0.15–1.84)	0.3 (0.07–1.15)	**0.12 (0.03–0.47)**	1			
J	0.48 (0.13–1.74)	0.43 (0.12–1.55)	0.39 (0.1–1.43)	0.46 (0.13–1.84)	0.26 (0.06–1.1)	**0.11 (0.03–0.43)**	0.91 (0.17–4.57)	1		
L	0.58 (0.17–2.09)	0.52 (0.16–1.92)	0.47 (0.13–1.71)	0.57 (0.16–2.1)	0.32 (0.08–1.35)	**0.13 (0.03–0.51)**	1.09 (0.22–5.35)	1.22 (0.25–6.06)	1	

	B	C	D	E	F	G	I	J	L	M
M	0.66 (0.42–1.05)	**0.59 (0.39–0.92)**	**0.53 (0.32–0.87)**	0.64 (0.38–1.06)	**0.37 (0.17–0.74)**	**0.15 (0.07–0.3)**	1.22 (0.4–3.84)	1.38 (0.42–4.41)	1.1 (0.34–3.45)	1

B: M-CSF + CA15–3, C: VEGF + CA15–3, D: VEGF + M-CSF + CA 15–3, E: VEGF+ M-CSF, F: p16+ c-MYC+ P53, G: CA15–3 + CEA, I: MSA + B2m, J: GATA3 + E-cadherin L: MSA + CA15–3 M = Mammography.

Table 4.
Relative effects and its 95% credible interval of all pairwise panels for accuracy based on Bayesian network meta-analysis method.

panel J, panel I (MSA + B2m) with a sensitivity of 90 and specificity of 90.3 and panel L (MSA + CA15–3) with a sensitivity of 84 and specificity of 100 had the best function in primary breast cancer detection than the rest of the panels. However, more experimental studies are required with larger samples, on different populations, and using other chemical measurement methods to verify these results.

Acknowledgements

This study was supported by Research Institute and Cancer Prevention Research Center, Isfahan University of Medical Sciences.

Author contributions

Vahid Raja had the idea for the research. The literature search was performed by Vahid Raja, Mohammad Sadegh Aboutalebi, and Rasool Nouri. The data analysis was performed by Marjan Mansourian and Khojaste Ghasemi. The article was drafted by Vahid Raja and Ziba Farajzadegan. The article was critically revised by Vahid Raja, Ziba Farajzadegan, and Fariborz Mokarian.

Conflict of interest

Not applicable.

Data availability

The data used to support the findings of this study are available from the corresponding author upon request.

Ethical statement

Our study did not require an ethical board approval because it did not contain human or animal trials.

Supplementary material

Including traditional meta-analysis of all panels, nod-splitting analysis of inconsistency for sensitivity, specificity and accuracy, ranking of different panels in sensitivity, specificity and accuracy, the search strategy for each data base, and 54 studies were identified relevant to our research question.

Author details

Vahid Raja[1*], Ziba Farajzadegan[2*], Marjan Mansourian[3], Khojaste Ghasemi[3], Mohammad Sadegh Aboutalebi[4], Rasool Nouri[5] and Fariborz Mokarian[6]

1 Clinical Laboratory Sciences, Amin Hospital, Isfahan University of Medical Sciences, Isfahan, Iran

2 Community and Preventive Medicine, Isfahan University of Medical Sciences, Isfahan, Iran

3 Department of Biostatistics and Epidemiology, School of Public Health, Isfahan University of Medical Sciences, Isfahan, Iran

4 Faculty of Nursing and Midwifery, Isfahan University of Medical Sciences, Isfahan, Iran

5 Department of Medical Library and Information Sciences, Isfahan University of Medical Sciences, Isfahan, Iran

6 Hematology and Oncology Department of Internal Medicine, Isfahan University of Medical Sciences, Isfahan, Iran

*Address all correspondence to: www.mahantajhizs@gmail.com
and farajzadegan@med.mui.ac.ir

References

[1] Raja V, Farajzadegan Z, Mansourian M, Ghasemi K, Aboutalebi MS, Nouri R, et al. Diagnostic value of nonacid nucleic blood tumor marker panels in early diagnosing breast cancer: A systematic review and network meta-analysis. Disease Markers. 2022;**2022**:15

[2] Sadler C, Goldfarb M. Comparison of primary and secondary breast cancers in adolescents and young adults. Cancer. 2015;**121**(8):1295-1302

[3] Zackrisson S, Cardoso F, Guidelines E. Clinical practice guidelines primary breast cancer: ESMO clinical practice Guidelines for diagnosis, treatment and follow-up† clinical practice guidelines. Annals of Oncology. 2015;**26**(5):8-30

[4] Moher D, Liberati A, Tetzlaff J, Altman DG, Group* P. Preferred reporting items for systematic reviews and meta-analyses: The PRISMA statement. Annals of internal medicine. 2009;**151**(4):264-269

[5] Pepe MS, Thompson ML. Combining diagnostic test results to increase accuracy. Biostatistics. 2000;**1**(2): 123-140

[6] Yankaskas BC, Haneuse S, Kapp JM, Kerlikowske K, Geller B, Buist DS, et al. Performance of first mammography examination in women younger than 40 years. JNCI: Journal of the National Cancer Institute. 2010;**102**(10):692-701

[7] Sinclair N, Littenberg B, Geller B, Muss H. Accuracy of screening mammography in older women. American Journal of Roentgenology. 2011;**197**(5):1268-1273

[8] Ontario HQ. Screening mammography for women aged 40 to 49 years at average risk for breast cancer: An evidence-based analysis. Ont Health Technol Assess Ser. 2007;**7**(1):1-32

[9] Zajkowska M, Głażewska EK, Będkowska GE, Chorąży P, Szmitkowski M, Ławicki S. Diagnostic power of vascular endothelial growth factor and macrophage colony-stimulating factor in breast cancer patients based on ROC analysis. Mediators of Inflammation. 2016;**2016**:8

[10] Sacks N, Stacker S, Thompson C, Collins J, Russell I, Sullivan J, et al. Comparison of mammary serum antigen (MSA) and CA15-3 levels in the serum of patients with breast cancer. British journal of cancer. 1987;**56**(6):820-824

[11] Liu Y, Liao Y, Xiang L, Jiang K, Li S, Huangfu M, et al. A panel of autoantibodies as potential early diagnostic serum biomarkers in patients with breast cancer. International Journal of Clinical Oncology. 2017;**22**(2):291-296

[12] Molina R, Jo J, Filella X, Zanon G, Pahisa J, Muñoz M, et al. c-erbB-2 oncoprotein, CEA, and CA 15.3 in patients with breast cancer: Prognostic value. Breast cancer research and treatment. 1998;**51**(2):109-119

[13] Ławicki S, Zajkowska M, Głażewska EK, Będkowska GE, Szmitkowski M. Plasma levels and diagnostic utility of VEGF, MMP-9, and TIMP-1 in the diagnosis of patients with breast cancer. Onco Targets and therapy. 2016;**9**:911

[14] Ławicki S, Zajkowska M, Głażewska EK, Będkowska GE, Szmitkowski M. Plasma levels and diagnostic utility of VEGF, MMP-2 and TIMP-2 in the diagnostics of breast cancer patients. Biomarkers. 2017;**22**(2): 157-164

[15] Tjandra J, McLaughlin P, Russell I, Collins J, McKenzie I. Comparison of mammary serum antigen (MSA) with β2-microglobulin (β2M) and carcinoembryonic antigen (CEA) assays in patients with breast cancer. European Journal of Cancer and Clinical Oncology. 1988;**24**(10):1633-1640

[16] Ławicki S, Będkowska G, Wojtukiewicz M, Szmitkowski M. Hematopoietic cytokines as tumor markers in breast malignancies. A multivariate analysis with ROC curve in breast cancer patients. Advances in Medical Sciences. 2013;**58**(2):207-215

[17] Ławicki S, Będkowska GE, Szmitkowski M. VEGF, M-CSF and CA 15-3 as a new tumor marker panel in breast malignancies: A multivariate analysis with ROC curve. Growth Factors. 2013;**31**(3):98-105

[18] Luo M, Huang Y, Huang J, Huang S, Wei L, Zhang Y, et al. Evaluation of the value of GATA3 combined with E-cadherin in the diagnosis of breast cancer. Journal of BU ON: Official Journal of the Balkan Union of Oncology. 2019;**24**(3):1038-1044

[19] Looi K, Megliorino R, Shi F-D, Peng X-X, Chen Y, Zhang J-Y. Humoral immune response to p16, a cyclin-dependent kinase inhibitor in human malignancies. Oncology Reports. 2006; **16**(5):1105-1110

[20] Guadagni F, Ferroni P, Carlini S, Mariotti S, Spila A, Aloe S, et al. A re-evaluation of carcinoembryonic antigen (CEA) as a serum marker for breast cancer: A prospective longitudinal study. Clinical Cancer Research. 2001; **7**(8):2357-2362

[21] Stellman SD. Book review: Epidemiology. In: Gordis L, editor. Gordis Epidemiology, 6th ed. Philadelphia, PA, US: Saunders; 2009. p. 2010. ISBN: 978-0-323-55229-5. Copyright © 2019 by Elsevier, Inc. All rights reserved

Chapter 12

Membrane-Bound Complement Regulatory Proteins in Breast Cancer: Are They Best Therapeutic Targets?

Sofia Álvarez-Lorenzo, Rebeca Elizabeth Montalvo-Castro, Jeannie Jiménez-López, María Adriana Medina-Mondragón and Nohemí Salinas-Jazmín

Abstract

Breast cancer is one of the most aggressive diseases in women, responsible for thousands of deaths annually and millions of new diagnoses; its treatment presents multiple obstacles due to late diagnosis and the various mechanisms of tumor resistance. In breast cancer the membrane-bound complement regulatory proteins (mCRP) have been proposed as biomarkers of malignant cellular transformation. These are molecules capable of inhibiting therapeutic efficacy, from both antibodies and cytotoxic drugs. Therefore, these proteins are potential targets to increase therapeutic efficacy and avoid cancer progression. We will gather information about mCRP: (i) structural features; (ii) expression levels in breast cancer and relationship with prognosis; (iii) therapeutic resistance mechanisms; and (iv) strategies to down-regulate mCRP in both activity and expression.

Keywords: breast cancer, mCRP, therapeutic resistance, therapeutic mAb, systemic treatments

1. Introduction

Cancer is one of the most fatal diseases in the world, and breast cancer is the most incidence and mortality in women [1]. Breast cancer is a highly heterogeneous disease with morphological features and variable clinical outcomes. The clinical course, prognosis, and responsiveness to breast cancer treatment depend on their specific biological characteristics or classification. The immunohistochemical classification is based on hormone receptor (HR) expression (estrogen receptor [ER] and progesterone receptor [PGR]) and amplification of the human epidermal growth factor receptor ERBB2/HER2-: the HR-positive (luminal A or B), the HER2-positive and triple-negative (TNBC) subtypes [2, 3].

Overall, the systemic therapy administered consists of endocrine therapy for all HR+ tumors, immunotherapy plus chemotherapy for all HER2-positive tumors, and cytotoxic chemotherapy plus immunotherapy for TNBC [4–7]. It has been reported that long exposure to therapeutic agents may generate an adaptive cellular response that results in the induction of acquired drug resistance. So, the use of combination chemotherapy potentially provides advantages such as chances for increasing or maintaining efficacy and reduced or delayed development of drug resistance [8].

However, there are many factors involved in the failure of treatment, such as the expression of complement regulatory proteins (mCRP). These proteins have been reported to be up-regulated in several cancer cells and tumor tissues, as a mechanism to evade elimination by the complement system [9–11].

High expression of mCRP by cancer cells confers resistance against antitumoral therapies by controlling the activation of the complement cascade and regulation of intracellular complement signaling in cancer cells [11–15].

Herein, we summarize evidence related to mCRP tumoral activity in cancer cells and discuss the implications of its biological actions in anticancer therapy. Therefore, we will gather information about mCRP: (i) structural features; (ii) expression levels in breast cancer and relationship with prognosis; (iii) therapeutic resistance mechanisms; and (iv) several strategies to down-regulate mCRP in both activity and expression.

2. The complement system and breast cancer

2.1 Breast cancer treatment

Breast cancer is the most frequently diagnosed cancer in women comprising 24.2% of total cancers, and is the leading cause of cancer mortality in women worldwide (15.5%), constituting a complex public health problem [16]. On the molecular level, breast cancer is a heterogeneous disease, and it has been classified according to gene expression patterns and the presence of specific molecular markers in tumors. The main molecular markers considered are the estrogen receptor (ER), progesterone receptor (PR), and the human epidermal growth factor receptor 2 (ERBB/HER2) because of their relevance in cancer pathogenesis and their prognostic value in treatment response. In clinical practice, the detection of these markers by immunohistochemistry (IHC) allows tumor classification. Tumors expressing ER and PR are considered hormone receptor-positive; those that exhibit HER2 amplification or overexpression are HER2-positive, and tumors lacking expression of ER, PR or HER2 are triple-negative [2, 4, 17].

Systemic therapy for breast cancer is determined by subtype; patients with HR-positive tumors receive endocrine therapy, and a minority also receive chemotherapy. Patients with HER2-positive tumors receive HER2-targeted monoclonal antibody (mAb) or small-molecule inhibitor therapy combined with chemotherapy, and patients with triple-negative tumors usually receive chemotherapy [4, 5]. Several antibody-based treatments targeting tumor antigens and tumor-promoting signaling pathways have been shown to rely on complement system activation for mAb-induced cytotoxicity, including the HER2-specific mAbs trastuzumab and pertuzumab (IgG1 isotype). Their Fc regions interact with the complement component C1q, inducing activation of the classical complement pathway. Moreover, the Fc regions can also interact with FcγRs of natural killer cells, macrophages, and neutrophils to induce antibody-dependent cellular cytotoxicity (ADCC). Phagocytosis of tumor cells by phagocytes is also enhanced by complement fragments such as C3b, in a mechanism referred to as complement-dependent cell-mediated cytotoxicity (CDCC) [10]. Not only trastuzumab and pertuzumab but also other mAbs such as sacituzumab-govitecan, an anti-Trop-2 IgG1 antibody used for the treatment of triple-negative breast cancer, follow these mechanisms of action [7].

Despite their efficacy, intrinsic or acquired resistance to mAbs-based treatments occurs frequently. For example, about 70% of HER2-positive breast cancer may have intrinsic resistance to trastuzumab, and most of those who respond to this treatment tend to develop acquired resistance within 1 or 2 years [18]. Several mechanisms may lead to antibody resistance, e.g. down-regulation of the target epitope, diminished ADCC or opsonization, or resistance to complement-mediated lytic attack. There is ample evidence that complement resistance of tumor cells is a widespread phenomenon, and therefore strategies to overcome this problem are needed [19].

2.2 The complement system

The complement system is part of the innate immune response, and it represents one of the first lines of defense against pathogens. However, it also plays crucial roles in maintaining homeostasis through mechanisms such as the removal of apoptotic cells, the regulation of coagulation, angiogenesis, lipid metabolism, and importantly, the surveillance of cancer cells [9]. Complement functions through a series of over 30 coordinated cascading proteins and zymogens to induce cellular lysis, opsonize pathogens, induce inflammation and interact with cells of adaptive immunity [20].

Depending on the activator, complement can be triggered by three different pathways: classical, lectin, and alternative (**Figure 1**).

- The classical pathway is activated by the binding of C1q, in complex with C1r and C1s serine proteases, to the Fc region of immunoglobulins (IgG or IgM) complexed with antigen. The binding of C1q to a ligand results in a conformational change leading to the sequential activation of C1r and C1s. Activated C1s cleaves C4 into C4a and C4b, and C2 into C2a and C2b. Subunits C4b and C2a form C4bC2a, a C3 convertase enzyme complex able to cleave C3.

- The lectin pathway is analogous to the classical one, but its activation is triggered by mannose-binding lectins (MBLs), collectins or ficolins that bind to carbohydrate ligands such as mannose, and together with MBL-associated serine proteases (MASP1,2) form a C1-like complex, leading to the formation of a C3 convertase.

- Activation of the alternative pathway occurs through spontaneous hydrolysis of C3 to C3(H20), often referred to as "tick-over mechanism" that leads to a constitutive low level of complement activation. C3(H20) binds to factor B (FB), which is then cleaved by Factor D, and the Bb fragment forms the C3(H20) Bb complex. This fluid phase complex cleaves plasma C3, resulting in C3b, which binds to cell surfaces and Bb, generating C3Bb, the C3 convertase of the alternative pathway.

In all pathways, the C3 convertase generates a C5 convertase by binding to C3b molecules. Then, C5 convertase cleaves C5 to create C5b which binds with C6, C7, C8, and multiple C9 to form the C5b-9 complex or membrane attack complex (MAC) which functions as a pore in the cell membrane that leads to cellular lysis [9, 19–21].

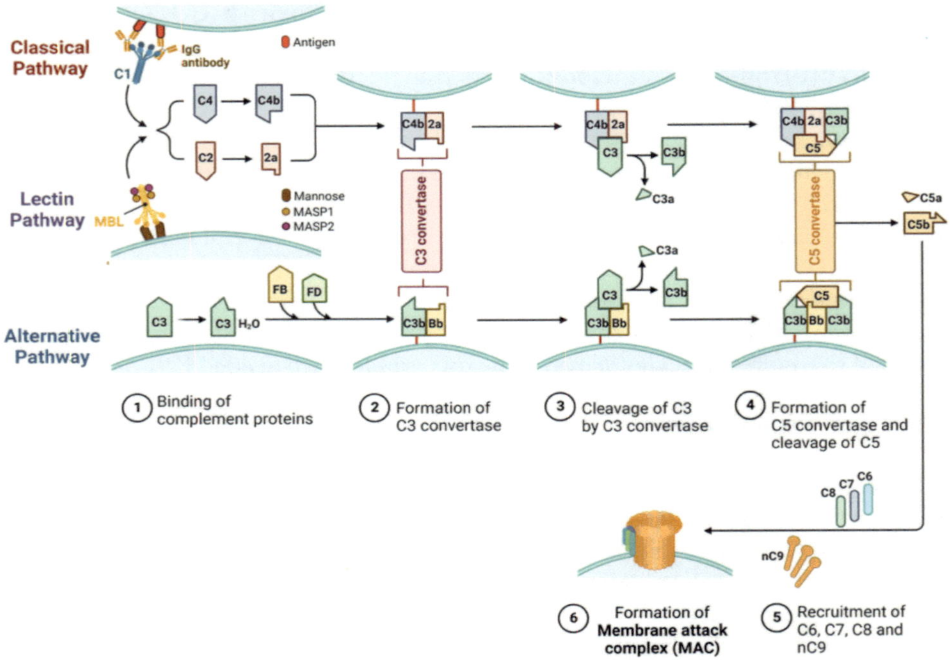

Figure 1.
The complement system activation pathways. Depending on the context, complement system can be initiated by three distinct pathways: classical, lectin, and alternative, each leading to lead to the formation of C3 and C5 convertases and the common terminal pathway, in which the formation of the membrane attack complex (MAC) leads to cellular lysis. Created with Biorender.

While inducing cell lysis through MAC is an important effector arm, the complement system can also trigger pro-inflammatory signaling and phagocytic functions that are equally important. C3a and C5a function as anaphylatoxins and are constantly released during complement activation. These molecules recruit and induce activation of immune cells expressing anaphylatoxin receptors (C3aR, C5aR1, C5aR2) such as neutrophils, monocytes, eosinophils, mast cells, and macrophages. Furthermore, C3b and C4b function as opsonins that aid in phagocytosis by binding to the target cells surface, allowing the elimination of pathogens and stressed cells [9, 21].

2.3 Complement activation by tumor cells

It has been recognized that cancer cells acquire several genetic and epigenetic abnormalities that induce the expression of tumor-associated antigens, which may target tumor cells for recognition by complement proteins. The classical pathway has been found to be activated by the recognition of post-transcriptionally modified tumor-specific antigens by natural antibodies. Natural antibodies are predominantly IgM isotype and are produced without prior antigenic stimulation against a variety of self and foreign antigens. Furthermore, IgM antibodies can effectively activate the classical complement pathway because, unlike IgG, a single molecule of IgM can bind to C1q and initiate the proteolytic cascade [9, 22]. However, the activation of the classical pathway through IgG antibodies in breast cancer is not excluded, as is the case with therapeutic antibodies [5, 12]. The presence of IgG, C3, and C4 together with deposits of C5b-9 complexes on tumor cell membranes, were observed in samples from breast cancer patients, indicating a persistent *in situ* complement activation [23]. In addition, altered glycosylation patterns reported in breast cancer cells, such as an increased expression of α2,3-sialic acid and α-L-fucose [24], are likely to induce activation of the complement via the lectin pathway.

Although complement activation may favor the elimination of tumor cells, the role of this system appears to be more complex in the context of the tumor microenvironment (TME). Recent studies demonstrate that the impact of complement in cancer is diverse, ranging from anti-tumor defense by killing antibody-coated tumor cells, to potent tumor promotion by supporting local chronic inflammation or interfering with anti-tumor T-cell responses. Indeed, complement molecules C3, C3a, and C5a are reported to play an important role in cancer progression. For example, in mice models of breast cancer, C3 expressed by CD8+ T cells inhibits their antitumor activity through an autocrine mechanism [25], whereas C5a/C5aR signaling promotes metastasis by the recruitment of myeloid-derived suppressor cells (MDSC) in premetastatic sites, causing suppression of effector CD8+ and CD4+ T cell responses [26]. In contrast, other complement components act as tumor-inhibiting factors. For example, C1q deficient mice exhibit accelerated tumor growth and an increased number of lung metastases, which are not directly related to absence of complement activation, but to the induction of angiogenesis and an increase in HER2 expression [27]. Taken together, studies suggest that opposing effects of complement in cancer are dependent upon the sites of activation, the composition of the TME, and the tumor cell sensitivity to complement attack [28].

3. Characterization of the mCRPs: structure, localization, and function

Complement activation must be a tightly coordinated orchestra through any of its pathways to avoid damage to its tissues. Multiple negative regulators are known as complement regulatory proteins (CRP); their function is to maintain homeostasis in the system. Among them, we can mention two main groups: (i) soluble complement regulatory proteins (sCRP), such as C1 inhibitor, C4b binding protein, and factors H, B, D, and I; and (ii) membrane-bound complement regulatory proteins (mCRP), which include CD35, CD46, CD55, and CD59 [9]. Mostly CD46, CD55, and CD59 have received more attention since they are overexpressed in tumor tissues, and their complement inhibitory functions have been proposed as resistance strategies applied by cancer cells [9, 11, 29, 30].

3.1 CD46

Membrane cofactor protein (MCP) known as CD46 is a type 1 transmembrane glycoprotein, with a molecular weight that varies between 48 and 68 kDa. Was discovered on peripheral blood cells in 1986 during a search for novel C3b-binding proteins [31] and renamed as "membrane cofactor protein" due to the growing structure/function information in 1991 [32]. This protein has a structural heterogeneity, partly explained by the expression of multiple cDNA/protein isoforms that arise by alternative splicing of serine/threonine/proline-rich exons (sites of heavy O-glycosylation) and cytoplasmic tails (**Figure 2**) [33]. CD46 is expressed in all nucleated cells, thus only erythrocytes lack CD46 expression [34]. The gene for this protein is encoded on chromosome 1q32.2 and its transcription depends on binding the activated transcription factor STAT3 to its promoter [35].

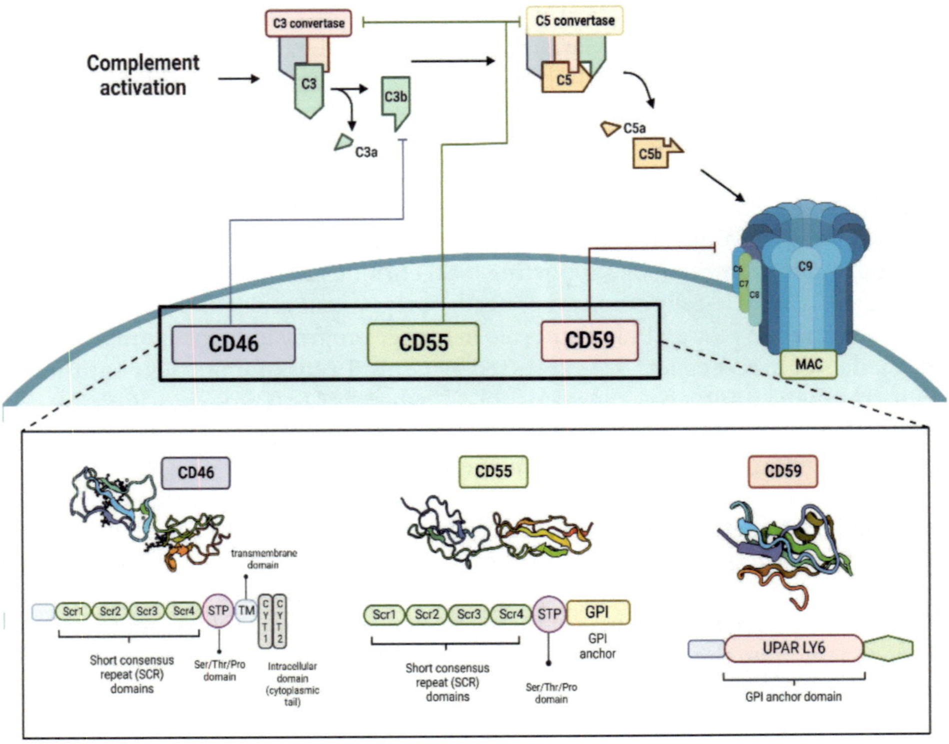

Figure 2.
Membrane-bound complement regulatory proteins: structure and function in the complement system inhibition. Created with Biorender.

CD46, belongs to the family of regulators of complement activation (RCA), elucidated since 1985. Its structure is common to all proteins expressed from the RCA family; it is mainly based on four short consensus repeat (SCR) domains that make up most of the extracellular region, the SCR repeats are connected to a hooking region rich in serine, threonine, and proline (STP region), a single membrane-spanning segment (transmembrane domain), and a cytoplasmic tail divided into two domains, identified as CYT1 and CYT2 [32, 36, 37]. CD46 inhibits the formation of complement C5 convertase by promoting the degradation of C3b and C4b by proteolytic cleavage [38, 39]. Biochemical mapping studies strongly implicate the SCR2, SCR3, and SCR4 domains in the interaction of this protein with complement cascade proteins (**Figure 2**) [40, 41].

CD46 can be proteolytically modified on cell membranes and released by a metalloproteinase from cancer cells as vesicles with a diameter of 200 nm. Both vesicular and soluble forms of CD46 are functional and promote C3b cleavage by factor I [42].

3.2 CD55

CD55, also known as Decay-accelerating factor (DAF), was first discovered in 1969 on the cell surface of an erythrocyte. It is a glycophosphatidylinositol (GPI)-anchored cell surface glycoprotein with a molecular weight that varies from between 50 and 100 kDa depending on cell type [43]. DAF is present in most cell types; its gene is encoded on chromosome 1q32.2 located adjacent to the genes comprising the RCA gene family, which includes as well CD46. Its expression is primarily modulated at the transcriptional level by a cAMP response element on its promoter and by the Sp1 transcription factor. The most abundant variant generated by alternative splicing is found in the membrane [44].

The main function of CD55 is to protect cells from autologous complement attacks. Its role as a complement regulator is accelerating the dissociation and disintegration of C3 convertase and preventing the formation of C5 convertase, avoiding cell damage due to the subsequent formation of the MAC [45, 46]. Mature CD55 has three domains: (i) consensus repeat domains consist of four short consensus repeat (SCR) domains e.g. SCR-1, SCR-2, SCR-3, and SCR-4; (ii) O-linked carbohydrate domain having a serine/threonine/proline-rich region, and (iii) GPI anchor [47]. The final GPI-anchored domain of CD55 binds the protein to the membrane's outer leaflet at dynamic structures composed of sphingolipid and cholesterol, called lipid raft microdomains (**Figure 2**). This segment is composed of about 30 amino acids cleaved post-translationally at the C-terminal signal peptide located at Ser352 during processing at the endoplasmic reticulum (ER) and its later modification in the Golgi apparatus before transporting to the cell membrane [48].

Has been reported that cell-surface CD55 is a ligand for CD97, a member of the epidermal growth factor seven-span transmembrane (EGF-7TM) receptor family; the binding of CD55 to CD97 can protect several cell types from complement-mediated damage, thus playing an important role in host defense and inflammation [43, 49]. Furthermore, CD55 can stimulate CD97 signaling and modulate cancer metastasis, as a mechanism dependent on the upregulation of MMP2 and MMP9 [50].

The CD55 signaling can be activated by growth factors, cytokines, and augment prostaglandins [43]. In Hep3B hepatoma cells, the exposition of cytokines such as TNF-α, IL-6, and IL-1β increased the expression of CD55 (three-fold) and CD59 (two-fold) and decreased the expression of CD46, demonstrating the relevance function of TME and inflammatory cytokines on the expression of mCRP [51]. Another example of the fine regulation of CD55 expression in HT-29 colon cancer cells depends on the activation via p42/44 MAPK pathway by the epidermal growth factor (EGF) [52].

3.3 CD59

CD59 or membrane attack complex inhibitor (MAC-i), is a glycoprotein of 20 kDa encoded on chromosome 11p13, expressed in most cells. It belongs to a protein superfamily characterized by the expression of a Ly-6/uPAR domain (**Figure 2**), which allows it to interact with complement proteins [53, 54]. This protein was first described in 1986 and multiple groups worked on its characterization; in 1988 was identified in human lymphoid cells and designed as a "membrane attack complex inhibiting protein" [45, 55]. Their role in the regulation of the complement system consists in inhibiting cell lysis by binding to the α chain of C8 and the β domain of C9 to prevent MAC formation in the membrane of cells, including cancer cells [56].

CD59 has three folded β sheets and one α helix; it has a cysteine-rich Ly6/uPAR three-finger domain, a characteristic pattern of disulfide bonds, and a unique group of amino acids susceptible to N- and O-glycosylation (Leu1-Asn77) that constitute the core of the molecule. It has been proposed that these glycosylations may influence its membrane distribution, limiting the spatial orientation of the extracellular domain to interact with membrane attack complex (MAC) proteins and preventing their digestion by proteases [54]. This protein requires the presence of detergent-insoluble glycolipid rafts (DGI) and the glycosylphosphatidylinositol (GPI) anchor to remain in the cell membrane [53]. Its membrane binding with GPI allows it to activate intracellular signaling to promote carcinogenesis, enhance cell adhesion, migration and signaling through binding to vitronectin and interactions with integrins in breast cancer cells [57].

Its expression takes place under different contexts: (i) constitutively regulated by the Sp1 transcription factor, (ii) induced under inflammatory conditions by scaffolds between NF-κB and CREB proteins bound to CBP/p300 [58], (iii) conditionally regulated by the transcription factor Smad3 induced by TGF-β during the epithelial-mesenchymal transition (EMT) [44], and (iv) selectively expressed by SOX2 in populations of cancer stem cells (CSC) [59].

4. mCRP expression in breast cancer and prognosis in patients

Expression of CD46, CD55, and CD59 in breast tumor samples, through PCR analysis, showed that CD46 is the most highly expressed mCRP in breast cancer [60]. In addition, IHC analysis confirmed the high expression of CD46 with both cytoplasmic and membrane staining; however, there are controversies regarding the expression of CD46 and its impact on prognosis [61, 62]. In samples of patients with primary invasive tumors, CD46 was highly expressed in most samples (99.4%), and the intensity of its expression has an inverse correlation with tumor grade histological, and tumor size. Furthermore, intense staining of CD46 was found in good prognosis-type tumors (tubulo-lobular, tubular, mucinous, and invasive cribriform types). In contrast, it was less common in poor prognosis types (ductal/NST, solid lobular, lobular mixed, mixed NST, and lobular types). Finally, older patients had a higher expression of CD46 [61]. However, another study showed that patients with CD46 negative tumor have a better prognosis, with an increased progression-free time and overall survival time compared to patients expressing CD46. All patients in this study underwent post-operative radiotherapy, while the patients in the first study did not. This could explain the different results between the two studies [62].

It has also been reported that ER-positive tumors overexpress CD46 and that its expression confers a loss of differentiation of tumors, a characteristic strongly related to aggressiveness. This is consistent with the report of Thorsteinsson et al. on the upregulation of CD46 during malignant progression [60, 63].

CD55 is also highly expressed in breast cancer: in a study with 74 samples, 50 of them (67.6%) were categorized as CD55-high and the remaining as CD55-low, with a strong positivity in stage II and III tumors. Immunohistochemistry analyses also showed a high expression of CD55 in the cytoplasm of the cells [64]. Furthermore, a strong correlation exists between patients with CD55-high tumors and a shorter relapse rate. Thus, CD55 could be a recurrence prognostic factor [64]. Madjd et al. report that after therapy, surviving cells may overexpress CD55 on breast tumors as a response to complement activation by the tumor environment [61]. On the other hand, a study of 480 cases of primary operable invasive breast carcinoma reported a higher expression of CD55 in grade 1 or 2 tumors, and this high CD55 expression correlates with a good prognosis [65]. This same study revealed that the loss of CD55 might also correlate with poor prognosis, which is consistent with another report that establishes that during malignant progression, there appears to be a downregulation of CD55. This could be due to the protein's role in regulating the immune response via interaction with its ligand, CD97 [63, 65].

An analysis of clinical specimens from 120 patients (58 with lung metastases and 62 without metastatic disease) revealed that patients with high CD59 expression

mCRP	Expression	Samples	Treatment	Prognosis
CD46	High	70	Chemotherapy + radiotherapy	Unfavorable [62]
		510	Chemotherapy	Good [61]
CD55	High	74	Only surgery	Poor: relapse [64]
		480	Radiotherapy +/− chemotherapy	Good [65]
CD59	High	120	—	Poor [66]
		520	No information	Good [67]

IHC: immunohistochemistry.

Table 1.
Comparison between different reports on mCRP expression and impact on prognosis in breast tumor samples evaluated by IHC.

might have a worse prognosis, as there was a positive association between CD59 expression and metastasis. Therefore, patients with high CD59 expression are more likely to develop metastases [66]. Kaplan-Meier analysis showed that the expression of CD59 in breast cancer patients correlates with a worse relapse-free survival rate and, furthermore, it appears that CD59 upregulation occurs during malignant progression. Thus, CD59 may be a prognostic biomarker of poor outcomes in patients with breast cancer [63, 66]. However, as with CD55, it has been reported that the loss of CD59 could be correlated with poor prognosis due to its role in regulating the immune response via interaction with its ligand, CD2. In addition, the same study revealed that high levels of CD55 are associated with a good prognosis of moderately differentiated tumors [67]. In contrast, another study revealed that breast cancer patients with CD55 or CD59 overexpression had a higher relapse rate than those with low CD55 expression. Similarly, the mean disease-free survival of patients with CD55 or CD59 overexpression was significantly shorter than that of patients with low CD55 expression. Multivariate analysis confirmed that CD55, but not CD59, was an independent risk factor of recurrence [68].

Due to conflicting results between different studies, it is essential to consider the differences between them: the sample size, the treatment prior analysis, and scoring criteria (**Table 1**). For instance, in some studies, to categorize each case as CD55-high or CD55-low, the grade of CD55 staining intensity in each tumor cell was multiplied by the proportion of CD55-positive cells among the total tumor cells. In contrast, other studies classified as high-CD55, those cases with >1% of tumor cells showing strong CD55 expression. Because only tumor cells with significantly strong CD55 staining were counted, the proportion of CD55-low cases was higher than in the previous study [64]. Another important factor is the subtypes of breast tumors, described previously, which have different characteristics that could affect either mCRP expression or its correlation with prognosis, and none of the studies defined the type of the samples they analyzed. This could also explain the differences in the results between studies.

5. mCRP and resistance mechanisms

For many decades, antitumor therapies have improved; however, despite significant progress in cancer therapy clinical oncologists often face a major impediment to anticancer drug resistance: intrinsic resistance from the start of therapy or after initial responses and in repeated courses of drug treatment, acquired resistance. Here, our contribution to understanding the underlying molecular basis of the role of mCRP in therapeutic resistance.

Some conditions might affect the expression levels of mCRP and, therefore, impact on the prognosis of patients. Some reports on how mCRP expression changes after chemotherapy and its relationship with resistance. Evidence indicates that mCRPs are involved in resistance to different therapeutic schemes in the treatment of patients with breast cancer. The associated mechanisms are still being studied, but it has been recognized that complement resistance conferred by mCRPs facilitates cell proliferation, survival of circulating metastatic tumor cells, poor immune response, and reduced efficacy of immunotherapy/chemotherapy.

5.1 Immunotherapy

Immune escape mechanisms limit the susceptibility of tumor cells to antibody-based therapy. The optimal efficacy of anticancer antibodies is limited by the resistance of tumor cells to complement-mediated attack, mainly through the overexpression of mCRPs [69]. Has been reported that 50% of women affected with HER2-positive breast cancer present or acquire resistance to trastuzumab.

Following the evidence that HER2-positive patients who did not respond to trastuzumab had elevated CD55 expression, CD55 and CD59 have been reported to be involved in resistance to trastuzumab or pertuzumab. Mechanistically, HER2 antibodies (trastuzumab or pertuzumab) contain IgG1 Fc that induces CDC in cancer cells by activating the classical complement pathway, thus canonical CD55 and CD59 signaling allow blockade of HER2 antibody-mediated complement regulation [13, 70]. This was studied in breast cancer cell lines by blocking CD55/CD59 activity using mAbs, modulating their expression via phosphatidylinositol-specific phospholipase C (PI-PLC) and silencing their expression using short hairpin RNA (shRNA). Results of trypan blue exclusion assays demonstrated that treatment of cells with trastuzumab incubated with pooled normal human serum (NHS) used as the source of complement, significantly enhanced CDC-dependent lysis of SK-BR3 and BT-474 cells in these three scenarios where the participation of the mCRP was inhibited [13, 68].

Another study evaluated the efficacy of trastuzumab or pertuzumab alone or in combination to induce C3 tumor cell opsonization in SK-BR3 and BT-474 cells. Enhanced deposition of activated C3 (C3d, used as a surrogate marker for the opsonization of C3b and iC3b molecules) was observed when tumor cells were incubated with trastuzumab and pertuzumab, accompanied by silencing of CD55 and CD46, but not CD59. Nevertheless, knockdown of all three mCRPs results in an optimal C3d deposition, enhanced CDC effect due to treatment with trastuzumab and pertuzumab with an overall cell lysis of 48 ± 11% in BT474 cells and 46 ± 6% in SK-BR-3 cells, as well as an increase in complement-dependent macrophage-mediated cytotoxicity of BT474 cells, analyzed by 51Cr release assay, in the presence of both trastuzumab and pertuzumab with C8 depleted human serum to avoid MAC formation [71]. These studies describe the mechanisms of resistance to immunotherapeutic antibodies due to the expression of mCRP in cancer cells. Mechanisms of resistance to Trastuzumab-emtansine, Trastuzumab-deruxtecan, and sacituzumab-govitecan due to mCRP expression have not yet been reported due to their recent approval.

5.2 Chemotherapy

After chemotherapy treatment, response rates range from 30 to 70%, but responses are often not durable as patients develop resistance [72, 73].

CD55 can also promote chemoresistance by suppressing antitumor immunity in response to neoadjuvant chemotherapy. A significantly increased tumor-infiltrating ICOSL+ B population was identified after neoadjuvant chemotherapy in samples from breast cancer patients. It has been described that tumor cell death induced by chemotherapy activates the complement system via the alternative pathway through phosphatidylserine (PS) and is responsible for inducing ICOSL+ B cells via complement receptor type 2 (CR2) [70]. CR2 recognizes complement C3 cleavage products (C3b, iC3b, and C3c) bound to antigens and acts with the B cell antigen receptor (BCR) to lower the activation threshold and overcome B cell anergy [74]. This ICOSL+CR2high B cell population can improve antitumor immune response by increasing the frequency of CD8+ T cells and Th1 cells expressing granzyme-B or perforin and decreasing Tregs in tumors. Moreover, it was identified that CD55 determines the opposite roles of B cells in chemotherapy. The role of this complement inhibitory protein in chemosensitivity and tumor immunity was evaluated in mice injected with E0771 cells (a Luminal B cell line) with or without CD55 overexpression. The results showed that doxorubicin increased tumor-infiltrating ICOSL+ B cells and effector T cells in mice bearing parental E0771 cells, but not in those bearing CD55-overexpressing cells. On the other hand, chemotherapy-induced complement C3 cleavage products analyzed by western blotting were reduced in CD55-overexpressing tumors treated with doxorubicin. Additionally, the effect of CD55 overexpression on chemosensitivity and T cell response was completely suppressed in C3−/− mice, suggesting that it is complement dependent. This evidence indicates that CD55 overexpression on breast cancer tumor cells decreases the efficacy of chemotherapy by inhibiting the induction of complement-dependent ICOSL+ B cells [75].

5.3 Endocrine therapy

Most ER+ breast cancer may initially respond to endocrine therapy, but 15–20% of tumors are intrinsically resistant to treatment, and another 30–40% acquire resistance [76].

Some conditions might affect the expression levels of mCRP and, therefore, have an impact on the prognosis of patients. There are some reports on how mCRP expression changes after chemotherapy and its relationship with resistance. On breast cancer cell lines (SK-Br3 and BT-474) it was found that tamoxifen inhibited both the protein and mRNA expression levels of CD55, potentiating the effect of trastuzumab, suggesting the combined use of trastuzumab and tamoxifen for HER2-positive breast cancer treatment [68].

A higher CD59 expression in tamoxifen-resistant breast cancer cells has been reported, both in protein and mRNA levels, suggesting that this mCRP may play a key role in tamoxifen resistance in MCF-7 cells, a luminal A cell line. Moreover, after RNAi-mediated attenuation of CD59, cells were able to overcome tamoxifen resistance, and CD59 silencing suppressed cell proliferation, indicating that CD59 plays an important role in the response of cells to tamoxifen: knockdown of CD59-induced apoptosis through changes in apoptosis-related genes: the active form of some cell programmed death factors (cleaved-caspase-8, cleaved-caspase-6, cleaved-caspase-3, cleaved-PARP proteins, and Bax/Bcl2 ratio) was increased in the CD59-silenced tamoxifen-resistant cells [15]. These findings evidence the participation of CD59 in the regulation of pro/antiapoptotic proteins and cell proliferation in response to tamoxifen treatment to promote drug resistance in breast cancer cells.

Evidence correlating the expression of these molecules and the prognosis of patients suggests that we still have much to understand about their functions, structure, and signaling in tumor cells. As a biomarker or therapeutic target, mCRP offers several pathways for cancer therapeutics.

5.4 mCRP-expression dependent resistance but drug non-related

5.4.1 Cancer stem cells related

It has also been suggested that the overexpression of mCRPs is associated with the presence of cancer stem cells (CSC), which indicate drug resistance. The function and differentiation state of CSC are substantially modulated by many interconnected signaling pathways including IL-6/JAK2/STAT3, Hedgehog, WNT, and Notch signaling. CSCs are considered resistant to apoptosis, can modulate survival pathways and have high cell plasticity; therefore, they could survive antitumoral therapy [77].

Xu et al. reported the use of CD55 as a biomarker for CSC, after determinate high level of CD55 on mammary carcinomas (MDA-MB-231 and MCF7), two colorectal carcinomas (Lovo, RCM-1), and one lung carcinoma cell line (A549). Sorting of the CD55-high population, identified as side-population (SP) cells, revealed that cells had *in vitro* colony formation, a high self-renewal potential, and were more resistant to apoptosis in two conditions: serum depletion and ceramide addition, such as what happens with cancer stem cells. They found that anti-apoptotic proteins such as Bcl-2 were overexpressed in both SP cells and $CD55^{high}$ cells, which explain why they are tolerant to apoptosis. Researchers validated the use of high CD55 expression as a surrogate marker for sorting SP cells, which function as an identifier for CSC and, consequently, as an indicator of poor therapeutic prognosis due to the intrinsic malignancy characteristics of CSC [78]. Therefore, the authors concluded that CD55 could be an important target for CSCs, although more studies, such as the evaluation of tumorigenicity are needed.

Chen et al., reported that CD59, but not other mCRPs, was upregulated to protect sphere-forming CSCs from complement-dependent cytotoxicity. Cetuximab, a chimeric monoclonal IgG1 antibody whose specific target is the epidermal growth factor receptor (EGFR), together with normal human serum (NHS) were used to test the resistance to CDC mediated by CD59 upregulation in CSCs of MCF-7 and Calu-3 cell lines. The LDH release assay results suggested that the cell death rate was conversely correlated with the expression level of CD59. Additionally, SOX2 could transcriptionally upregulate the expression of CD59, but not the expression of CD46 and CD55, in epithelial CSCs and this mechanism protects cancer cells from complement destruction. After overexpressing SOX2 in MCF-7 and Calu-3 cells a CDC assay was conducted to test the effect of upregulated CD59 by SOX2 functionally; the results demonstrated that SOX2-overexpressing MCF-7 and Calu-3 cells are more resistant than control cells to cetuximab-mediated complement damage [59]. The antitumoral effect of this mAb is abolished by overexpression of CD59 in lung and breast cancer cells, even when this mAb is not used for breast cancer treatment, this mCRP affects its possible repositioning.

Other studies have reported that enrichment of CSCs in the tumor population can confer resistance to therapy, providing worse scenarios for the prognosis of patients. In tumor cells (CaSki, H1299, HCT116, and HEK293), NANOG increased CD59 expression, contributing to the resistance of tumor cells against complement-dependent cytotoxicity (CDC) [79]. Another example is the role of CD55 in the maintenance of CSCs by regulating self-renewal and cisplatin resistance. CSCs have been implicated in tumor recurrence and treatment resistance, and cisplatin is used for endometrioid tumors and breast cancer. CD55 regulates self-renewal and core pluripotency genes via ROR2/JNK signaling and, in parallel, cisplatin resistance via lymphocyte-specific protein tyrosine kinase (LCK) signaling, which induces the expression of DNA repair genes. Overexpression of CD55 in non-CSCs increased NANOG and SOX2 mRNA levels (core pluripotency genes). It led to significantly higher self-renewal and stem cell frequencies, with lower levels of caspase 3/7 activity upon cisplatin treatment [14].

5.4.2 Signaling pathways

Many studies have established that the transcription factor STAT3 is constitutively activated in various human cancer cells and tumor tissues compared with their normal counterparts. Different signaling pathways involving persistent STAT3 activation have been related to modulating the cancer stem cell phenotype in breast cancer [80, 81]. The role of tumor cell STAT3 signaling in immune evasion has also been described by negatively regulating cellular and innate immune responses [82]. A potential mechanism has been suggested by which oncogenic signaling contributes to tumor cell evasion of antibody-mediated immunity. Buettner et al. demonstrated that activation of STAT3 signaling induces the CD46 promoter and protects human cancer cells from complement-dependent cytotoxicity. Using microarray gene expression profiling, the CD46 gene was identified as a target for activated STAT3 signaling in human breast (MDA-MB-435 s cell line) and prostate cancer cells (DU145 cell line). Moreover, in luciferase reporter assays, CD46 promoter activity was induced by STAT3 activation and blocked by STAT3β, a dominant negative form of STAT3. Finally, inhibition of cell surface expression of CD46 mediated by inhibition of STAT3 signaling sensitized prostate cancer cells to cytotoxicity in an *in vitro* complement lysis assay using rabbit anti-DU145 antiserum, as a source of antibodies, and rabbit complement where cell death was measured by lactate dehydrogenase release [35]. This study shows that STAT3 can contribute to protecting cancer cells from complement system attack, at least through the upregulation of CD46. Still, the regulation of others mCRPs, such as CD55 and CD59, could also be evaluated.

Another mechanism of CDC resistance in breast cancer cells has been described. One study found that Mammalian hepatitis B X-interacting protein (HBXIP), a novel oncoprotein, upregulates mCRPs through ERK1/2/NF-κB signaling to protect breast cancer cells from complement attack [83]. The results showed that HBXIP decreased the sensitivity of MCF-7 cells to CDC; then, CDC susceptibility was rescued when mCRPs were blocked with antibodies against CD46, CD55, and CD59. Furthermore, overexpression of HBXIP was able to upregulate the expression of these mCRPs in levels of promoter activity, mRNA and protein expression in MCF-7 and MDA-MB-231 cells. Finally, the inhibition of ERK1/2 and NF-κB was able to sensitize the MCF-7 cells with HBXIP overexpression to CDC; this was examined by trypan blue absorbance assay after treatment with PD98059 (an inhibitor of MEK) or PDTC (an inhibitor of NF-κB). Thus, the role of HBXIP in regulating mCRPs has been suggested as a complement resistance mechanism in breast cancer cells.

6. Therapeutic strategies and future challenges to regulate mCRP in breast cancer

Here we have exposed that the function of mCRP on complement has been widely explored. But these proteins also can regulate non-complement signaling in promoting cancer proliferation, chemoresistance, and metastasis. We proposed a model of signaling pathways activated by mCRP [12] and recently Bharti et al. also proposed a series of pathways intracellularly by CD55 [43]. Due to their relevance in the potential of anticancer antibodies, they have been proposed and studied mCRP as therapeutic targets through various models and strategies: small interfering RNAs (siRNA) [69, 71, 84, 85], antibodies anti-mCRP [13], and enzyme-peptide [13, 86]. Although there are multiple studies in the preclinical stage and in development, none are exclusive for each mCRP and neither has reached clinical use.

Geis et al. designed siRNAs for post-transcriptional gene knockdown of CD46, CD55, and CD59 aiming to sensitize tumor cells lines (BT474 (breast) and K562 (erythroleukemia) and Du145 (prostate)) to better for tumor cell destruction by complement. Interestingly, the breast carcinoma cells BT474 were predominantly sensitized to CDC upon inhibiting CD46 expression. In contrast, suppression of CD55 and CD59 had no or only a minor effect, suggesting that CD46 is more critical in regulating complement activity [69]. But it is necessary to identify the activity intracellular to all mCRP in this context.

Other authors also used siRNAs anti-mCRP, but the delivery of chemically was stabilized siRNAs using cationic lipoplexes (AtuPLEXes). Their results suggest that siRNA-induced inhibition of mCRP expression enhances complement and macrophage-mediated anti-tumor activity of trastuzumab and pertuzumab on HER2-positive tumor cells [71].

To increase the selectivity of silencing, other authors used siRNAs encapsulated in transferrin-coupled lipoplexes for the specific targeted and delivery to transferrin receptor CD71high expressing BT474 tumor cells. The mCRP knockdown led to a significant increase of CDC in BT474; it was also observed that the downregulation of CD46 and CD55 significantly increased C3 opsonization in these tumor cells [84].

The inhibition of mCRP with siRNA has been used to study the relevance of this molecule in other tumors [87, 88]. In general, silencing can sensitize tumor cells to CDC and ADCC *in vitro*. Although siRNA is an attractive strategy, in vivo data will be needed to validate the therapeutic potential.

Wang et al. explored three different strategies to inhibit the activity of mCRP. One strategy consisted of inhibiting the expression of mCRP using shRNA (short hair-pin RNA). Other approach blocked the function of CD55 and CD59 using targeted monoclonal antibodies; the third consisted of treatment with a phosphatidylinositol-specific phospholipase C (PI-PLC), which caused a significant decrease in the surface area of CD55 and CD59. These strategies significantly improved cell lysis of SK-BR-3 and BT474 cells with trastuzumab [13].

The use of monoclonal antibodies anti-mCRP or bispecific antibodies (bsAbs) has also been evaluated in other types of cancer, demonstrating that the efficacy of therapeutic antibodies can be increased by blocking these proteins [89–96].

Ad35K++ that binds with high affinity to CD46 and is one of the most advanced strategies to block CD46 activity. This peptide has been evaluated in lymphoma model and the preclinical studies Ad35K++ have been demonstrated safety and efficacy. Intravenous Ad35K++ injection triggers the shedding of the CD46 extracellular domain in xenograft mouse tumor models and in macaques. The authors suggest their study is the basis for an investigational new drug application for the use of Ad35K++ in combination with rituximab in the treatment of patients with B-cell malignancies [86, 97]. The first studies with this peptide were evaluated in cancer lines cells (Raji lymphoma cells and BT474-M) using alemtuzumab and trastuzumab, in both case increased CDC [86].

7. Conclusions

The molecular mechanisms of mCRP in the drug resistance of breast cancer cells are still poorly understood. Few investigations have focused in study on the relationship between mCRP and drug resistance. Also, we must learn how mCRP activates intracellular pathways and relate its domains and interactions with other proteins to perform non-complement dependent functions. Therefore, we suggest:

- Future research ought on the role of mCRP in the resistance of breast cancer cells to therapy available, including chemotherapeutic agents and mAb.

- Direct our efforts to understand mCRP signaling in breast cancer and its activity-structure relationship to offer opportunities for regulation or silencing.

- We need rigorous investigation of the pathways activated by mCRP to develop better cancer therapy and improve the efficacy of existing treatments.

- Identify the signaling pathways activated by mCRP. If a previously studied signaling pathway is identified, we could use the drugs developed to regulate the activity of its components. This would lead to new therapeutic applications of the drugs evaluated or to identify the relevance of the signaling pathway activated by mCRP.

- Explorer whether the combined use of tamoxifen and trastuzumab for the treatment of HER2-positive breast cancer enhances the antitumor effects of trastuzumab as suggested the evidence.

- Demonstrate whether therapeutic agents can directly regulate mCRP expression or do so by activating signaling pathways.

Acknowledgements

This work was supported by UNAM-PAPIIT (IA205421 and IA204323). M.A.M-M was recipient of a M. Sc fellowship from CONACYT (1101500). The images were generated with Biorender.com.

Conflict of interest

The authors declare no conflict of interest.

Author details

Sofia Álvarez-Lorenzo[1,2], Rebeca Elizabeth Montalvo-Castro[1,2], Jeannie Jiménez-López[1,2], María Adriana Medina-Mondragón[1,2] and Nohemí Salinas-Jazmín[1*]

1 Department of Pharmacology, School of Medicine, National Autonomous University of Mexico (UNAM), Mexico City, Mexico

2 School of Chemistry, National Autonomous University of Mexico (UNAM), Mexico City, Mexico

*Address all correspondence to: nohemysj@unam.mx

References

[1] Kashyap D, Pal D, Sharma R, Garg VK, Goel N, Koundal D, et al. Global increase in breast cancer incidence: Risk factors and preventive measures. BioMed Research International. 2022;**2022**:1-16. DOI: 10.1155/2022/9605439

[2] Vučković L, Klisic A, Raonić J, Vućinić J. Comparative study of immunohistochemical determination of breast cancer molecular subtypes on Core biopsy and surgical specimens. European Review for Medical and Pharmacological Sciences. 2021;**25**:3990-3996. DOI: 10.26355/eurrev_202106_26039

[3] Hammerl D, Smid M, Timmermans AM, Sleijfer S, Martens JWM, Debets R. Breast cancer genomics and immuno-oncological markers to guide immune therapies. Seminars in Cancer Biology. 2018;**52**:178-188. DOI: 10.1186/s12943-017-0621-z

[4] Waks AG, Winer EP. Breast cancer treatment: A review. JAMA. 2019;**321**:288-300. DOI: 10.1001/JAMA.2018.19323

[5] Kerr AJ, Dodwell D, McGale P, Holt F, Duane F, Mannu G, et al. Adjuvant and neoadjuvant breast cancer treatments: A systematic review of their effects on mortality. Cancer Treatment Reviews. 2022;**105**:1-12. DOI: 10.1016/j.ctrv.2022.102375

[6] Bardia A, Hurvitz SA, Tolaney SM, Loirat D, Punie K, Oliveira M, et al. Sacituzumab Govitecan in metastatic triple-negative breast cancer. The New England Journal of Medicine. 2021;**384**:1529-1541. DOI: 10.1056/nejmoa2028485

[7] Nagayama A, Vidula N, Ellisen L, Bardia A. Novel antibody-drug conjugates for triple negative breast cancer. Therapeutic Advances in Medical Oncology. 2020;**12**:1-12. DOI: 10.1177/1758835920915980

[8] Fisusi FA, Akala EO. Drug combinations in breast cancer therapy. Pharmaceutical Nanotechnology. 2019;**7**:3-23. DOI: 10.2174/2211738507666190122111224

[9] Geller A, Yan J. The role of membrane bound complement regulatory proteins in tumor development and cancer immunotherapy. Frontiers in Immunology. 2019;**10**:1-13. DOI: 10.3389/fimmu.2019.01074

[10] O'brien RM, Cannon A, Reynolds JV, Lysaght J, Lynam-Lennon N. Complement in tumourigenesis and the response to cancer therapy. Cancers (Basel). 2021;**13**:1209-1241. DOI: 10.3390/cancers13061209

[11] Golay J, Taylor RP. The role of complement in the mechanism of action of therapeutic anti-cancer MAbs. Antibodies. 2020;**9**:58. DOI: 10.3390/antib9040058

[12] Montalvo-Castro RE, Salinas-Jazmín N. Relationship between the expression of complement inhibitory proteins and therapeutic efficacy of antibodies in breast cancer. Gaceta Médica de México. 2022;**158**:141-149. DOI: 10.24875/GMM.M22000657

[13] Wang Y, Yang YJ, Wang Z, Liao J, Liu M, Zhong XR, et al. CD55 and CD59 expression protects HER2-overexpressing breast cancer cells from Trastuzumab-induced complement-dependent cytotoxicity. Oncology Letters. 2017;**14**:2961-2969. DOI: 10.3892/ol.2017.6555

[14] Saygin C, Wiechert A, Rao VS, Alluri R, Connor E, Thiagarajan PS, et al. CD55 regulates self-renewal and cisplatin resistance in endometrioid tumors. The Journal of Experimental Medicine. 2017;**214**:2715-2732. DOI: 10.1084/jem.20170438

[15] Xiong H, Jin X, You C. Expression of the CD59 glycoprotein precursor is upregulated in an Estrogen receptor-alpha (ER-α)-negative and a tamoxifen-resistant breast cancer cell line in vitro. Medical Science Monitor. 2018;**24**:7883-7890. DOI: 10.12659/MSM.910647

[16] Global Cancer Observatory. Available from: https://gco.iarc.fr/ [Accessed: 22 December 2022]

[17] Harbeck N, Penault-Llorca F, Cortes J, Gnant M, Houssami N, Poortmans P, et al. Breast cancer. Nature Reviews Disease Primers. 2019;**5**:66. DOI: 10.1038/s41572-019-0111-2

[18] Mohit E, Hashemi A, Allahyari M. Breast cancer immunotherapy: Monoclonal antibodies and peptide-based vaccines. Expert Review of Clinical Immunology. 2014;**10**:927-961. DOI: 10.1586/1744666X.2014.916211

[19] Mamidi S, Höne S, Kirschfink M. The complement system in cancer: Ambivalence between tumour destruction and promotion. Immunobiology. 2017;**222**:45-54. DOI: 10.1016/j.imbio.2015.11.008

[20] Revel M, Daugan MV, Sautés-Fridman C, Fridman WH, Roumenina LT. Complement system: Promoter or suppressor of cancer progression? Antibodies. 2020;**9**:57-78. DOI: 10.3390/antib9040057

[21] Merle NS, Church SE, Fremeaux-Bacchi V, Roumenina LT. Complement system part I—Molecular mechanisms of activation and regulation. Frontiers in Immunology. 2015;**6**:1-30. DOI: 10.3389/fimmu.2015.00262

[22] Manson JJ, Mauri C, Ehrenstein MR. Natural serum IgM maintains immunological homeostasis and prevents autoimmunity. Springer Seminars in Immunopathology. 2004;**26**:425-432. DOI: 10.1007/S00281-004-0187-X

[23] Niculescu F, Rus HG, Retegan M, Vlaicu R. Persistent complement activation on tumor cells in breast cancer. The American Journal of Pathology. 1992;**140**:1039

[24] Coulibaly FS, Youan BBC. Current status of lectin-based cancer diagnosis and therapy. AIMS Molecular Science. 2017;**4**:1-27. DOI: 10.3934/MOLSCI.2017.1.1

[25] Wang Y, Sun SN, Liu Q, Yu YY, Guo J, Wang K, et al. Autocrine complement inhibits IL10-dependent T-cell-mediated antitumor immunity to promote tumor progression. Cancer Discovery. 2016;**6**:1022-1035. DOI: 10.1158/2159-8290.CD-15-1412/42468/AM/AUTOCRINE-COMPLEMENT-INHIBITS-IL10-DEPENDENT-T

[26] Vadrevu SK, Chintala NK, Sharma SK, Sharma P, Cleveland C, Riediger L, et al. Complement C5a receptor facilitates cancer metastasis by altering T-cell responses in the metastatic niche. Cancer Research. 2014;**74**:3454-3465. DOI: 10.1158/0008-5472.CAN-14-0157

[27] Bandini S, Macagno M, Hysi A, Lanzardo S, Conti L, Bello A, et al. The non-inflammatory role of C1q during Her2/Neu-driven mammary carcinogenesis. Oncoimmunology. 2016;**5**:1-13. DOI: 10.1080/2162402X.2016.1253653

[28] Roumenina LT, Daugan MV, Petitprez F, Sautès-Fridman C,

Fridman WH. Context-dependent roles of complement in cancer. Nature Reviews. Cancer. 2019;**19**:698-715. DOI: 10.1038/S41568-019-0210-0

[29] Fishelson Z, Donin N, Zell S, Schultz S, Kirschfink M. Obstacles to cancer immunotherapy: Expression of membrane complement regulatory proteins (MCRPs) in tumors. Molecular Immunology. 2003;**40**:109-123. DOI: 10.1016/S0161-5890(03)00112-3

[30] Wu J, Liu Q, Wang C, Tao M, Liu C, Lu F, et al. Targeting complement regulatory proteins in tumor immunotherapy. International Journal of Clinical and Experimental Medicine. 2019;**12**:3083-3094

[31] Cole JL, Housley GA, Dykman TR, MacDermott RP, Atkinson JP. Identification of an additional class of C3-binding membrane proteins of human peripheral blood leukocytes and cell lines. Proceedings of the National Academy of Sciences of the United States of America. 1985;**82**:859-863. DOI: 10.1073/PNAS.82.3.859

[32] Liszewski MK, Post TW, Atkinson JP. Membrane cofactor protein (MCP or CD46): Newest member of the regulators of complement activation gene cluster. Annual Review of Immunology. 1991;**9**:431-455. DOI: 10.1146/ANNUREV.IY.09.040191.002243

[33] Liszewski MK, Atkinson JP. Membrane cofactor protein (MCP; CD46). Isoforms differ in protection against the classical pathway of complement. Journal of Immunology. 1996;**156**:4415-4421

[34] McNearney T, Ballard L, Seya T, Atkinson JP. Membrane cofactor protein of complement is present on human fibroblast, epithelial, and endothelial cells. The Journal of Clinical Investigation. 1989;**84**:538-545. DOI: 10.1172/JCI114196

[35] Buettner R, Huang M, Gritsko T, Karras J, Enkemann S, Mesa T, et al. Activated signal transducers and activators of transcription 3 signaling induces CD46 expression and protects human cancer cells from complement-dependent cytotoxicity. Molecular Cancer Research. 2007;**5**:823-832. DOI: 10.1158/1541-7786.MCR-06-0352

[36] Persson BD, Schmitz NB, Santiago C, Zocher G, Larvie M, Scheu U, et al. Structure of the extracellular portion of CD46 provides insights into its interactions with complement proteins and pathogens. PLoS Pathogens. 2010;**6**:1-12. DOI: 10.1371/journal.ppat.1001122

[37] Liszewski MK, Atkinson JP. Membrane Cofactor Protein BT - Membrane Defenses Against Attack by Complement and Perforins. In: Parker CJ, editor. Berlin, Heidelberg: Springer Berlin Heidelberg; 1992. pp. 45-60. ISBN 978-3-642-77014-2

[38] Johnstone RW, Loveland BE, Mckenzie IFC. Identification and quantification of complement regulator CD46 on normal human tissues. Immunology. 1993;**79**:341

[39] Liszewski MK, Atkinson JP. Membrane cofactor protein. In: Barnum S, Schein T, editors. In Factsbook. The Complement FactsBook. 2nd ed. Academic Press; 2018. pp. 271-281. ISBN 9780128104200. DOI: 10.1016/B978-0-12-810420-0.00026-2

[40] Kathryn, Liszewski M, Atkinson JP. Complement regulator CD46: Genetic variants and disease associations. Human Genomics. 2015;**9**:1-13. DOI: 10.1186/S40246-015-0029-Z

[41] Yamamoto H, Fara AF, Dasgupta P, Kemper C. CD46: The “multitasker” of complement proteins. The International

Journal of Biochemistry & Cell Biology. 2013;**45**:2808-2820. DOI: 10.1016/J. BIOCEL.2013.09.016

[42] Hakulinen J, Junnikkala S, Sorsa T, Meri S. Complement inhibitor membrane cofactor protein (MCP; CD46) is constitutively shed from cancer cell membranes in vesicles and converted by a metalloproteinase to a functionally active soluble form. European Journal of Immunology. 2004;**34**:2620-2629. DOI: 10.1002/EJI.200424969

[43] Bharti R, Dey G, Lin F, Lathia J, Reizes O. CD55 in cancer: Complementing functions in a non-canonical manner. Cancer Letters. 2022;**551**:1-8. DOI: 10.1016/j.canlet.2022.215935

[44] Christy JM, Toomey CB, Cauvi DM, Pollard KM. Decay-Accelerating Factor. In: Barnum S, Schein T, editors. In Factsbook. The Complement FactsBook. 2nd ed. Academic Press; 2018. pp. 261-270. ISBN 9780128104200. DOI: 10.1016/ B978-0-12-810420-0.00025-0

[45] Lublin DM, Atkinson JP. Decay-accelerating factor: Biochemistry, molecular biology, and function. Annual Review of Immunology. 1989;7:35-58. DOI: 10.1146/ANNUREV. IY.07.040189.000343

[46] Lukacik P, Roversi P, White J, Esser D, Smith GP, Billington J, et al. Complement regulation at the molecular level: The structure of decay-accelerating factor. Proceedings of the National Academy of Sciences of the United States of America. 2004;**101**:1279-1284. DOI: 10.1073/PNAS.0307200101

[47] He Y, Lin F, Chipman PR, Bator CM, Baker TS, Shoham M, et al. Structure of decay-accelerating factor bound to echovirus 7: A virus-receptor complex. Proceedings of the National Academy of Sciences of the United States of America. 2002;**99**:10325-10329. DOI: 10.1073/ PNAS.152161599

[48] Lingwood D, Simons K. Lipid rafts as a membrane-organizing principle. Science (80-.). 2010;**327**:46-50. DOI: 10.1126/SCIENCE.1174621

[49] Niu M, Xu S, Yang J, Yao D, Li N, Yan J, et al. Structural basis for CD97 recognition of the decay-accelerating factor CD55 suggests mechanosensitive activation of adhesion GPCRs. The Journal of Biological Chemistry. 2021;**296**:100776. DOI: 10.1016/J. JBC.2021.100776

[50] Yin Y, Xu X, Tang J, Zhang W, Zhangyuan G, Ji J, et al. CD97 promotes tumor aggressiveness through the traditional G protein-coupled receptor-mediated signaling in hepatocellular carcinoma. Hepatology. 2018;**68**:1865-1878. DOI: 10.1002/HEP.30068

[51] Spiller OB, Criado-García O, Rodríguez De Córdoba S, Morgan BP. Cytokine-mediated up-regulation of CD55 and CD59 protects human hepatoma cells from complement attack. Clinical and Experimental Immunology. 2000;**121**:234-241. DOI: 10.1046/J.1365-2249.2000.01305.X

[52] Takeuchi K, Mizuno M, Uesu T, Nasu J, Kawada M, Hori S, et al. Epidermal growth factor induces expression of decay-accelerating factor in human colonic cancer cells via the mitogen-activated protein kinase pathway. The Journal of Laboratory and Clinical Medicine. 2001;**138**:186-192. DOI: 10.1067/MLC.2001.117405

[53] Petranka J, Zhao J, Norris J, Tweedy NB, Ware RE, Sims PJ, et al. Structure-function relationships of the complement regulatory protein, CD59. Blood Cells, Molecules, and Diseases. 1996;**22**:281-296. DOI: 10.1006/ bcmd.1996.0111

[54] Kong HK, Park JH. Characterization and function of human Ly-6/UPAR molecules. BMB Reports. 2012;**45**:595-603. DOI: 10.5483/BMBREP.2012.45.11.210

[55] Davies A, Simmons DL, Hale G, Harrison RA, Tighe H, Lachmann PJ, et al. CD59, an LY-6-like protein expressed in human lymphoid cells, regulates the action of the complement membrane attack complex on homologous cells. The Journal of Experimental Medicine. 1989;**170**:637-654. DOI: 10.1084/JEM.170.3.637

[56] Hussein NH, Amin NS, El Tayebi HM. GPI-AP: Unraveling a new class of malignancy mediators and potential immunotherapy targets. Frontiers in Oncology. 2020;**10**:1-18. DOI: 10.3389/FONC.2020.537311

[57] Van Veen M, Matas-Rico E, van de Wetering K, Leyton-Puig D, Kedziora KM, de Lorenzi V, et al. Negative regulation of Urokinase receptor activity by a GPI-specific phospholipase C in breast cancer cells. eLife. 2017;**6**:1-20. DOI: 10.7554/ELIFE.23649

[58] Mikesch J-H, Buerger H, Simon R, Brandt B. Decay-accelerating factor (CD55): A versatile acting molecule in human malignancies. Biochimica et Biophysica Acta. 2006;**1766**:42-52. DOI: 10.1016/j.bbcan.2006.04.001

[59] Chen J, Ding P, Li L, Gu H, Zhang X, Zhang L, et al. CD59 regulation by SOX2 is required for epithelial cancer stem cells to evade complement surveillance. Stem Cell Reports. 2017;**8**:140-151. DOI: 10.1016/j.stemcr.2016.11.008

[60] Rushmere NK, Knowlden JM, Gee JMW, Harper ME, Robertson JF, Morgan BP, et al. Analysis of the level of MRNA expression of the membrane regulators of complement, CD59, CD55 and CD46, in breast cancer. International Journal of Cancer. 2004;**108**:930-936. DOI: 10.1002/IJC.11606

[61] Madjd Z, Durrant LG, Pinder SE, Ellis IO, Ronan J, Lewis S, et al. Do poor-prognosis breast tumours express membrane cofactor proteins (CD46)? Cancer Immunology, Immunotherapy. 2005;**54**:149-156. DOI: 10.1007/s00262-004-0590-0

[62] MacIejczyk A, Szelachowska J, Szynglarewicz B, Szulc R, Szulc A, Wysocka T, et al. CD46 expression is an Unfavorable prognostic factor in breast cancer cases. Applied Immunohistochemistry & Molecular Morphology. 2011;**19**:540-546. DOI: 10.1097/PAI.0b013e31821a0be9

[63] Thorsteinsson L, O'Dowd GM, Harrington PM, Johnson PM. The complement regulatory proteins CD46 and CD59, but not CD55, are highly expressed by glandular epithelium of human breast and colorectal tumour tissues. APMIS. 1998;**106**:869-878. DOI: 10.1111/J.1699-0463.1998.TB00233.X

[64] Ikeda J, Morii E, Liu Y, Qiu Y, Nakamichi N, Jokoji R, et al. Prognostic significance of CD55 expression in breast cancer. Clinical Cancer Research. 2008;**14**:4780-4786. DOI: 10.1158/1078-0432.CCR-07-1844

[65] Madjd Z, Durrant LG, Bradley R, Spendlove I, Ellis IO, Pinder SE. Loss of CD55 is associated with aggressive breast tumors. Clinical Cancer Research. 2004;**10**:2797-2803. DOI: 10.1158/1078-0432.CCR-1073-03

[66] Ouyang Q, Zhang L, Jiang Y, Ni X, Chen S, Ye F, et al. The membrane complement regulatory protein CD59 promotes tumor growth and predicts poor prognosis in breast cancer.

International Journal of Oncology. 2016;**48**:2015-2024. DOI: 10.3892/IJO.2016.3408

[67] Madjd Z, Pinder SE, Paish C, Ellis IO, Carmichael J, Durrant LG. Loss of CD59 expression in breast tumours correlates with poor survival. The Journal of Pathology. 2003;**200**:633-639. DOI: 10.1002/PATH.1357

[68] Liu M, Yang YJ, Zheng H, Zhong XR, Wang Y, Wang Z, et al. Membrane-bound complement regulatory proteins are prognostic factors of operable breast cancer treated with adjuvant Trastuzumab: A retrospective study. Oncology Reports. 2014;**32**:2619-2627. DOI: 10.3892/or.2014.3496

[69] Geis N, Zell S, Rutz R, Li W, Giese T, Mamidi S, et al. Inhibition of membrane complement inhibitor expression (CD46, CD55, CD59) by SiRNA sensitizes tumor cells to complement attack in vitro. Current Cancer Drug Targets. 2010;**10**:922-931. DOI: 10.2174/156800910793357952

[70] Wang Y, Liao J, Yang YJ, Wang Z, Qin F, Zhu SM, et al. Effect of membrane-bound complement regulatory proteins on tumor cell sensitivity to complement-dependent cytolysis triggered by heterologous expression of the α-gal xenoantigen. Oncology Letters. 2018;**15**:9061-9068. DOI: 10.3892/OL.2018.8478

[71] Mamidi S, Cinci M, Hasmann M, Fehring V, Kirschfink M. Lipoplex mediated silencing of membrane regulators (CD46, CD55 and CD59) enhances complement-dependent anti-tumor activity of trastuzumab and pertuzumab. Molecular Oncology. 2013;7:580-594. DOI: 10.1016/j.molonc.2013.02.011

[72] Rivera E, Gomez H. Chemotherapy resistance in metastatic breast cancer: The evolving role of Ixabepilone. Breast Cancer Research. 2010;**12**:1-12. DOI: 10.1186/BCR2573/FIGURES/1

[73] Prihantono, Faruk M. Breast cancer resistance to chemotherapy: When should we suspect it and how can we prevent it? Annals of Medicine and Surgery. 2021;**70**:102793. DOI: 10.1016/J.AMSU.2021.102793

[74] Carroll MC, Isenman DE. Regulation of humoral immunity by complement. Immunity. 2012;**37**:199-207. DOI: 10.1016/J.IMMUNI.2012.08.002

[75] Lu Y, Zhao Q, Liao JY, Song E, Xia Q, Pan J, et al. Complement signals determine opposite effects of B cells in chemotherapy-induced immunity. Cell. 2020;**180**:1081-1097.e24. DOI: 10.1016/J.CELL.2020.02.015

[76] Lei JT, Anurag M, Haricharan S, Gou X, Ellis MJ. Endocrine therapy resistance: New insights. Breast. 2019;**48**:S26. DOI: 10.1016/S0960-9776(19)31118-X

[77] Safa AR. Resistance to cell death and its modulation in cancer stem cells. Critical Reviews in Oncogenesis. 2016;**21**:203-219. DOI: 10.1615/CRITREVONCOG.2016016976

[78] Xu JX, Morii E, Liu Y, Nakamichi N, Ikeda J, Kimura H, et al. High tolerance to apoptotic stimuli induced by serum depletion and ceramide in side-population cells: High expression of CD55 as a novel character for side-population. Experimental Cell Research. 2007;**313**:1877-1885. DOI: 10.1016/J.YEXCR.2007.03.006

[79] Son SW, Cho E, Cho H, Woo SR, Lee HJ, Oh SJ, et al. NANOG confers resistance to complement-dependent cytotoxicity in immune-edited tumor cells through up-regulating CD59.

Scientific Reports. 2022;**12**:1-10. DOI: 10.1038/S41598-022-12692-6

[80] Marotta LLC, Almendro V, Marusyk A, Shipitsin M, Schemme J, Walker SR, et al. The JAK2/STAT3 signaling pathway is required for growth of $CD44^{+}CD24^{-}$ stem cell-like breast cancer cells in human tumors. The Journal of Clinical Investigation. 2011;**121**:2723-2735. DOI: 10.1172/JCI44745

[81] Ibrahim SA, Gadalla R, El-Ghonaimy EA, Samir O, Mohamed HT, Hassan H, et al. Syndecan-1 is a novel molecular marker for triple negative inflammatory breast cancer and modulates the cancer stem cell phenotype via the IL-6/STAT3, notch and EGFR signaling pathways. Molecular Cancer. 2017;**16**:1-19. DOI: 10.1186/S12943-017-0621-Z

[82] Wang T, Niu G, Kortylewski M, Burdelya L, Shain K, Zhang S, et al. Regulation of the innate and adaptive immune responses by Stat-3 signaling in tumor cells. Nature Medicine. 2004;**10**:48-54. DOI: 10.1038/NM976

[83] Cui W, Zhao Y, Shan C, Kong G, Hu N, Zhang Y, et al. HBXIP upregulates CD46, CD55 and CD59 through ERK1/2/NF-KB signaling to protect breast cancer cells from complement attack. FEBS Letters. 2012;**586**:766-771. DOI: 10.1016/J.FEBSLET.2012.01.039

[84] Cinci M, Mamidi S, Li W, Fehring V, Kirschfink M. Targeted delivery of SiRNA using transferrin-coupled lipoplexes specifically sensitizes CD71 high expressing malignant cells to antibody-mediated complement attack. Targeted Oncology. 2015;**10**:405-413. DOI: 10.1007/S11523-014-0345-6/FIGURES/4

[85] Mamidi S, Gies N, Kirschfink M, Li W. Specific SiRNA targeting of the membrane complement regulator CD59 with Herceptin® immunoliposomes sensitize breast carcinoma cells to complement mediated cytotoxicity. Clinical Immunology. 2010;**135**:S55-S56. DOI: 10.1016/j.clim.2010.03.169

[86] Beyer I, Cao H, Persson J, Wang H, Liu Y, Yumul R, et al. Transient removal of CD46 is safe and increases B-cell depletion by rituximab in CD46 transgenic mice and macaques. Molecular Therapy. 2013;**21**:291-299. DOI: 10.1038/mt.2012.212

[87] Bellone S, Roque D, Cocco E, Gasparrini S, Bortolomai I, Buza N, et al. Downregulation of membrane complement inhibitors CD55 and CD59 by SiRNA sensitises uterine serous carcinoma overexpressing Her2/Neu to complement and antibody-dependent cell cytotoxicity in vitro: Implications for trastuzumab-based immunotherapy. British Journal of Cancer. 2012;**106**:1543-1550. DOI: 10.1038/bjc.2012.132

[88] Kesselring R, Thiel A, Pries R, Fichtner-Feigl S, Brunner S, Seidel P, et al. The complement receptors CD46, CD55 and CD59 are regulated by the tumour microenvironment of head and neck cancer to facilitate escape of complement attack. European Journal of Cancer. 2014;**50**:2152-2161. DOI: 10.1016/j.ejca.2014.05.005

[89] Kuliczkowski K. Expression of complement regulatory proteins : CD46 , CD55 , and CD59 and response to rituximab in patients with CD20 (+) Non-Hodgkin ' s. Lymphoma. 2010;**20**:743-746. DOI: 10.1007/s12032-009-9278-9

[90] Macor P, Tripodo C, Zorzet S, Piovan E, Bossi F, Marzari R, et al. In vivo targeting of human neutralizing antibodies against CD55 and CD59 to lymphoma cells increases the

antitumor activity of rituximab. Cancer Research. 2007;**59**:10556-10564. DOI: 10.1158/0008-5472.CAN-07-1811

[91] Ziller F, Macor P, Bulla R, Sblattero D, Marzari R, Tedesco F. Controlling complement resistance in cancer by using human monoclonal antibodies that neutralize complement-regulatory proteins CD55 and CD59. European Journal of Immunology. 2005;**35**:2175-2183. DOI: 10.1002/EJI.200425920

[92] Gorter A, Blok VT, Haasnoot WHB, Ensink NG, Daha MR, Fleuren GJ. Expression of CD46, CD55, and CD59 on renal tumor cell lines and their role in preventing complement-mediated tumor cell lysis. Laboratory Investigation. 1996;**74**:1039-1049

[93] Shao F, Gao Y, Wang W, He H, Xiao L, Geng X, et al. Silencing EGFR-upregulated expression of CD55 and CD59 activates the complement system and sensitizes lung cancer to checkpoint blockade. Nature Cancer. 2022;**3**(10):1192-1210. DOI: 10.1038/s43018-022-00444-4

[94] Macor P, Secco E, Mezzaroba N, Zorzet S, Durigutto P, Gaiotto T, et al. Bispecific antibodies targeting tumor-associated antigens and neutralizing complement regulators increase the efficacy of antibody-based immunotherapy in mice. Leukemia. 2015;**29**:406-414. DOI: 10.1038/LEU.2014.185

[95] Gelderman KA, Blok VT, Fleuren GJ, Gorter A. The inhibitory effect of CD46, CD55, and CD59 on complement activation after immunotherapeutic treatment of cervical carcinoma cells with monoclonal antibodies or bispecific monoclonal antibodies. Laboratory Investigation. 2002;**82**:483-493. DOI: 10.1038/LABINVEST.3780441

[96] Ullenhag GJ, Spendlove I, Watson NFS, Indar AA, Dube M, Robins RA, et al. A neoadjuvant/adjuvant randomized trial of colorectal cancer patients vaccinated with an anti-Idiotypic antibody, 105AD7, mimicking CD55. Clinical Cancer Research. 2006;**12**:7389-7396. DOI: 10.1158/1078-0432.CCR-06-1003

[97] Richter M, Yumul R, Saydaminova K, Wang H, Gough M, Baldessari A, et al. Preclinical safety, pharmacokinetics, pharmacodynamics, and biodistribution studies with Ad35K++ protein: A novel rituximab cotherapeutic. Molecular Therapy—Methods & Clinical Development. 2016;**3**:16013. DOI: 10.1038/MTM.2016.13

Section 2

Treatments

Chapter 13

Minimally Invasive Surgery in Breast Reconstruction: The Past and Future

Elizabeth A. Bailey and Sarah N. Bishop

Abstract

Restoring breast aesthetics and minimizing morbidity while providing excellent oncologic control has been the driving force in the evolution of both breast cancer and breast reconstructive surgery. This chapter will discuss recent developments using minimally invasive techniques to further move the needle towards even better patient outcomes. We outline the technical considerations and evidence behind minimally invasive breast reconstructive procedures including laparoscopic deep inferior epigastric perforator (DIEP) flap harvest, robotic DIEP flap harvest, and robotic latissimus dorsi flap harvest. We also introduce minimally invasive breast cancer surgery including robotic mastectomy. Finally, this chapter discusses future applications of emerging technology and the controversies surrounding the widespread adoption of minimally invasive techniques in breast cancer and breast reconstructive surgery.

Keywords: breast reconstruction, robotic surgery, mastectomy, DIEP flap, minimally invasive surgery

1. Introduction

Breast cancer surgery has dramatically evolved since Halstead first described the radical mastectomy in 1894 [1]. Over time, radical mastectomy with resection of the entire breast, chest wall musculature, and axillary nodes, was abandoned due to its high morbidity and failure to achieve superior oncologic outcomes compared to less aggressive resections. Since then, the field has recognized the importance of achieving excellent cancer outcomes while also minimizing morbidity and preserving breast aesthetics. Skin-sparing mastectomy, breast conservation surgery, sentinel lymph node biopsy, and now nipple-sparing mastectomy (NSM) in the appropriate patient have become the standard of care.

While initially avoided for fear of the loss of local control, breast reconstruction is now considered part of routine breast cancer care. The late 1800s and first half of the twentieth century are spotted with case reports and small case series of autologous tissue reconstruction; however, autologous reconstruction really took hold in the 1970s [2]. The advent of the silicone breast implant in the 1960s also ushered breast reconstruction into the modern age.

Breast reconstruction using autologous flaps gained acceptance following descriptions of the pedicled latissimus dorsi flap in 1977 [2]. The flap was refined to allow for a single-stage reconstruction of breast defects; however, the volume was often insufficient to be used alone and thus the flap was paired with an implant. To replace the entire volume of the breast mound, surgeons turned to abdominal tissue. The pedicled transverse rectus abdominis myocutaneous (TRAM) flap was introduced by Hartrampf, Schelfan, and Black in 1982 [2]. The TRAM flap revolutionized breast cancer reconstruction as it allowed for a complete autologous reconstruction with an acceptable donor scar and body contouring effect similar to abdominoplasty. Unfortunately, the blood supply-to-tissue ratio from the superiorly-based pedicle contributed to high incidence of fat necrosis and harvest of the rectus abdominis muscle led to significant abdominal wall weakness. Initially described in 1979, the free TRAM uses microsurgical technique to transfer the disconnected abdominal tissue and connect the TRAM blood supply to distantly located recipient vessels. The free TRAM is based on the deep inferior epigastric vessels rather than the superior epigastric vessels that supply the pedicled TRAM. The deep inferior epigastric vessels are noted to be more robust and provide improved blood supply to the TRAM flap compared to the superior epigastric system. Therefore, the free TRAM optimizes the blood flow to the flap which reduces fat necrosis compared to the pedicled TRAM. The free TRAM did not, however, decrease abdominal wall morbidity compared to the pedicled TRAM. To address this, plastic surgeons adapted the dissection technique to reduce damage to the rectus abdominis muscle, first with the muscle-sparing TRAM (ms-TRAM) then the deep inferior epigastric artery perforator (DIEP) flap. Considered by most to be the current gold standard in autologous tissue reconstruction, the DIEP flap

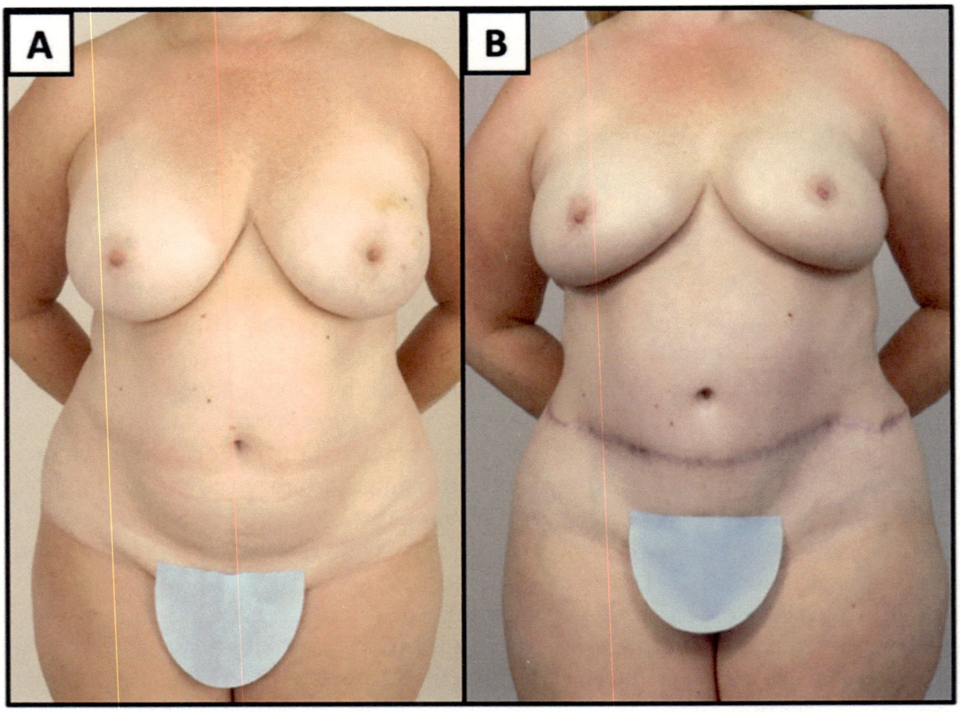

Figure 1.
(A) Preoperative (B) following bilateral nipple-sparing mastectomies and DIEP flap reconstruction.

minimizes muscle sacrifice by carefully dissecting the muscle away from the vasculature (**Figure 1**). Additional soft tissue donor sites have been introduced including the thighs, gluteal region, and lower back, yet the DIEP flap remains the preferred operative approach for autologous tissue reconstruction for the majority of patients.

As illustrated above, restoring breast aesthetics and minimizing morbidity while treating the patient's underlying cancer has been a driving force in the evolution of both breast cancer and breast reconstructive surgery. This chapter will discuss recent developments using minimally invasive techniques to further move the needle towards even better patient outcomes.

2. Minimally invasive surgery in breast reconstruction

Donor site concerns including the risk of hernia or abdominal bulge following DIEP flap reconstruction have driven plastic surgeons to explore minimally invasive options for flap harvest. Hernia, muscle-bulging, and decreased core strength are the most significant donor site complications that minimally invasive surgery seeks to correct. Multiple studies have shown decreased abdominal wall morbidity as muscle preserving techniques increase [3–10]. The increased abdominal wall morbidity is typically attributed to 3 factors: weakened musculature, denervated musculature, and violation of the anterior sheath. The first, inclusion of the rectus abdominus in the flap design (TRAM or ms-TRAM) may be minimized by performing a true perforator flap with perforators selected to minimize muscular disruption. The second, denervation of the rectus abdominus can be reduced by selecting medial row perforators when suitable and using a nerve-sparing or at least nerve-repairing technique for any motor nerves encountered during pedicle dissection [11]. The final factor associated with abdominal wall morbidity is the violation of the anterior sheath that occurs during dissection of the deep inferior epigastric vessels from the level of the perforating vessels to their origin off the external iliac artery and vein (**Figure 2**). The anterior rectus sheath is the primary strength layer of the abdominal wall, especially below the arcuate line where the only barrier between the rectus abdominis and the peritoneal cavity is the thin transversalis fascia and peritoneum.

To limit the fascial incision, short pedicle techniques were described by Saint-Cyr [12]. However, as the pedicle is shortened, the caliber of the artery and vein decrease. Additionally, the degrees of surgical freedom when performing the microsurgical anastomoses are reduced which can lead to increased microscopic complications in less experienced hands. Furthermore, visualization of the vessels is limited with a small fascial incision. These challenges have inspired plastic surgeons to innovate using minimally-invasive tools commonly used in other surgical disciplines.

2.1 Laparoscopic DIEP flap harvest

In 2017, a group in France published the first feasibility study of a laparoscopic technique for DIEP flap harvest [13]. They utilized a preperitoneal or total extraperitoneal (TEP) laparoscopic technique. The TEP technique uses insufflation to bluntly open the space between the posterior sheath/transversalis fascia and the posterior surface of the rectus abdominus muscles. Once this plane is separated, the vessels can be easily seen and dissected free of the muscles from the level of external iliacs to the perforating vessels without entering the abdominal cavity. The vessels are clipped and divided at their origin, and the entire length is extracted through a minimal fascial

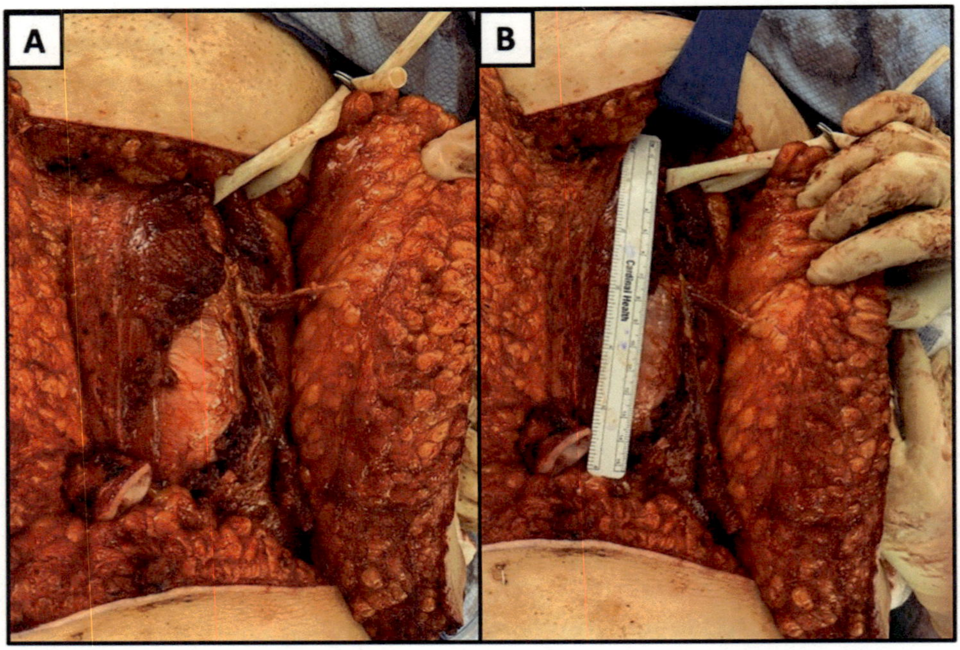

Figure 2.
(A) Traditional harvest of open DIEP flap with longitudinal splitting of muscle and fascia. (B) Ruler illustrates the nearly 15 cm incision of the anterior sheath required for pedicle dissection.

incision created during the open perforator dissection. In their series of 5 cadavers (10 hemiabdominal dissections), they were able to achieve a mean anterior fascial incision length of 3 cm compared to 12 cm for the traditional approach.

Laparoscopic DIEP flap harvest has subsequently been adopted by other groups. In 2020, a group at the University of Pennsylvania reported the then largest clinical series of patients who underwent laparoscopically-assisted harvest of DIEP vessels [14]. They reported a novel variation on previously published techniques to maximize flap blood flow while simultaneously reducing abdominal wall morbidity. They utilize a two-stage surgical delay technique to optimize the perforator most suitable for laparoscopic harvest. Prior to the initial procedure, a single perforator is selected not based on caliber but rather on location (low, central) and a short intramuscular course as seen on CT angiogram. At the initial operation, all other perforators and the superficial inferior epigastric artery and vein are ligated. This prompts the remaining perforator to dilate in response to relative tissue ischemia. At the second stage 2 weeks later, the single perforator is dissected through a minimal fascial incision and the pedicle is mobilized using a preperitoneal (TEP) approach similar to the description above. In their case series of 33 patients (57 flaps), the mean fascial incision length was 2 cm with 2 pedicle transections occurring during dissection which required repair.

2.2 Robotic DIEP flap harvest

Since the first robotic cholecystectomy was performed in 1997, the da Vinci surgical robot (Intuitive Surgical) has revolutionized the field of minimally invasive surgery. Indeed, use of the robotic platform has become the preferred approach over laparoscopy for many surgical procedures [15]. By 2018, cadaveric studies and case reports of robotic DIEP flap harvest began to arise in the plastic surgery literature [16]. In 2019, Jesse Selber at the University of Texas MD Anderson Cancer Center published his approach to robotic unilateral DIEP flap harvest [17]. He performs the procedure in a single step although usually delayed from the time of mastectomy. Similar to Kanchwala et al., the perforator is chosen preoperatively based on its short intramuscular course on CT angiography (**Figure 3**). Suprafascial dissection begins in standard fashion with the target perforator isolated and circumferentially dissected down to the posterior sheath via a small fascial incision (**Figure 4**). Robotic ports are then placed through the fascia of the contralateral hemiabdomen and the pedicle is mobilized from an intra-abdominal or transabdominal preperitoneal (TAPP approach) (**Figure 5**). The pedicle is then exteriorized and the fascia closed (Video 1, **Figure 6**).

Other groups have reported success with other approaches including use of a single port site and TEP approach [18, 19]. Many initial case series have focused on unilateral flap harvest; however, surgeons have begun to adapt the technique to allow bilateral flap dissection [20]. A group in Pittsburgh, has presented their technique for bilateral robotic DIEP pedicle harvest using a TAPP approach and 3 8 mm ports placed to target the pelvis. This allows access to both flap pedicles without undocking the robot or placing additional ports. They also report utilizing the da Vinci Firefly fluorescence technology following indocyanine green injection to better visualize the course of the vessels. In their cohort of 10 patients (20 flaps), the mean fascial incision length was 4.5 cm with an average of 1.9 perforators included in the flap design. Mesh was not required to reinforce the abdominal wall in any case. No pedicle or bowel injuries occurred during intraabdominal dissection [21].

2.3 Robotic latissimus flap harvest

For patients who have failed or are not candidates for implant-only reconstruction and who prefer to avoid free-flap breast reconstruction, a pedicled latissimus dorsi (LD) flap often combined with a tissue expander is a viable option for reconstruction. Traditional harvest technique for this flap requires a long posterior incision that

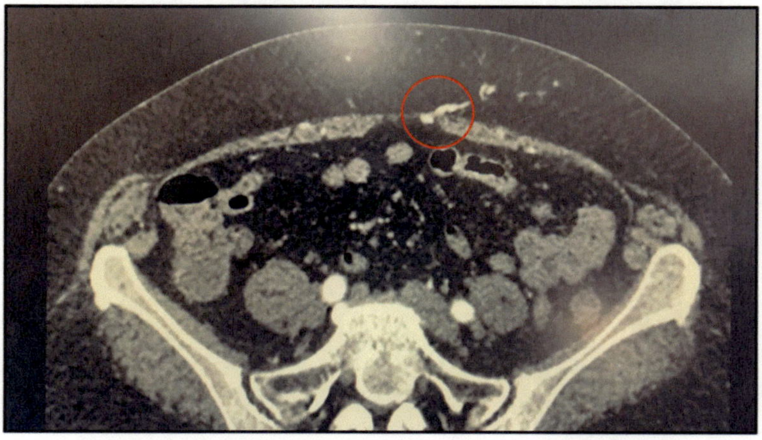

Figure 3.
CT angiography identifies dominant DIEP medial perforator (red circle) with minimal intramuscular course. This anatomy makes the patient an ideal candidate for robotic DIEP flap harvest.

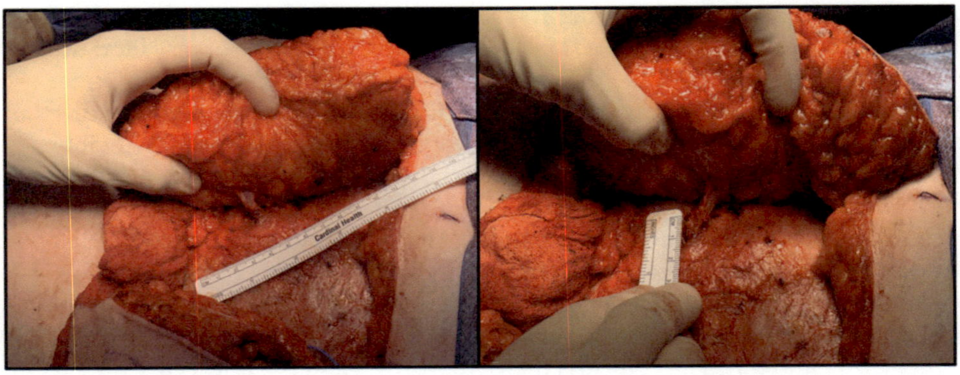

Figure 4.
Robotic DIEP flap with perforator dissection performed via 1 cm fascial opening.

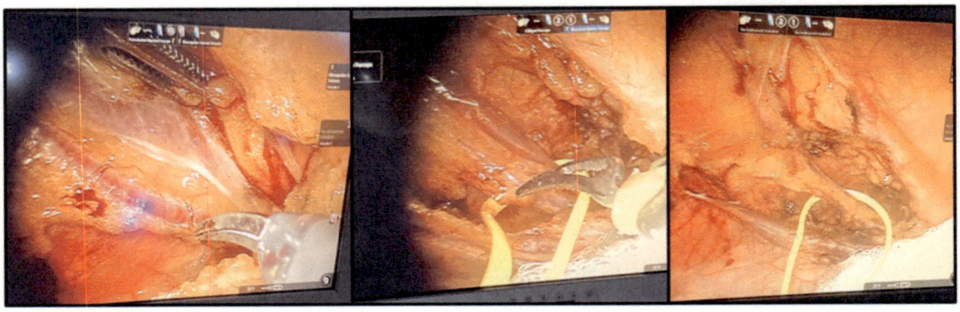

Figure 5.
Robotic mobilization of the deep inferior epigastric inferior vessels.

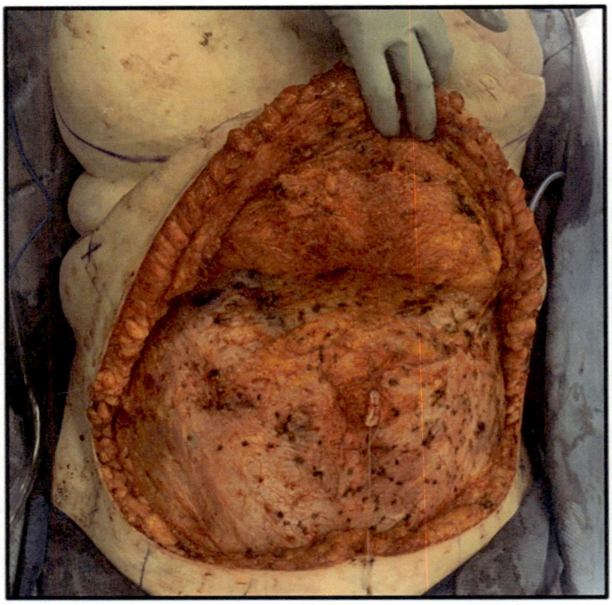

Figure 6.
Abdominal wall after fascial closure following robotic DIEP approach.

presents an aesthetic challenge for many patients. While this may not be avoidable if a fasciocutaneous flap is used, an unsightly scar can be avoided using minimally invasive techniques if a muscle-only flap is desired.

While endoscopic harvest has been attempted, this approach is constrained by the curvature of the chest wall which limits the ability to maintain satisfactory visualization. More recently, several centers have begun to use the surgical robot for muscle-only LD muscle harvest. The first clinical case series was published by Selber et al. in 2013 [22]. To compete the dissection, three robotic ports are used. One may be placed in an already existing axillary incision if concurrent sentinel node biopsy or axillary node dissection is performed. The anterior border of the muscle is marked. The axillary incision is used to identify and isolate the thoracodorsal artery. Using a lighted retractor, the subcutaneous space anterior to the border of the muscle is opened to allow placement of 2 additional ports. The deep surface of the muscle is dissected first followed by the superficial surface. Finally, the inferior and posterior borders of the muscle are released. Once freed, the flap can be brought up through the axillary incision and transposed into the mastectomy space.

Subsequent reports of robotic latissimus flap harvest have been largely positive. A literature review performed in 2020 identified 32 cases in 5 studies of robotically harvested pedicled LD flaps for implant-based breast reconstruction [23]. All cases were completed successfully without conversion to an open approach. Only 1 study compared complication rates in robotic (n = 12) versus open harvest (n = 64). The authors found a lower rate of complications including seroma, infection, delayed wound healing, and capsular contracture in the robotic group although this was not statistically significant [24]. In all studies, patients were noted to have an excellent aesthetic result.

3. Minimally invasive surgery in breast cancer surgery

As reconstructive surgeons have begun to use minimally invasive surgery to minimize donor site morbidity, breast surgeons have also begun to push the envelope to optimize patient aesthetic concerns.

3.1 Robotic mastectomy

In 2016, Toesca et al. in Milan, Italy published the first robotic-assisted nipple sparing mastectomy (rNSM) [25]. Their technique utilized a single port with 4 working channels inserted through a 3 cm incision placed in the midaxillary line within the axillary fossa. Through this single site, the entire gland was dissected and implant-based reconstruction performed in either the subpectoral or prepectoral plane.

Since their initial feasibility and safety study, the Milan group has published their outcomes comparing standard nipple sparing mastectomy (sNSM) to rNSM [26]. They performed a randomized non-blinded clinical trial of patients with breast cancer or a genetic predisposition to cancer who were eligible for NSM by standard criteria. Eighty patients were included, 40 in each group. They found that, while rNSM took on average 78 minutes longer to complete compared to sNSM, there were lower rates of surgical complications in the robotic group although this was not statically significant. No ischemic complications were seen in the robotic group while

2 patients in the sNSM group had nipple alveolar complex (NAC) ischemia and 5 had skin flap necrosis. Additionally, Breast-Q scores reflecting satisfaction with breasts, psychosocial, and physical and sexual well-being were significantly higher in the rNSM group.

Other groups have pioneered similar techniques although the use of the surgical robot for mastectomy remains off-label according to the FDA. In response, an expert panel from the International Endoscopic and Robotic Breast Surgery Symposium released a consensus statement to provide guidance regarding the safe practice of robotic mastectomy [27]. The panel sited advantages to the technique including easy visualization and improved surgeon ergonomics. Disadvantages included prolonged operative time and increased cost and limited availability of the surgical platform. They noted the procedure was safe with notably low NAC necrosis rates. They ultimately produced 12 statements to guide patient selection, technique, and selection of surgical, oncologic, and aesthetic outcomes. They conclude that "robotic mastectomy is a promising technique and could well be the future of minimally invasive breast surgery."

4. Future possibilities

As techniques continue to be refined for both minimally invasive mastectomy and minimally invasive flap harvest, the next natural step may be to combine the two. In 2020, French surgeons published their experience with combined robotic mastectomy and robotic pedicled LD flap harvest [28]. In their cohort, 35 patients underwent both robotic NSM and robotic LD flap harvest. Similar to the technique outlined above, they used a gel mono-trocar device placed via a 4-6 cm incision in the anterior axillary line. They dissected and removed the breast parenchyma then repositioned and used the same incision and trocar to mobilize the latissimus muscle. The muscle was then transposed and appropriately fixated the chest wall within the mastectomy cavity with or without an underlying implant.

Another permutation of this could combine robotic mastectomy with free flap breast reconstruction. A major limitation to this approach is the requirement for the surgical robot to have the capability to perform microvascular anastomosis. Currently, the dominant robotic system, the da Vinci surgical system, has optics and instruments that were not designed for tissue handling at this scale. Recently two robotic systems dedicated to microsurgery have been developed: MUSA by MicroSure and Symani by MMI [29]. These robots have the ability to handle delicate tissue all while eliminating tremor and providing motion scaling. This is a crucial advance, not only for microsurgery, but for the ability to perform supermicrosurgery which is defined as connecting vessels between 0.3 and 0.8 mm, commonly required during lymphedema surgery. Preclinical studies of the MUSA system illustrated that it is possible to use this platform to perform microsurgical anastomosis although overall time for anastomosis completion was longer and dexterity scores were lower using the robot compared to manual microsurgical anastomosis [30].

The first-in-human use of MUSA system to perform supermicrosurgical lymphovenous anastomosis (LVA) for the treatment of lymphedema was reported by a group in the Netherlands in 2020 [31]. They randomized 20 patients to robotic versus manual LVA. In this initial study, time to perform supermicrosurgical anastomosis was shorter in the manual group; however, they did note a steep decline in the time required for robotic-assisted LVA during the course of the study. All LVA's were patent at the end of the procedure. Additionally, no adverse events occurred attributable to use of the surgical robot during the procedure; therefore, the authors concluded that use of the platform for supermicrosurgical anastomosis was feasible and safe. Subsequent studies by other groups using the Symani robot have seen similar promising results [32].

Whether these microsurgical robots will be integrated into simultaneous robotic mastectomy and breast reconstruction remains to be seen. Unlike the da Vinci surgical robot, they were designed to maximize surgeon precision while operating on minute and delicate structures rather than to minimize the invasiveness of the procedure. Thus, in their current iteration, they are ideal for open surgery, but their utility may be limited in a deep body cavity.

5. Conclusions

While initial studies evaluating minimally invasive techniques for breast cancer surgery and breast reconstruction illustrate their feasibility, their use remains controversial. Studies of rNSM consistently report low rates of mastectomy flap compromise and high patient satisfaction, yet the primary goal of the operation is oncologic control. At this time, the number of patients who have undergone this procedure is low and the length of follow-up short. Further studies will be needed to decisively establish the oncologic safety of this approach [33]. Similarly, larger studies and longer follow-up will be required to fully see the effect of minimally invasive flap harvest on donor site morbidity.

Another concern is the cost associated with the use of the surgical robot. This includes the cost of the console, disposable instrumentation, service contracts, and the operative time associated with a longer operative procedure. These costs may be offset by shortened hospital length of stay, but that has yet to be seen in any of the studies cited above. Laparoscopy is less expensive compared to the surgical robot; however, laparoscopy is more difficult in a small operative space as the instruments only provide 4-degrees of freedom of movement compared to the 7-degrees of freedom afforded by the da Vinci platform.

There is a learning curve that will have to be addressed prior to any surgeon attempting to perform these minimally invasive techniques. As most plastic surgery trainees complete integrated residency programs, they seldom encounter cases using laparoscopy or the surgical robot beyond the early years of their training, thus they are unlikely to have the opportunity to become proficient. Even breast surgeons, who must complete a residency in general surgery, may have variable exposure as robotic skills as these are not currently required for board certification unlike laparoscopy and endoscopy. This challenge is not insurmountable as numerous studies have shown rapid skill acquisition and validated tools have been developed to assess robotic microsurgical skill [25, 34].

In summary, minimally invasive breast cancer surgery and breast reconstruction is currently only offered at select centers. Further studies regarding the safety and efficacy of these techniques as well as surgeon training will be required before they are likely to gain widespread adoption. If this occurs, minimally invasive breast cancer surgery and reconstruction can truly serve as the next step in the quest for a further reduction in surgical morbidity and improved patient outcomes beyond the current standard of care.

Conflict of interest

The authors declare no conflict of interest.

Video link

https://youtu.be/kaw-uAXpGuw.

Author details

Elizabeth A. Bailey and Sarah N. Bishop*
Cleveland Clinic Foundation, Cleveland, OH, USA

*Address all correspondence to: bishops@ccf.org

References

[1] Ghossain A, Ghossain MA. History of mastectomy before and after Halsted. J Med Lib. 2009;**57**:65-71

[2] Uroskie TW, Colen LB. History of breast reconstruction. Seminars in Plastic Surgery. 2004;**18**:65-69. DOI: 10.1055/s-2004-829040

[3] Blondeel N, Vanderstraeten GG, Monstrey SJ, et al. The donor site morbidity of free DIEP flaps and free TRAM flaps for breast reconstruction. British Journal of Plastic Surgery. 1997;**50**:322-330. DOI: 10.1016/s0007-1226(97)90540-3

[4] Bonde CT, Lund H, Fridberg M, Danneskiold-Samsoe B, Elberg JJ. Abdominal strength after breast reconstruction using a free abdominal flap. Journal of Plastic, Reconstructive & Aesthetic Surgery. 2007;**60**:519-523. DOI: 10.1016/j.bjps.2006.07.003

[5] Egeberg A, Rasmussen MK, Sørensen JA. Comparing the donor-site morbidity using DIEP, SIEA or MS-TRAM flaps for breast reconstructive surgery: A meta-analysis. Journal of Plastic, Reconstructive & Aesthetic Surgery. 2012;**65**:1474-1480. DOI: 10.1016/j.bjps.2012.07.001

[6] Man LX, Selber JC, Serletti JM. Abdominal wall following free TRAM or DIEP flap reconstruction: A meta-analysis and critical review. Plastic and Reconstructive Surgery. 2009;**124**:752-764. DOI: 10.1097/PRS.0b013e31818b7533

[7] Wu LC, Bajaj A, Chang DW, Chevray PM. Comparison of donor-site morbidity of SIEA, DIEP, and muscle-sparing TRAM flaps for breast reconstruction. Plastic and Reconstructive Surgery. 2008;**122**:702-709. DOI: 10.1097/PRS.0b013e3181823c15

[8] Atisha D, Alderman AK. A systematic review of abdominal wall function following abdominal flaps for postmastectomy breast reconstruction. Annals of Plastic Surgery. 2009;**63**:222-230. DOI: 10.1097/SAP.0b013e31818c4a9e

[9] Selber JC, Nelson J, Fosnot J, et al. A prospective study com-paring the functional impact of SIEA, DIEP, and muscle-spar-ing free TRAM flaps on the abdominal wall: Part I. unilateral reconstruction. Plastic and Reconstructive Surgery. 2010;**126**:1142-1153. DOI: 10.1097/PRS.0b013e3181f02520

[10] Selber JC, Fosnot J, Nelson J, et al. A prospective study com-paring the functional impact of SIEA, DIEP, and muscle-sparing free TRAM flaps on the abdominal wall: Part II. Bilateral reconstruction. Plast Reconstr Surg. 2010;**126**:1438-1453. DOI: 10.1097/PRS.0b013e3181ea42ed

[11] Hembd A, Teotia SS, Zhu H, et al. Optimizing perforator selection: A multivariable analysis of predictors for fat necrosis and abdominal morbidity in DIEP flap breast reconstruction. Plastic and Reconstructive Surgery. 2018;**142**:583-592. DOI: 10.1097/PRS.0000000000004631

[12] Colohan S, Maia M, Langevin CJ, et al. The short- and ultrashort-pedicle deep inferior epigastric artery perforator flap in breast reconstruction. Plastic and Reconstructive Surgery. 2012;**129**(2):331-340. DOI: 10.1097/PRS.0b013e31823ae9a3

[13] Hivelin M, Soprani A, Schaffer N, et al. Minimally invasive laparoscopically

dissected deep inferior epigastric artery perforator flap: An anatomical feasibility study and a first clinical case. Plastic and Reconstructive Surgery. 2018;**141**:33-39. DOI: 10.1097/PRS.0000000000003989

[14] Shakir S, Spencer AB, Kozak GM, et al. Laparoscopically assisted DIEP flap harvest minimizes fascial incision in autologous breast reconstruction. Plastic and Reconstructive Surgery. 2020;**146**(3):265e-275e. DOI: 10.1097/PRS.0000000000007048

[15] Lane T. A short history of robotic surgery. Annals of the Royal College of Surgeons of England. 2018;**100**:5-7. DOI: 10.1308/rcsann.supp1.5

[16] Gundlapalli VS, Ogunleye AA, Scott K, et al. Robotic-assisted deep inferior epigastric artery perforator flap abdominal harvest for breast reconstruction: A case report. Microsurgery. 2018;**38**(6):702-705. DOI: 10.1002/micr.30297

[17] Selber JC. The robotic DIEP flap. Plastic and Reconstructive Surgery. 2020;**145**(2):340-343. DOI: 10.1097/PRS.0000000000006529

[18] Choi JH, Song SY, Park HS, et al. Robotic DIEP flap harvest through a totally Extraperitoneal approach using a single-port surgical robotic system. Plastic and Reconstructive Surgery. 2021;**148**(2):304-307. DOI: 10.1097/PRS.0000000000008181

[19] Manrique OJ, Bustos SS, Mohan AT, et al. Robotic-assisted DIEP flap harvest for autologous breast reconstruction: A comparative feasibility study on a cadaveric model. Journal of Reconstructive Microsurgery. 2020;**36**(5):362-368. DOI: 10.1055/s-0040-1701666

[20] Daar DA, Anzai LM, Vranis NM, et al. Robotic deep inferior epigastric perforator flap harvest in breast reconstruction. Microsurgery. 2022;**42**(4):319-325. DOI: 10.1002/micr.30856

[21] Bailey EA, Chen B, Nelson W, et al. Robotic versus standard harvest of deep inferior epigastric artery perforator flaps: Early outcomes. Plas Reconstr Surg Glob Open. 2022;**10S**:64-65. DOI: 10.1097/01.GOX.0000898644.00762.77

[22] Selber JC, Baumann DP, Holsinger FC. Robotic latissimus dorsi muscle harvest: A case series. Plastic and Reconstructive Surgery. 2012;**129**(6):1305-1312. DOI: 10.1097/PRS.0b013e31824ecc0b

[23] Vourtsis SA, Paspala A, Lykoudis PM, et al. Robotic-assisted harvest of latissimus dorsi muscle flap for breast reconstruction: Review of the literature. Journal of Robotic Surgery. 2022;**16**(1):15-19. DOI: 10.1007/s11701-021-01232-5

[24] Clemens MW, Kronowitz S, Selber JC. Robotic-assisted latissimus dorsi harvest in delayed-immediate breast reconstruction. Seminars in Plastic Surgery. 2014;**28**(1):20-25. DOI: 10.1055/s-0034-1368163

[25] Toesca A, Peradze N, Manconi A, et al. Robotic nipple-sparing mastectomy for the treatment of breast cancer: Feasibility and safety study. Breast. 2017;**31**:51-56. DOI: 10.1016/j.breast.2016.10.009

[26] Toesca A, Sangalli C, Maisonneuve P, et al. A randomized trial of robotic mastectomy versus open surgery in women with breast cancer or BrCA mutation. Annals of Surgery. 2022;**276**(1):11-19. DOI: 10.1097/SLA.0000000000004969

[27] Lai HW, Toesca A, Sarfati B, et al. Consensus statement on robotic

mastectomy-expert panel from international endoscopic and robotic breast surgery symposium (IERBS) 2019. Annals of Surgery. 2020;**271**(6):1005-1012. DOI: 10.1097/SLA.0000000000003789

[28] Houvenaeghel G, Cohen M, Ribeiro SR, et al. Robotic nipple-sparing mastectomy and immediate breast reconstruction with robotic latissimus Dorsi flap harvest: Technique and results. Surgical Innovation. 2020;**27**(5):481-491. DOI: 10.1177/1553350620917916

[29] Innocenti M. Back to the future: Robotic microsurgery. Archives of Plastic Surgery. 2022;**49**(3):287-288. DOI: 10.1055/s-0042-1748020

[30] van Mulken TJM, Boymans CAEM, Schols RM, et al. Preclinical experience using a new robotic system created for microsurgery. Plastic and Reconstructive Surgery. 2018;**142**(5):1367-1376. DOI: 10.1097/PRS.0000000000004939

[31] van Mulken TJM, Schols RM, Scharmga AMJ, et al. First-in-human robotic supermicrosurgery using a dedicated microsurgical robot for treating breast cancer-related lymphedema: A randomized pilot trial. Nature Communications. 2020;**11**(1):757. DOI: 10.1038/s41467-019-14188-w

[32] Lindenblatt N, Grünherz L, Wang A, et al. Early experience using a new robotic microsurgical system for lymphatic surgery. Plastic and Reconstructive Surgery. Global Open. 2022;**10**(1):e4013. DOI: 10.1097/GOX.0000000000004013

[33] Morrow M. Robotic mastectomy: The next major advance in breast cancer surgery? The British Journal of Surgery. 2021;**108**(3):233-234. DOI: 10.1093/bjs/znab010

[34] Selber JC, Alrasheed T. Robotic microsurgical training and evaluation. Seminars in Plastic Surgery. 2014;**28**(1): 5-10. DOI: 10.1055/s-0034-1368161

Chapter 14

Solutions in Breast Reconstruction

Perçin Karakol, Mert Noyan Dabak and Ömer Büyükkaya

Abstract

Breast reconstruction, after cancer surgery, is not only a reconstructive surgery but also an esthetic surgery. No woman should be expected to give up the breast tissue, which is the symbol of female identity, easily. The reconstruction stage after breast cancer is difficult enough in the early and late stages. It is generally not possible to cover the defect and to equalize the two breasts in a single step. General surgery and plastic surgery should work together. Recently, innovative solutions have been offered in breast reconstruction. Starting from skin grafts and local flaps, various flap options, dermal equivalents, fat transfer, and tissue expansion operations are among the options. Breast reconstruction is difficult enough in breasts that have undergone radiotherapy, and reconstruction with autologous tissue is preferred.

Keywords: breast reconstruction, breast surgery, oncoplastic surgery

1. Introduction

Breast reconstruction has become an important part of breast cancer treatment today. Its application with increasing frequency brings with it many innovations. Today, many techniques have been described in breast reconstruction. These techniques range from simple local flaps and implant reconstruction to free tissue transplants. The advantages and disadvantages of each technique bring many discussions on the subject. The timing of treatment is also an important issue of debate. In this study, we aim to present the current treatment options and the latest developments in breast reconstruction.

2. Autologous breast reconstruction

The main purpose of a reconstruction is to restore the damaged tissue as functionally and cosmetically as possible. Satisfactory results can be obtained by using autology tissues to attain this restoration. The main purpose is to restore the lost breast volume in patients who have undergone mastectomy, creating a new NAC if the NAC is not preserved, and creating a breast similar in shape to the other breast. Very satisfactory results can be obtained by using autologous tissues to provide it.

In general, breast-conserving surgery can be recommended for patients having tumors smaller than 3 cm. The treatment option is mastectomy in masses larger than 3 cm [1]. Removal of more than 10% of breast tissue has been determined to be associated with poor cosmetic results. In addition, masses in the central and lower quadrants have also been associated with poor cosmetic results [2]. Therefore, additional procedures may be required in cases in which more than 10–20% of breast tissue is removed.

We can consider our basic options in autologous breast reconstruction under the headings of local options, pedicle tissue transplantation, perforator flaps, and free tissue transplantation.

2.1 Local and pedicled flaps

Restoration by using existing breast tissues can be defined as local option. Breast tissue can be shaped or the missing breast volume can be completed, through local flaps or oncoplastic reduction [2]. Patient satisfaction can be increased by surgical procedures to be applied on the contralateral breast to ensure symmetry.

The first two flaps that come to mind are latissimus dorsi and TRAM flaps when it comes to pedicled flaps in breast reconstruction. The pedicled rectus abdominis muscle-skin flap in breast reconstruction was first described by Hartrampf et al. [3]. In this flap, the rectus abdominis muscle and the skin island on it are transferred to the defected area on the breast tissue over the superior epigastric artery. The biggest handicap of the flap is that the feeding of the superior epigastric artery is not occasionally sufficient [4]. Another handicap of the flap is weakness in the abdominal wall and long-term anterior wall hernias can be observed because the rectus abdominis muscle is used [5]. To overcome this situation, muscle-sparing TRAM flap, techniques in which anterior rectus sheath is preserved [6, 7] and DIEP [8] flaps are described. Studies have demonstrated that DIEP and muscle-sparing TRAM flaps have similar herniation rates [9]. However, there are also publications indicating that the DIEP flap has lower total-partial necrosis rates, and it is more reliable [10].

One of the biggest contraindications of the use of TRAM flap in breast reconstruction is that it got damaged to the internal mammary artery during mastectomy or it got injured previously. The superior epigastric artery is the continuation of this artery [11] and if it is damaged, the use of the superior pedicled rectus abdominis flap will not be possible. Likewise, if there are previous operations in the superior abdomen, it should be carefully investigated whether these arteries are damaged, and if there is damage, other alternatives should be considered.

TRAM flap continues to be a good pedicled tissue transplantation option, especially in patients for whom free tissue transplantation is not considered appropriate, since the tissue volume and skin island it provides are sufficient, it is a well-known and relatively safe flap, and it is simpler and more applicable than free tissue transplants.

Another frequently used option in pedicle tissue transplantation is the latissmus dorsi muscle flap. The flap, first discovered by Iginio Tansini in 1906, still maintains its popularity today [12]. This flap receives its blood supply from the thoracodorsal artery, which is the terminal branch of the subscapular artery [13]. This flap can only be used as a muscle flap or with the skin island on it as a muscle skin flap.

Unlike the TRAM flap in breast defects that require volume due to insufficient soft tissue volume, its use alone does not make it possible to achieve the desired results. That is why this flap is mostly used in combination with breast implants. However, it should not be overlooked that it can provide sufficient volume alone in cases such as small breast resections.

This flap with a pedicle of approximately 11 cm has a sufficient range of motion to close the breast tissues [14]. Another advantage of the flap is that it has a large surface area. The skin island can be designed in different sizes according to the needs [15]. It does not cause significant functional loss when the muscle is sacrificed [16]. It can be a good option for both simultaneous and late repairs.

Today, the frequency of use has decreased along with the development of microsurgery. However, it is still the most important option as a salvage flap in cases in which primary treatment fails. Therefore, it is important to preserve the thoracodorsal artery and the latissimus dorsi muscle as much as possible during breast reconstructions to have a safe second option in case of a possible complication. The fact that the learning curve is simple and it is an applicable flap easily is still a reason to be preferred by many surgeons.

2.2 Perforator flaps

Since it was defined by Koshima and Soeda [17] in 1989, perforator flaps have become one of the most popular topics in plastic surgery and their use is becoming more common day by day. Although its use in breast reconstruction is not as common as pedicled and free tissue transplants, its use in this field is also increasing. The biggest advantage of perforator flaps is that they do not require artery and vein anastomosis compared to free tissue transplants, so the application is easier and safer, and the donor site comorbidities are lower. However, the learning curve is longer than pedicled flaps and the surgical technique is more difficult. As they contain lower volume, they are generally more suitable for partial breast defects. Today, the most commonly used perforator flaps in breast reconstruction are the lateral intercostal artery perforator (LICAP) flap, thoracodorsal artery perforator flap (TDAP), anterior intercostal artery perforator flap (AICAP), and internal mammary artery perforator flap (IMAP) [18].

The LICAP flap is a good alternative, especially for use in lateral breast defects. Contrary to the TDAP flap, it is an important advantage to protect the pedicle of the latissimus dorsi while harvesting the flap. Some patients may have perforators arising from anastomoses between the intercostal artery and the serratus anterior muscle. If these serratus anterior perforators are used, a longer pedicle length can be achieved compared to LICAP [19]. The most dominant lateral intercostal artery perforators are usually observed in the 4–7 intercostal regions [20]. The flap skin island can be modified according to the existing defect, however, the borders of the 6 ribs and the inferior mammarian fold usually constitute the borders of this flap. The perforator is generally located at the level of the sixth rib and 2–3 cm posterior to the anterior axillary line [21]. In some patients, a vascular network consisting of intercostal artery perforators may appear in the dissection area. Pedicle dissection is typically more difficult in such patients [21]. The major disadvantage of the LICAP flap is that the donor site scar is visible in the lateral chest wall [21].

The TDAP flap is the most commonly used perforator flap in breast reconstruction [18]. It was first described in 1995 by Angrigiani et al. [22]. The TDAP flap has the same pedicle as the latissimus dorsi muscle flap. However, since the skin is only lifted over the perforator and the muscle is left intact, donor site complications are less [23]. It is a more difficult surgery compared to the latissimus dorsi flap, and its learning curve is longer than the latissimus dorsi flap. The borders of the latissimus dorsi muscle and the axillary artery are determined for the TDAP flap. Then, the perforators are marked with the help of a handheld doppler, and flaps are designed over the marked perforators. Skin island up to 15×25 cm can be included in the flap [24]. The thoracodorsal artery relatively always divides into two parts horizontal and lateral branches, approximately 4 cm distal to the inferior scapular border and 2.5 cm medial to the lateral border of the latissimus. The perforators leave these branches and reach the skin. Therefore, the design of the skin island on the lateral and upper border of the latissimus muscle facilitates the inclusion of perforators in the skin island while designing the flap [25].

The AICAP flap is harvested over the perforators of the anterior intercostal arteries. It is a relatively new flap. Its use in breast reconstruction was first described by Tenna et al. [26] in 2017. Intercostal artery perforators are commonly found in the thoracic region and supply the thoracic skin. There are more dominant perforators in the lateral thorax region. They were sparser and smaller caliber medially. Anterior intercostal perforators may be sufficient to feed a fasciocutaneous flap [27]. While designing the flap, the donor site scar can be designed to be hidden in the inframammarian fold [28]. In this way, a less visible donor site scar can be obtained. AICAP flap can be preferred especially in medial and inferior quadrant breast defects where LICAP flap is not preferred.

The IMAP flap is harvested over the perforator of the internal mammarian artery. The internal mammarian artery is mostly used as a recipient artery in breast reconstruction with free flaps. The IMAP flap can be lifted in dimensions up to 20 × 13 cm. The perforator emerging from the second intercostal space is usually the most dominant. If this perforator is small, usually one of the 1st and 3rd intercostal perforators is large enough to compensate for this [29]. There are few articles in the literature about IMAP flaps. In current articles, the use of this flap in thoracic wall reconstruction has been discussed [30, 31]. However, IMAP flap is an option that can be considered in medial quadrant defects.

2.3 Free tissue transplantation

With the development of microsurgical techniques and the increase in success rates, free tissue transplants are increasingly used in all areas of reconstruction. Today, one of the most preferred methods of breast reconstruction is free tissue transplantation. The most popular free tissue options for breast reconstruction are DIEP (deep inferior epigastric artery perforator) and TRAM (transverse rectus abdominis muscle) flaps. DIEP flap was described in 1989 by Koshima et al. [17]. Unlike the TRAM flap, its most important advantage is that it does not contain the rectus muscle. It is a less invasive technique because it does not involve the rectus muscle, and it is generally accepted among surgeons that it has lower donor site morbidity [32].

There are very detailed anatomical studies on DIEA perforators [33, 34]. According to these studies, DIEA perforators can be considered medial row and lateral row perforators. Medial row perforators are DIEA perforators that are close to the midline and have a wide perfusion field. These perforators are of a larger caliber than lateral perforators and can feed the contralateral medial half as well as the ipsilateral hemi-abdomen. Lateral row perforators typically lack anastomoses reaching the contralateral region and can feed the ipsilateral hemiabdomen. Therefore, larger DIEP flaps can be harvested by using medial row perforator [35]. Including more than one perforator in the flap may increase the success rate of the flap. It has been observed that fat necrosis is less common in DIEP flaps in which more than one perforator is included [36].

Flap size is another important parameter. As we mentioned earlier, different perforators have different perfusion patterns and are important in determining the boundaries of the flap to be removed. However, it is difficult to determine the exact borders of the flap due to the variations that can be seen in each patient. With the Indocyanine green angiography (SPY Elite System, Novadaq Technologies Inc., Toronto, Canada) method, the perfused parts of the lifted flap can be determined precisely and complications such as partial flap loss and fat necrosis can be prevented in the future [37]. With this method, Regardless of the perforasome concept, perfused flap tissues can be identified and modified as necessary before or after the flap is adapted to the recipient site.

Abdominal tissues are the gold standard in breast reconstruction with free tissue transplantation. However, in some cases, the use of abdominal tissues may not be possible. In such cases, we need to consider alternative flap options.

Superior and inferior gluteal artery perforator flap (SGAP-IGAP) is an important alternative in breast reconstruction. The SGAP flap is a flap that is harvested over the perforator of the superior gluteal artery, which is the terminal branch of the internal iliac artery [38]. These perforators are usually located on the imaginary line drawn from the posterior superior iliac crest to the greater trochanter. Perforators on this line can be found with the help of a handheld doppler and a flap can be designed to contain these perforators. Pedicle length can reach up to 12 cm [39].

The IGAP flap is also raised from the perforators of the inferior gluteal artery. The inferior gluteal artery, like the superior gluteal artery, is the terminal branch of the internal iliac artery. While the superior branch passes superiorly to the piriformis muscle, the inferior branch passes through the inferior border of this muscle [40]. While designing the IGAP flap, care is taken to conceal the donor site scar in the inferior gluteal fold. The perforators in this region are found and marked with the help of a handheld doppler. The flap is then designed so that the scar fits into the inferior gluteal fold and contains the perforators [39].

The most important advantages of these flaps are the absence of donor site scarring in visible areas and low donor site morbidity. Patients can be mobilized in the early period [39, 40]. They have sufficient pedicle length and volume. With all these advantages, the gluteal region is a good alternative to the abdominal region as a donor site.

Profunda femoris perforator flap (PAP) is another alternative for breast reconstruction. The profunda femoris artery passes between the adductor longus and pectineus muscles and reaches the posterior thigh, where it divides into two medial and lateral branches. The perforators of this artery are located on an imaginary line drawn from the ischium to the lateral femoral condyle [41]. While designing the flap, the superior border is drawn 1 cm below the inferior gluteal fold, and the inferior border is drawn approximately 7 cm below it. In this way, the donor site scar can be hidden in the inferior gluteal fold region [42]. The PAP flap is similar to the IGAP flap, but the longer pedicle and larger caliber make microsurgery easier [43].

Lumbar artery perforator (LAP) flap is another option. These perforators emerge between the erector spinal and quadratus lumborum muscles and feed the skin over them. This corresponds to approximately 5–9 cm lateral from the midline [44, 45]. Pedicle length may vary between 4.5 and 7 cm [46]. After deciding on the appropriate perforator, the axis extending from this perforator to the anterior iliac spine forms the axis of our flap, and a flap can be designed on this axis [47]. The pedicle of the flap is shorter than its alternatives, and its caliber is smaller than the internal mammarian artery, which is usually used as the recipient artery. Dissection is relatively challenging. However, donor site morbidity is low and can be removed as a sensate flap [46].

The Transverse Upper Gracilis (TUG) flap is a frequently used DIEP alternative flap. The pedicle of this flap is the gracilis branch, which leaves the profunda femoris artery. The anatomy of this branch is relatively stable and preoperative imaging is not recommended as standard. Dissection is easy. While designing the flap, the superior border of the flap is drawn 1–2 cm inferior to the inguinal crease to hide the donor site scar from the inguinal crease and inferior gluteal crease. Then, according to the pinch test, the inferior border is drawn to allow the primary closure of the donor site [48]. The most important disadvantage of this flap is that it has a higher donor site morbidity than perforator flaps [49].

3. Breast reconstruction with implant

Among the breast reconstruction options after mastectomy, the most commonly used method is implant-based reconstruction (alloplastic). In 2020, approximately 75% of reconstructive breast operations in the USA were performed through an implant [50]. Although the developing technology and surgical techniques have strengthened the surgeon's hand in reconstruction, these developments have also brought many questions to the agenda, such as stages of the operation (direct-two stages), implant type (silicone, saline, round, anatomical, polyurethane coated ...), anatomical plan (total-partial submuscular, prepectoral), and use of ADM. To obtain superior esthetic results and successful surgical results in implant-based breast reconstruction, these questions should be evaluated and planned separately for each patient.

3.1 Direct-to-implant/2 stages

The traditional approach in implant-based breast reconstruction is the two-stage technique. In the first stage, controlled tissue expansion is completed after the placement of a temporary expander. Then, with the second operation, the expander is replaced with a permanent prosthesis. However, in recent years, the single-stage direct-to-implant method has come to the fore with surgical techniques, such as skin and nipple-sparing mastectomy, and especially with technological developments like the discovery of ADM [51]. The reason why this method is popular is the improvement of esthetic results with the use of ADM is the completion of the reconstruction process in one step with the direct placement of the permanent implant in the same session as the mastectomy. It is more cost-effective because it does not require additional surgical sessions [52].

Although the complication rates of the direct-to-implant method were previously thought to be higher, according to recent studies, no significant differences were observed in terms of complications when the two methods were compared [53, 54].

Candidates suitable for direct-to-implant reconstruction are patients with preoperative small-medium-sized symmetrical breasts and those who want the same breast size postoperatively. The most important criterion for a successful direct-to-implant repair is a good and robust blood supply of the skin flaps after mastectomy. If the skin flaps have insufficient blood supply or if a significant change in pre-postop breast size is planned, two-stage reconstruction should be considered [55].

3.2 Anatomical plan and soft tissue support

Preferable placements to place implants or expanders:

Prepectoral (subcutaneous).

Total submuscular.

Partial submuscular (dual plan).

The subpectoral placement was first preferred with the discovery of implants and their use in breast reconstruction [56], but over time due to the excess of major complications such as capsular contracture and implant loss, this was abandoned and the submuscular location was started to be used frequently [57]. In total submuscular placement, the pectoral muscle covers most of the implant, while the serratus muscle and/or fascia covers the lateral of the implant, and the rectus abdominis fascia covers the inferior depending on the need. The leading advantages of this technique include adequate soft tissue support and a well-blooded dressing, but animation deformity, muscle spasm, and associated chronic muscle pain are the negative aspects of total submuscular placement [58].

The discovery of supporting materials such as acellular dermal matrix and mashes made partial submuscular (dual plane) placement possible. After the pectoral muscle is dissected from its inferior and lateral borders and is elevated, the lower and lateral edges of the implant are covered with ADM. This method provides better esthetic results by providing adequate tissue support for the upper pole while allowing adequate expansion of the lower pole (**Figure 1**).

The prepectoral pocket has gained popularity again with the development of highly cohesive implants and ADM/meshes, by obtaining thicker skin flaps with better blood supply after changing mastectomy methods, and with improvements in autologous fat graft techniques [59]. The advantages of prepectoral placement include minimal animation deformity, less implant malposition, and less pain [58].

Although there are many studies on the advantages and disadvantages of pocket selection in the literature, a complete consensus has not been obtained. However,

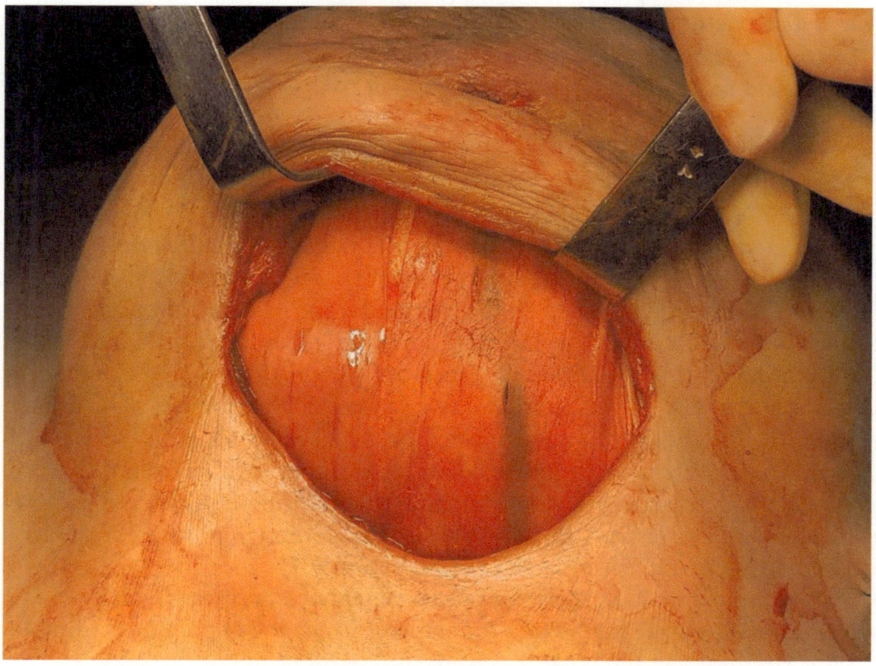

Figure 1.
Acelluler dermal matrix coverage on the inferior pole of the implant.

recent studies indicate that prepectoral pocket selection is similar to submuscular pocket selection in terms of complication rates. In a study by Ostapenko et al., prepectoral placement was demonstrated to be superior to subpectoral in complications such as capsule contracture, implant loss, and animation deformity, while complication rates such as infection, hematoma, and seroma were similar in prepectoral and subpectoral breast reconstructions [60]. According to another study by Bekisz et al., no significant difference was detected in the rates of complications such as skin flap necrosis, minor infection requiring antibiotics, hematoma, and the need for implant replacement in terms of prepectoral, dual plan, and total submuscular pocket choices [61]. According to a comprehensive meta-analysis study by Saldanha et al., the superiority of subpectoral-prepectoral and dual planes to each other in terms of complications could not be demonstrated in implant placement. There was only weak evidence that subpectoral and prepectoral location was associated with infection [62]. It is estimated that the breast reconstruction option with subpectoral implant placement will gradually increase in popularity due to the increase in studies that do not have a significant difference in terms of complications and shorter operation times.

3.3 Acellular dermal matrix

Implant-based breast reconstruction has gained a new concept with the use of biological and synthetic mashes. Acellular dermal matrix (ADM), a type of biological mash, was first used in direct-to-implant breast reconstruction in 2005 and has been increasingly preferred in breast reconstruction surgeries since then [63]. ADM can be used in direct-to-implant or two-stage expander/implant surgeries with submuscular or prepectoral placement. Many studies have indicated that the ADM is used as an inferolateral extension of the pectoralis muscle, by creating additional space and soft tissue support for the implant, filling the gap between the muscle and fascia, and creating a more natural IMF and a more esthetic lower pole [64]. In prepectoral repair, ADM is used to cover the anterior surface of the implant or to cover both the anterior and posterior surfaces of the implant to provide long-term soft tissue support [55].

In a 10-year prospective study by Ellsworth et al., breast reconstruction surgeries performed with ADM and without ADM were compared, and it has been observed that the use of ADM reduces capsular contracture, the amount of seroma is higher in patients who used ADM in the first year, and the rate of seroma between the two groups is similar on the 5th year. However, higher rates of infection were observed in repair with ADM [65]. According to another study, the use of ADM leads to an increase in complications such as infection, implant loss, reoperation, and re-admission to the hospital. Additionally, according to the same study, smoking, high BMI, operation time, and RT history are risk factors that increase complications in ADM use [66]. Another complication that should be known about ADM is Red Breast Syndrome. This syndrome is a clinical condition thought to arise from a hypersensitivity reaction characterized by non-infectious self-limiting erythema in patients undergoing breast reconstruction using ADM [67]. Although it usually resolves with time, it should be well differentiated from infection [67].

As a result, when we look at the literature, potential advantages include creating an additional implant cover, supporting the implant in the lower pole, providing faster expansion, emphasizing the breast contours and borders, and effects on capsule formation [68]. Although there are different findings, one of the most important factors for success in the use of ADM is the right patient selection.

3.4 Implant selection

Breast prostheses are classified as saline/silicone gel according to their content, anatomical/round according to their shape, and smooth/rough/polyurethane-coated according to the sheath properties, and all of them can be used in breast reconstruction. Implant selection is made according to many factors such as desired breast size, pocket dissection, existing soft tissue support, and the dimensions of the contralateral breast if unilateral repair is to be made. Whether anatomical or round-shaped prosthesis will be chosen, the decision should be made by considering the width of the breast base, the shape of the chest wall, and the breast footprint on the chest wall when deciding on the size of the prosthesis, and the pocket dissection should be made to fit the selected implant exactly. This approach is essential for a successful reconstruction with a low complication rate.

Today, except for rare cases, silicon gel implants are generally used. Because anatomical highly cohesive gel implants have a higher ability to resist the forces exerted by the tissue, less rippling is observed [6]. These implants give better esthetic results, especially in prepectoral placement [55]. Many studies are comparing the advantages and disadvantages of anatomical-textured and round-smooth implants. In a prospective study conducted by Khavanin et al. [69], the use of anatomical and round implants in breast reconstruction was compared. According to this study, while the infection rates were found to be higher in patients who used anatomical implants, there was no significant difference between the two implant types in complications such as seroma, hematoma, capsule contracture, and explantation [69]. According to the same study, it has been shown that the use of round implants in unilateral repairs requires more operations to provide symmetry in the contralateral breast [69]. Anatomical implants provide better expansion and contour in the lower pole, better symmetry, and esthetics in the submammary fold, while round implants are better in providing upper pole fullness [70]. In terms of patient satisfaction, anatomical implants came to the fore with their more natural appearance and were evaluated negatively as being stiff and palpable, and round implants were found to be more satisfactory in terms of softness and volume [70]. Although it promises superior esthetic results, the biggest disadvantage of textured implants is the possibility of the development of implant-related anaplastic large cell (BIA-ALCL) lymphoma. This disease, a type of T-cell lymphoma, has been associated with implants with a textured surface [71]. In this disease, which presents symptoms such as late seroma, capsular contracture, pericapsular mass, and LAP, treatment consists of implant removal, mass eradication, capsulectomy, and chemotherapy in addition to surgery in some patients [72].

Another implant option in breast reconstruction is polyurethane-coated implants. The main advantage of polyurethane-coated implants is that the probability of developing capsular contracture is lower than with other implant coatings [73]. It is known that post-mastectomy radiotherapy is particularly associated with capsular contracture, and it has been shown that PU-coated prostheses have a low incidence of capsular contracture in patients receiving radiotherapy [73]. Another advantage of PU-coated prostheses is that they should adhere to the tissue. This is especially advantageous in breast reconstruction surgeries with prepectoral implants, in fixing the implant to the chest wall without the need for extra mechanical support [74]. As a result, although each implant type has advantages and disadvantages, the patient should be informed about the implant and the decision should be made by discussing it with each patient within the framework of expectations, possible adjuvant theory, and patient characteristics.

3.5 Tissue expanders

Reconstruction with the two-stage expander/implant method after mastectomy is the most commonly used breast reconstruction method [50]. In conventional tissue expanders, expansion is based on the inflation of the expander by serial percutaneous saline injections. This procedure, which can be performed in outpatient conditions, is uncomfortable for the patient, requires frequent hospital visits, and increases the susceptibility to infection. However, a new tissue expander system based on CO_2 has received FDA approval. In this system, the patient provides controlled inflation without the need for a needle by triggering the release of CO_2 from an internal reservoir with a wireless system with a remote control [75]. This new system has been shown to reduce the number of visits, the time required for full expansion, and the complication rates [75].

3.6 Conclusion

Implant-based breast reconstruction is still the most commonly used breast reconstruction method and will continue to be popular. It is possible to achieve all the aims of the reconstruction more esthetically, while changes are occurring in the surgical approaches established with the developing surgical techniques and medical devices.

3.7 Tissue engineering

Mastectomy and any surgical procedure that causes deformity in the breast leads to the idea that the woman is psychologically less sexual. The method of reducing this load is to provide reconstruction with a tissue close to the normal contour in form.

Tissue engineering and cell-based breast reconstruction options, when combined with surgery, are pleasing to the patient and physician.

It is especially enriched with stem cells and stromal vascular fraction (SVF), increasing the permanence of the fat, SVF; endothelial stem cells include pluripotent vascular progenitor cells, preadipocytes, and macrophages. Increasing skin quality with repeated applications is a desired result, especially in thinned skin after tissue expanders. It is a big problem that after the prosthesis, especially in breasts receiving radiotherapy, unwanted, third- and fourth-degree contractions around the prosthesis, impaired healing, lymphedema, and mastectomy flaps disrupt circulation and cause necrosis. For these reasons, cases of implant exposure are very common (**Figure 2**). In this way, it is possible to maintain the breast contour and keep the prosthesis in the proper position after the permanent implant is placed [76, 77].

As it is known, it is not always possible to replace a tissue loss with autologous tissue. The idea of reproducing that tissue using autologous cells was based on complications such as donor site problems and capsule contraction. In cases where reconstruction cannot be planned with sufficient and appropriate autologous tissue, products that resemble tissues and replace damaged tissue are used with innovative tissue engineering. The microenvironment and extracellular matrix (ECM) are important for stem cells [78]. In terms of ECM, platelet rich plasma (PRP) contains especially sufficient growth factors. In summary, with the signaling of growth factors, proliferation and differentiation between cells begin. Aside from the use of recombinant proteins as scaffolds in tissue engineering, it is only possible in cellular-based productions without a scaffold [79]. Cellular-only approaches without a biocompatible scaffold have a low chance of success [77]. Because, with the ideal scaffold

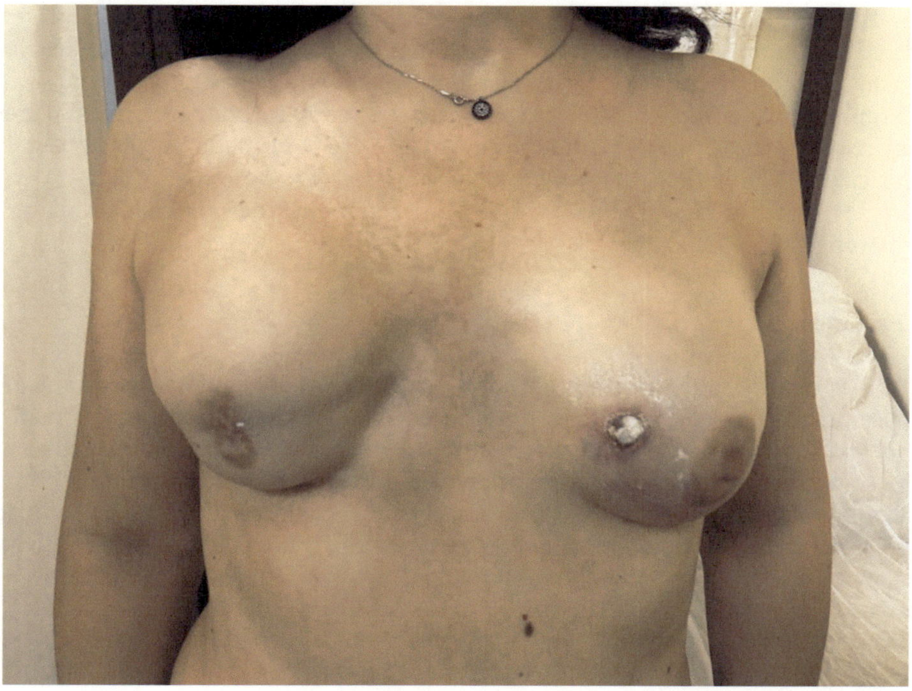

Figure 2.
Exposed implant on the left breast.

selection, natural tissues can be created that accurately mimic tissue in vivo, allow vascular ingrowth, and allow a porous and 3-dimensional microenvironment. In this way, biomaterials that remain intact until tissue is formed for a sufficient period but degrade at the appropriate time can be developed [77, 80]. Degradation must occur at the right time for tissue regeneration and the formation of new ECM [81].

Biomaterials can be obtained not only from humans but also from animal or natural sources. They are distinguished from synthetic materials in that they are incorporated into the host tissue during the natural degradation process. The main task of biomaterials is to act as a biophysical and chemical medium to enable cellular response. As biocompatibility increases, biointegration and vascularization increase. In the same environment, cells adhere, multiply, and differentiate appropriately. Anti-inflammatory cytokines are still released but result in a minimal foreign body reaction [82, 83]. Natural biomaterials used in adipose tissue engineering are primarily silk, alginate, collagen, and gelatin. Natural biomaterials can be combined with various biomaterials and their mechanical properties can be formed with different forms of cross-linking. Among the synthetic biomaterials, polyglycolic acid, polylactic acid, and polycaprolactone can be listed [83]. It is easy to add ECM and growth factors to synthetic components, so their use in tissue engineering is gaining momentum. Scaffolds in general; hydrogels, sponges, bioprinted or 3D structures, or electrospun scaffolds [83, 84]. The fact that the scaffold is hard is important in terms of providing structural integrity and imitating the natural tissue it has changed and being porous in terms of removing cellular wastes. The biggest problem in scaffolds consisting of synthetic components is the removal of harmful by-products formed after decomposition. Therefore, hybrid scaffold models containing both synthetic and natural components have been recently started to be studied to benefit from the strengths of both sides. Biological interactions are required to facilitate the natural secretion of proteases and cell migration [85]. Studies are showing that there may be a connection between these mechanical properties of scaffold and mesenchymal cell differentiation.

Nipple areolar complex (NAC), reconstruction; women's body image and patient satisfaction are more difficult, and the advantages of 3D-printed NAC have been emphasized recently [86]. In terms of adipose tissue regeneration, especially hydrogels are advantageous because their ability to mimic the extracellular matrix is very strong [80, 87].

3.8 Fat injection

As it is known, breast tissue is a common component of glandular tissue and adipose tissue. The most important problem encountered in replacing the formed defect with only fat is the inability to maintain resorption and adequate volume. Adipose-derived stem cell (ADSC) is widely used in breast reconstruction for both the awakening of autologous tissue sensation and contour correction after implant placement. When fat is enriched with ADSC, these cells can transform into new adipocytes, thus producing biocompatible, nonimmunological tissues. Likewise, studies are showing that the addition of SVF further increases angiogenesis in terms of interaction between endothelial precursor cells (**Figures 3–6**) [80, 88].

Studies continue to determine whether these cells increase the risk and recurrence of cancer with their secondary paracrine and autocrine effects after fat injection into the breast, which has become increasingly popular because it is more physiological [76, 78]. Insufficient follow-up time and the lack of clinical cases due to biases are among the study barriers.

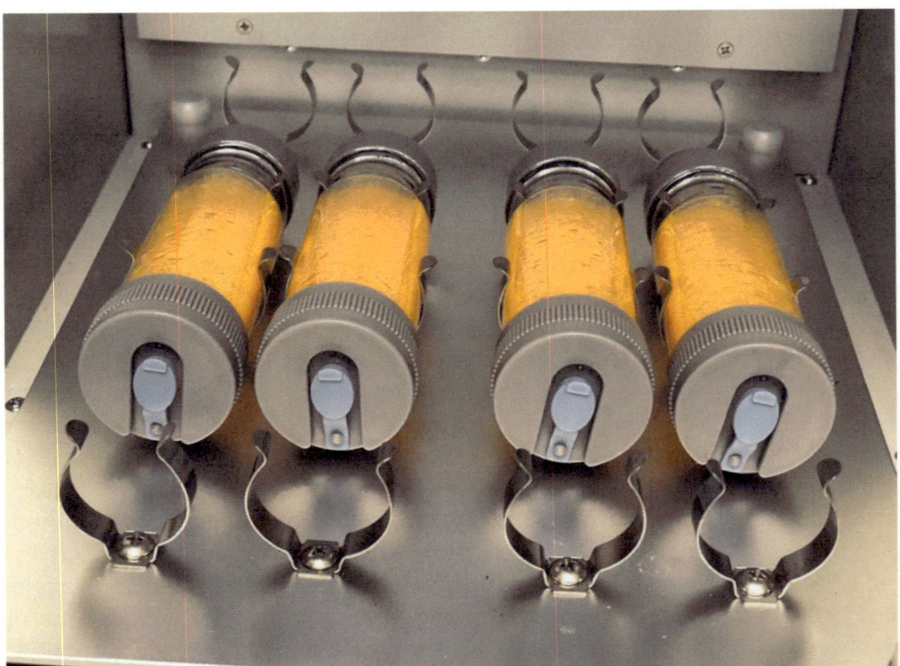

Figure 3.
Fat ready for injection after centrifugation.

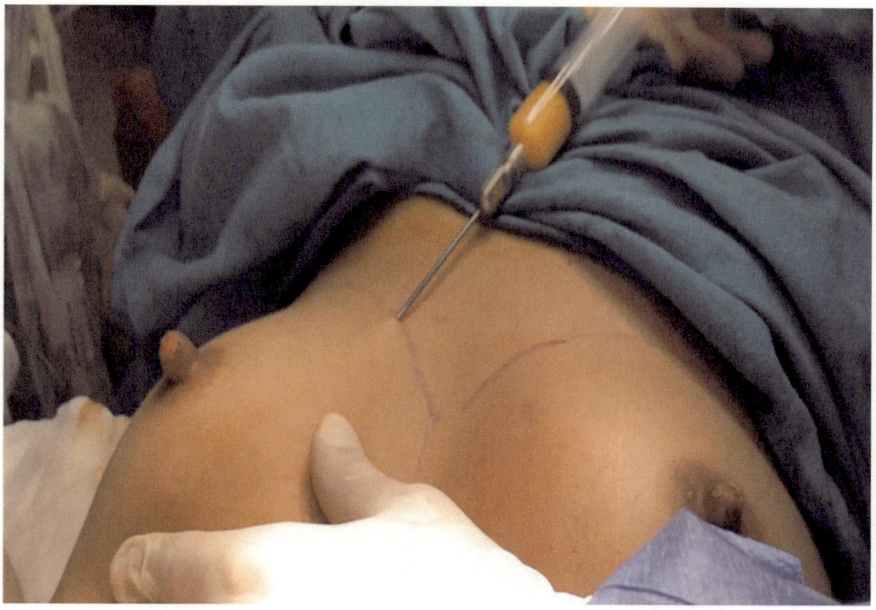

Figure 4.
Fat injection into the breast.

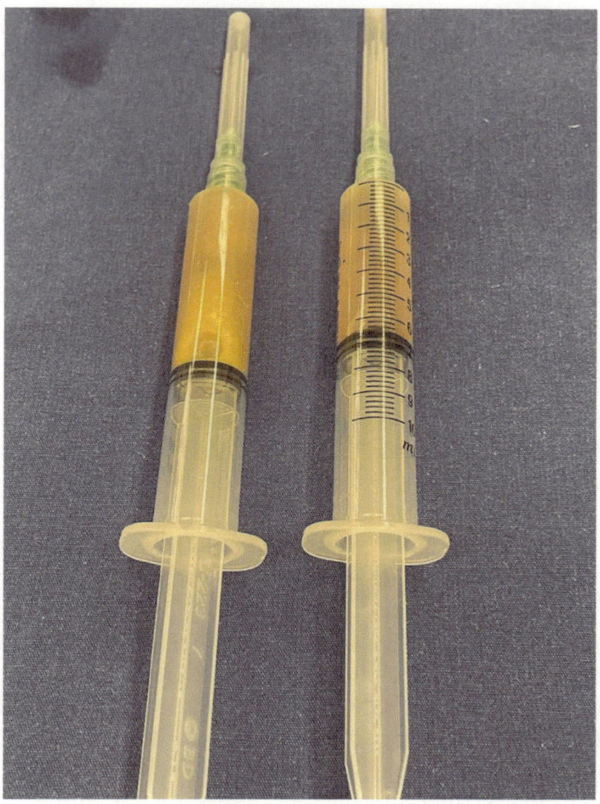

Figure 5.
Fat enriched with the stromal vascular fraction.

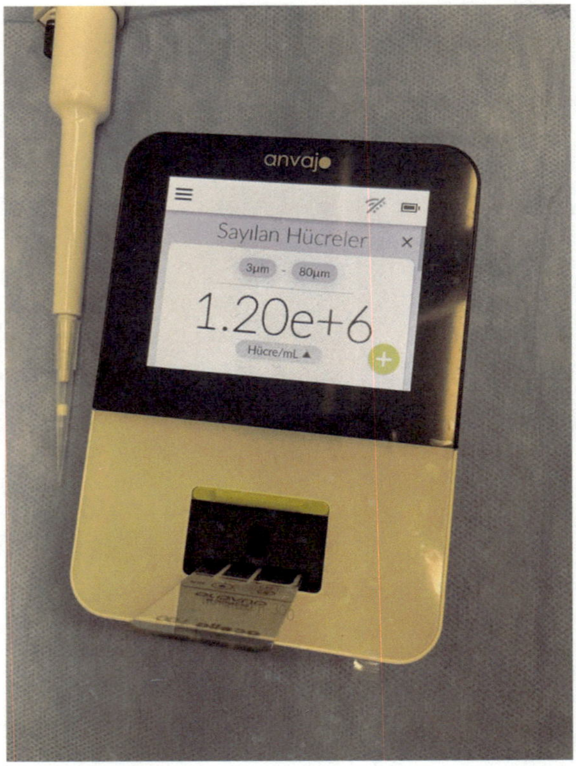

Figure 6.
Cell counter device.

It is accepted that fat injection should be done in the form of repetitive injections, rather than a sufficient amount in a single session in breast reconstruction. It should be kept in mind that the formation of sebaceous cysts and microcalcifications after excessive injections may lead to misleading results in the follow-up of malignancy [76, 80, 89].

3.9 Acellular dermal matrix

The main use of ADM in breast reconstruction is to provide more support and to minimize ripling and implant exposure. Especially in post-tissue expander implant applications, wrapping the implant with ADM reduces the frequency of complications compared to the traditional technique.

The aim is to improve scaffold fabrication techniques, increase tissue similarity and compatibility, and find inexpensive means of obtaining and selling. In this way, the frequency of use can be increased.

Concurrent contralateral mastectomy rates have also increased with breast-conserving surgery. In general, the favorite approach is to place the implant in the pouch designed in the subpectoral plane, still in the reconstruction phase. In this way, while sufficient muscle tissue covers the upper pole of the implant, the implant contacts the skin at the inferior pole, and after a while, the expansion mechanism thins the skin and prepares the ground for exposure [90]. In addition to the development of implant technologies in recent years, the use of ADM has decreased the exposure rate by increasing the safety of the implanted pouch. At the same time, it supports single-session approaches by providing contour regularity [91]. Closing the subpectorally placed implants by suturing ADM to the inferior wall of the pectoral muscle provided more esthetically meaningful results. Another advantage of ADM in

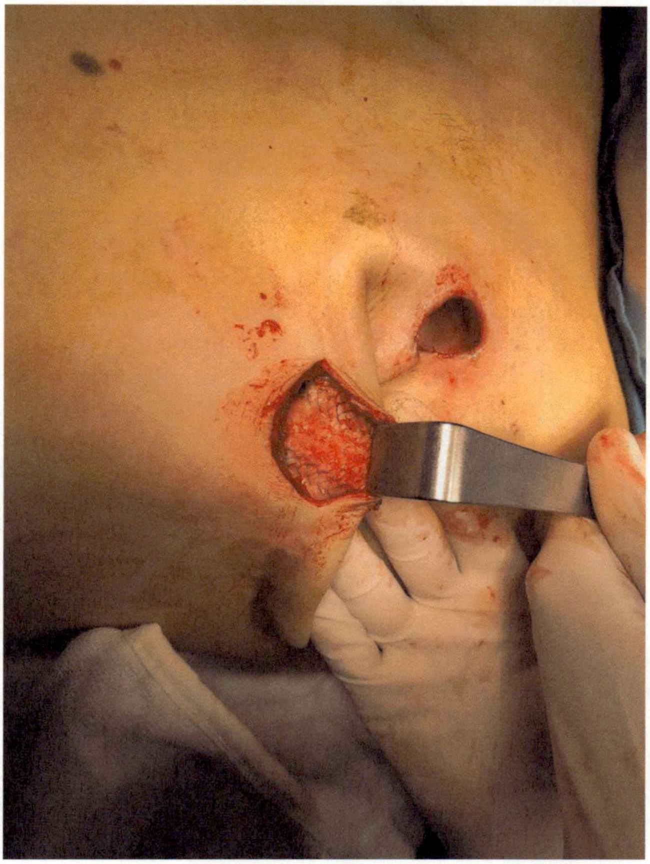

Figure 7.
Prevention of expansion with polypropylene mesh.

Product	Material	Company	FDA
Alloderm	Human	Life Cell Corp.	Approved
Allomax	Human	CR Bard/Davol Inc.	Not approved
Dermacell	Human	LifeNet Health Inc.	Not approved
Flex HD	Human	Ethicon Inc	Approved
Permacol	Porcine	Medtronic	Approved
Strattice	Porcine	Allergan	Approved
Surgimend	Bovine	Integra Life Scienes	Approved
Veritas	Bovine	Synovis	Approved
Vicryl Mesh	Polyglactin	Ethicon Inc	Approved

Table 1.
ADM products in breast reconstruction.

breast reconstruction is improved tissue expansion and increased volume. In addition, ADM itself can produce a fibrotic reaction. Studies on the reasons for this focus on dead space between the flap and ADM, formation of seroma, placement in an infected area, or insufficient perfusion [84]. In titanium-coated polypropylene meshes, the chance of tissue expansion is lower due to the stretch of the polypropylene (**Figure** 7) (**Table 1**).

4. Conclusion

After breast cancer and nipple-sparing surgical approaches became active, cosmetic expectations have increased even more. The introduction of ADM, especially in the sense of emergency breast reconstruction, has been groundbreaking. Despite its complications such as infection and seroma, ADM is successful in its use with well-fed flaps that cover it. The main problem is economic, although it is human-induced, which is more flexible in the choice of ADM.

In terms of psychological recovery and patient satisfaction, the use of ADM and biomaterials among the reconstruction options close to breast normal tissue and appearance is becoming more common with contributions to the literature. It is possible to contribute to breast volume and increase skin quality in the early and late periods with fat injection into the breast. What is discussed at this stage is what can be done additionally for fat survival.

3D printer technology aims to produce serial and personalized bioprints at low cost and to make them widely used in clinics. With biomaterials produced in this way, it may be possible to minimize volume loss by increasing the vitality and vascularity of fat cells injected for breast reconstruction.

5. Reconstruction: when and how?

One of the most controversial issues in reconstructions after breast cancer diagnosis is the timing of surgery. In any case, the most important issue to be considered is that the patient can start oncological treatment as soon as possible if needed. It is recommended to start adjuvant radiotherapy within 8–12 weeks after the surgery. Late radiotherapy is determined to have a risk of recurrence [92].

This situation leads us to the following question: Would the reconstruction be performed together with tumor surgery or the reconstruction after the completion of oncological treatment (especially chemoradiotherapy) would be more appropriate?

The most important factor in choosing early or late treatment is whether the patient needs radiotherapy or not. Some of the publications in the literature state that the complication and success rates in patients who underwent simultaneous repair and received RT are close to or at an acceptable level when compared to late repair [93–96]. There are some publications stating that early repair has more successful results [97]. However, many publications show that simultaneous repair is associated with a higher risk of complications than late repair in patients who will receive radiotherapy [98–101].

When the advantages of early treatment are stated, one of these advantages is that it does not require additional surgery, and it is a relatively easy surgery because it is performed before the tissue damage is caused by radiotherapy. The most important disadvantages are that a possible complication may delay the patient's receiving radiotherapy and additional complications may occur with radiotherapy. The general belief is that although there may be a delay in initiating RT treatment due to complications from time to time, the simultaneous repair usually does not cause a delay in initiating RT [102]. Simultaneous repair may be a good alternative, especially when autologous reconstruction options are preferred [93, 96].

The biggest advantage of the delayed treatment is that RT treatment has been completed and the reconstruction can be spread throughout the process. The most important problem is that the tissues damaged after RT make surgery significantly more difficult, and patients who have had mastectonia spend a long time until they have definitive reconstructive surgery.

In the statement published by the Oncoplastic Breast Consortium [103], some current recommendations were included.

If late repair is performed, definitive surgery should be performed at least 6–12 months later.

Waiting 6–12 months for fat graft applications.

Concomitant repair may affect the onset of RT in some patients, however, it generally does not cause a delay in the onset of therapy.

RT is not an absolute contraindication for simultaneous implant repair, but it has a higher risk of complications.

The fact that the patient will receive chemotherapy is another factor affecting the chance of success. Different chemotherapeutic drugs have been demonstrated to have different complication rates [104].

If the patient has advanced breast cancer such as inflammatory breast cancer, it would be better for patient safety to wait at least 1 year from the completion of treatment and confirm that there is no recurrence [105].

Many surgeons also have reservations about fat graft applications. The idea that the adipose stem cells contained in the fat graft may stimulate the proliferation of cancer cells makes many surgeons hesitant in the application of fat grafts. However, studies indicate that fat graft applications do not increase recurrence and metastasis [106].

Another drawback of fat grafting is that it may complicate the radiological follow-up of the patient. However, in general, the abnormal radiological images encountered in these patients are observed far from areas containing fat grafts, and it is most likely due to changes that occur as a result of surgery rather than fat grafting [107].

Conflict of interest

The authors declare no conflict of interest.

Author details

Perçin Karakol*, Mert Noyan Dabak and Ömer Büyükkaya
Department of Plastic, Reconstructive and Aesthetic Surgery, SBÜ Hamidiye Etfal Training Hospital, İstanbul, Turkey

*Address all correspondence to: ppercin@gmail.com

References

[1] Cochrane RA, Valasiadou P, Wilson ARM, Al-Ghazal SK, Macmillan RD. Cosmesis and satisfaction after breast-conserving surgery correlates with the percentage of breast volume excised. Journal of British Surgery. 2003;**90**(12):1505-1509

[2] Losken A, Smearman EL, Hart AM, Broecker JS, Carlson GW, Styblo TM. The impact oncoplastic reduction has on long-term recurrence in breast conservation therapy. Plastic and Reconstructive Surgery. 2022;**149**(5): 867e-875e

[3] Hartrampf CR, Scheflan M, Black PW. Breast reconstruction with a transverse abdominal island flap. Plastic and Reconstructive Surgery. Feb 1982; **69**(2):216-225

[4] Moon HK, Taylor GI. The vascular anatomy of rectus abdominis musculocutaneous flaps based on the deep superior epigastric system. Plastic and Reconstructive Surgery. 1988;**82**(5): 815-829

[5] Kroll SS, Schusterman MA, Reece GP, Miller MJ, Robb G, Evans G. Abdominal wall strength, bulging, and hernia after TRAM flap breast reconstruction. Plastic and Reconstructive Surgery. 1995;**96**(3): 616-619

[6] Erni D, Harder YD. The dissection of the rectus abdominis myocutaneous flap with complete preservation of the anterior rectus sheath. British Journal of Plastic Surgery. 2003;**56**(4): 395-400

[7] Nahabedian MY, Dooley W, Singh N, Manson PN. Contour abnormalities of the abdomen after breast reconstruction with abdominal flaps: The role of muscle preservation. Plastic and Reconstructive Surgery. 2002;**109**(1):91-101

[8] Allen RJ, Treece P. Deep inferior epigastric perforator flap for breast reconstruction. Annals of Plastic Surgery. 1994;**32**(1):32-38

[9] Espinosa-de-Los-Monteros A, Frias-Frias R, Alvarez-Tostado-Rivera A, Caralampio-Castro A, Llanes S, Saldivar A. Postoperative abdominal bulge and hernia rates in patients undergoing abdominally based autologous breast reconstruction: Systematic review and meta-analysis. Annals of Plastic Surgery. 2021;**86**(4): 476-484

[10] Man LX, Selber JC, Serletti JM. Abdominal wall following free TRAM or DIEP flap reconstruction: A meta-analysis and critical review. Plastic and Reconstructive Surgery. 2009;**124**(3): 752-764

[11] Miller LB, Bostwick J III, Hartrampf CR, Hester TR, Nahai F. The superiorly based rectus abdominis flap: Predicting and enhancing its blood supply based on an anatomic and clinical study. Plastic and Reconstructive Surgery. 1988;**81**(5):711-712

[12] Tansini I. Sopra il mio nuovo processo di amputazione della mammella. Gazzetta Medica Italiana. 1906;**57**(57):141

[13] Schneider WJ, Hill HL Jr, Brown RG. Latissimus dorsi myocutaneous flap for breast reconstruction. British Journal of Plastic Surgery. 1977;**30**(4):277-281

[14] Bartlett SP, May JW Jr, Yaremchuk MJ. The latissimus dorsi muscle: A fresh cadaver study of the

primary neurovascular pedicle. Plastic and Reconstructive Surgery. 1981;**67**(5): 631-636

[15] Pacella SJ, Vogel JE, Locke MB, Codner MA. Aesthetic and technical refinements in latissimus dorsi implant breast reconstruction: A 15-year experience. Aesthetic Surgery Journal. 2011;**31**(2):190-199

[16] Sood R, Easow JM, Konopka G, Panthaki ZJ. Latissimus dorsi flap in breast reconstruction: Recent innovations in the workhorse flap. Cancer Control. 2018;**25**(1):1073

[17] Koshima I, Soeda S. Inferior epigastric artery skin flaps without rectus abdominis muscle. British Journal of Plastic Surgery. 1989;**42**(6):645-648

[18] Chartier C, Safran T, Alhalabi B, Murphy A, Davison P. Locoregional perforator flaps in breast reconstruction: An anatomic review & quadrant algorithm. Journal of Plastic, Reconstructive & Aesthetic Surgery. Apr 2022;**75**(4):1328-1341

[19] Hamdi M, Spano A, van Landuyt K, D'Herde K, Blondeel P, Monstrey S. The lateral intercostal artery perforators: Anatomical study and clinical application in breast surgery. Plastic and Reconstructive Surgery. 2008;**121**(2): 389-396

[20] Jeon EY, Cho YK, Yoon DY, Seo YL, Lim KJ, Yun EJ. Angiographic analysis of the lateral intercostal artery perforator of the posterior intercostal artery: Anatomic variation and clinical significance. Diagnostic and Interventional Radiology. 2015;**21**(5):415

[21] Kim JB, Eom JR, Lee JW, Lee J, Park HY, Yang JD. Utility of two surgical techniques using a lateral intercostal artery perforator flap after breast-conserving surgery: A single-center retrospective study. Plastic and Reconstructive Surgery. 2019;**143**(3): 477e-487e

[22] Angrigiani C, Grilli D, Siebert J. Latissimus dorsi musculocutaneous flap without muscle. Plastic and Reconstructive Surgery. 1995;**96**(7): 1608-1614

[23] Gatto A, Parisi P, Brambilla L, Simonelli I, Vestri A, Torto FL, et al. Thoracodorsal artery perforator flap, muscle-sparing latissimus dorsi, and descending-branch latissimus dorsi: A multicenter retrospective study on early complications and meta-analysis of the literature. Journal of Plastic, Reconstructive & Aesthetic Surgery. Nov 2022;**75**(11):3979-3996

[24] Thomas BP, Geddes CR, Tang M, Williams J, Morris SF. The vascular basis of the thoracodorsal artery perforator flap. Plastic and Reconstructive Surgery. 2005;**116**(3):818-822

[25] Heitmann C, Guerra A, Metzinger SW, Levin LS, Allen RJ. The thoracodorsal artery perforator flap: Anatomic basis and clinical application. Annals of Plastic Surgery. 2003;**51**(1): 23-29

[26] Tenna S, Brunetti B, Coppola MM, Persichetti P. The anterior intercostal artery perforator flap: Clinical applications in partial breast reconstruction. Plastic and Reconstructive Surgery. 2017;**140**(5): 746e-747e

[27] Carrasco-López C, Ibañez JFJ, Vilà J, Rodriguez-Baeza A, Carrera-Burgaya A, Reina-De-La-Torre F, et al. The anterior intercostal artery flap: Anatomical and radiologic study. Plastic and Reconstructive Surgery. 2017; **139**(3):613e-619e

[28] Adler N, Carmon E, Chapchay K, Billig A. Anterior intercostal artery perforator flap for immediate reconstruction following breast conservation surgery. Microsurgery. Jan 2023;**43**(1):20-26

[29] Schmidt M, Aszmann OC, Beck H, Frey M. The anatomic basis of the internal mammary artery perforator flap: A cadaver study. Journal of Plastic, Reconstructive & Aesthetic Surgery. 2010;**63**(2):191-196

[30] Faini G, Pierazzi DM, Arleo S, Calabrese S, Alfieri EP, Cigna E. Internal mammary artery perforator flap for anterior thoracic and upper abdominal wall reconstruction: 16 case series. Journal of Plastic, Reconstructive & Aesthetic Surgery. 2022;**75**(7):2387-2440

[31] Koulaxouzidis G, Orhun A, Stavrakis T, Witzel C. Second intercostal internal mammary artery perforator (IMAP) fasciocutaneous flap as an alternative choice for the treatment of deep sternal wound infections (DSWI). Journal of Plastic, Reconstructive & Aesthetic Surgery. 2015;**68**(9):1262-1267

[32] Tokumoto H, Akita S, Arai M, Kubota Y, Kuriyama M, Mitsukawa N. A comparison study of deep muscle sparing transverse rectus abdominis musculocutaneous flap for breast reconstruction. Microsurgery. 2019; **39**(7):583-589

[33] Schaverien M, Saint-Cyr M, Arbique G, Brown SA. Arterial and venous anatomies of the deep inferior epigastric perforator and superficial inferior epigastric artery flaps. Plastic and Reconstructive Surgery. 2008; **121**(6):1909-1919

[34] Rozen WM, Ashton MW, le Roux CM, Pan W, Corlett RJ. The perforator angiosome: A new concept in the design of deep inferior epigastric artery perforator flaps for breast reconstruction. Microsurgery. 2010; **30**(1):1-7

[35] Wong C, Saint-Cyr M, Mojallal A, Schaub T, Bailey SH, Myers S, et al. Perforasomes of the DIEP flap: Vascular anatomy of the lateral versus medial row perforators and clinical implications. Plastic and Reconstructive Surgery. 2010;**125**(3):772-782

[36] Li Y, Long X. Optimizing perforator selection: A multivariable analysis of predictors for fat necrosis and abdominal morbidity in DIEP flap breast reconstruction. Plastic and Reconstructive Surgery. 2019;**143**(6): 1307e-1308e

[37] Ludolph I, Bettray D, Beier JP, Horch RE, Arkudas A. Leaving the perfusion zones? Individualized flap design in 100 free DIEP and ms-TRAM flaps for autologous breast reconstruction using indocyanine green angiography. Journal of Plastic, Reconstructive & Aesthetic Surgery. 2022;**75**(1):52-60

[38] Allen RJ, Tucker C Jr. Superior gluteal artery perforator free flap for breast reconstruction. Plastic and Reconstructive Surgery. 1995;**95**(7): 1207-1212

[39] Zoccali G, Mughal M, Giwa L, Roblin P, Farhadi J. Breast reconstruction with superior gluteal artery perforator free flap: 8 years of experience. Journal of Plastic, Reconstructive & Aesthetic Surgery. 2019;**72**(10):1623-1631

[40] Guerra AB, Metzinger SE, Bidros RS, Gill PS, Dupin CL, Allen RJ. Breast reconstruction with gluteal artery perforator (GAP) flaps: A critical

analysis of 142 cases. Annals of Plastic Surgery. 2004;**52**(2):118-125

[41] Ahmadzadeh R, Bergeron L, Tang M, Geddes CR, Morris SF. The posterior thigh perforator flap or profunda femoris artery perforator flap. Plastic and Reconstructive Surgery. 2007;**119**(1):194-200

[42] Allen RJ, Haddock NT, Ahn CY, Sadeghi A. Breast reconstruction with the profunda artery perforator flap. Plastic and Reconstructive Surgery. 2012;**129**(1):16e-23e

[43] Murphy DC, Razzano S, Wade RG, Haywood RM, Figus A. Inferior gluteal artery perforator (IGAP) flap versus profunda artery perforator (PAP) flap as an alternative option for free autologous breast reconstruction. Journal of Plastic, Reconstructive & Aesthetic Surgery. 2022;**75**(3):1100-1107

[44] Myers PL, Nelson JA, Allen RJ Jr. Alternative flaps in autologous breast reconstruction. Gland Surgery. 2021; **10**(1):444

[45] Offman SL, Geddes CR, Tang M, Morris SF. The vascular basis of perforator flaps based on the source arteries of the lateral lumbar region. Plastic and Reconstructive Surgery. 2005;**115**(6):1651-1659

[46] Peters KT, Blondeel PN, Lobo F, van Landuyt K. Early experience with the free lumbar artery perforator flap for breast reconstruction. Journal of Plastic, Reconstructive & Aesthetic Surgery. 2015;**68**(8):1112-1119

[47] de Weerd L, Elvenes OP, Strandenes E, Weum S. Autologous breast reconstruction with a free lumbar artery perforator flap. British Journal of Plastic Surgery. 2003;**56**(2): 180-183

[48] Dayan JH, Allen RJ Jr. Lower extremity free flaps for breast reconstruction. Plastic and Reconstructive Surgery. 2017;**140**(5S): 77S-86S

[49] Craggs B, Vanmierlo B, Zeltzer A, Buyl R, Haentjens P, Hamdi M. Donor-site morbidity following harvest of the transverse myocutaneous gracilis flap for breast reconstruction. Plastic and Reconstructive Surgery. 2014;**134**(5): 682e-691e

[50] Statistics P. American Society of Plastic Surgeons. Plastic Surgery Statistics Report. 2018

[51] Chun YS, Verma K, Rosen H, Lipsitz S, Morris D, Kenney P, et al. Implant-based breast reconstruction using acellular dermal matrix and the risk of postoperative complications. Plastic and Reconstructive Surgery. 2010;**125**(2):429-436

[52] Krishnan NM, Fischer JP, Basta MN, Nahabedian MY. Is single-stage prosthetic reconstruction cost effective? A cost-utility analysis for the use of direct-to-implant breast reconstruction relative to expander-implant reconstruction in postmastectomy patients. Plastic and Reconstructive Surgery. 2016;**138**(3):537-547

[53] Srinivasa DR, Garvey PB, Qi J, Hamill JB, Kim HM, Pusic AL, et al. Direct-to-implant versus two-stage tissue expander/implant reconstruction: 2-year risks and patient-reported outcomes from a prospective, multicenter study. Plastic and Reconstructive Surgery. 2017;**140**(5):869

[54] Dimovska EOF, Chen C, Chou H, Lin Y, Cheng M. Outcomes and quality of life in immediate one-stage versus two-stage breast reconstructions without an acellular dermal matrix: 17-years of

experience. Journal of Surgical Oncology. 2021;**124**(4):510-520

[55] Colwell AS, Taylor EM. Recent advances in implant-based breast reconstruction. Plastic and Reconstructive Surgery. 2020;**145**(2): 421e-432e

[56] Snyderman RK, Guthrie RH. Reconstruction of the female breast following radical mastectomy. Plastic and Reconstructive Surgery. 1971;**47**(6): 565-567

[57] Weinzierl A, Schmauss D, Brucato D, Harder Y. Implant-based breast reconstruction after mastectomy, from the subpectoral to the prepectoral approach: An evidence-based change of mind? Journal of Clinical Medicine. 2022; **11**(11):3079

[58] Kraenzlin F, Chopra K, Kokosis G, Venturi ML, Mesbahi A, Nahabedian MY. Revision breast reconstruction with prepectoral pocket conversion of submuscular breast implants. Plastic and Reconstructive Surgery. 2021;**147**(5):743e-748e

[59] ter Louw RP, Nahabedian MY. Prepectoral breast reconstruction. Plastic and Reconstructive Surgery. 2017;**140** (5S):51S-59S

[60] Ostapenko E, Nixdorf L, Devyatko Y, Exner R, Wimmer K, Fitzal F. Prepectoral versus subpectoral implant-based breast reconstruction: A systemic review and meta-analysis. Annals of Surgical Oncology. 2022;**2022**: 1-11

[61] Bekisz JM, Salibian AA, Frey JD, Choi M, Karp NS. Picking the right plane: A comparison of total submuscular, dual-plane, and prepectoral implant–based breast reconstruction. Plastic and Reconstructive Surgery. 2022;**150**(4): 737e-746e

[62] Saldanha IJ, Broyles JM, Adam GP, Cao W, Bhuma MR, Mehta S, et al. Implant-based breast reconstruction after mastectomy for breast cancer: A systematic review and meta-analysis. Plastic and Reconstructive Surgery Global Open. 18 Mar 2022;**10**(3):e4179

[63] Rolph R, Farhadi J. Breast reconstruction with biological and non-biological meshes and matrices. In: Breast Cancer. Springer International Publishing; 2017. pp. 513-520

[64] Logan Ellis H, Asaolu O, Nebo V, Kasem A. Biological and synthetic mesh use in breast reconstructive surgery: A literature review. World Journal of Surgical Oncology. 2016;**14**(1):1-9

[65] Ellsworth WA 4th, Hammer J, Luo L, Schumacher A. Acellular dermal matrices in breast reconstruction: CARE trial 5-year outcomes data for more than 9500 patients. Plastic and Reconstructive Surgery Global Open. 14 Apr 2022;**10**(4): e4258

[66] Potter S, Conroy EJ, Cutress RI, Williamson PR, Whisker L, Thrush S. Breast reconstruction research collaborative. Short-term safety outcomes of mastectomy and immediate implant-based breast reconstruction with and without mesh (iBRA): A multicentre, prospective cohort study. The Lancet Oncology. 2019;**20**(2): 254-266

[67] Wu PS, Winocour S, Jacobson SR. Red breast syndrome: A review of available literature. Aesthetic Plastic Surgery. 2015;**39**(2):227-230

[68] Brown M, Namnoum JD. Indications and controversies for implant-only based

breast reconstruction. Clinics in Plastic Surgery. 2018;**45**(1):47-54

[69] Khavanin N, Clemens MW, Pusic AL, Fine NA, Hamill JB, Kim HM, et al. Shaped versus round implants in breast reconstruction: A multi-institutional comparison of surgical and patient-reported outcomes. Plastic and Reconstructive Surgery. 2017;**139**(5): 1063

[70] Buonomo OC, Morando L, Materazzo M, Vanni G, Pistilli G, Palla L, et al. Comparison of round smooth and shaped micro-textured implants in terms of quality of life and aesthetic outcomes in women undergoing breast reconstruction: A single-Centre prospective study. Updates in Surgery. 2020;**72**(2):537-546

[71] Doren EL, Miranda RN, Selber JC, Garvey PB, Liu J, Medeiros LJ, et al. US epidemiology of breast implant–associated anaplastic large cell lymphoma. Plastic and Reconstructive Surgery. 2017;**139**(5):1042-1050

[72] Campanale A, Spagnoli A, Lispi L, Boldrini R, Marletta M. The crucial role of surgical treatment in BIA-ALCL prognosis in early-and advanced-stage patients. Plastic and Reconstructive Surgery. 2020;**146**(5):530e-538e

[73] Loreti A, Siri G, de Carli M, Fanelli B, Arelli F, Spallone D, et al. Immediate breast reconstruction after mastectomy with polyurethane implants versus textured implants: A retrospective study with focus on capsular contracture. The Breast. 2020; **54**:127-132

[74] Coyette M, Coulie J, Lentini A, Gerdom A, Lengelé B. Prepectoral immediate breast reconstruction with polyurethane foam-coated implants: Feasibility and early results in risk-reducing and therapeutic mastectomies. Journal of Plastic, Reconstructive & Aesthetic Surgery. 2021;**74**(11): 2876-2884

[75] Kraenzlin FS, Darrach H, Chopra K, Rosson GD, Broderick KP, Sacks JM. Prepectoral 2-stage breast reconstruction with carbon dioxide tissue expansion. Plastic and Reconstructive Surgery Global Open. 27 May 2020;**8**(5):e2850

[76] Bayram Y, Sezgic M, Karakol P, Bozkurt M, Filinte GT. The use of autologous fat grafts in breast surgery: A literature review. Archives of Plastic Surgery. 2019;**46**(06):498-510

[77] O'Halloran N, Courtney D, Kerin MJ, Lowery AJ. Adipose-derived stem cells in novel approaches to breast reconstruction: Their suitability for tissue engineering and oncological safety. Breast Cancer (Auckl.). 2017;**11**: 1178

[78] Techanukul T, Lohsiriwat V. Stem cell and tissue engineering in breast reconstruction. Gland Surgery. 2014; **3**(1):55

[79] Mahmoodi M, Ferdowsi S, Ebrahimi-Barough S, Kamian S, Ai J. Tissue engineering applications in breast cancer. Journal of Medical Engineering & Technology. 2020;**44**(4): 162-168

[80] Conci C, Bennati L, Bregoli C, Buccino F, Danielli F, Gallan M, et al. Tissue engineering and regenerative medicine strategies for the female breast. Journal of Tissue Engineering and Regenerative Medicine. 2020;**14**(2): 369-387

[81] Donnely E, Griffin M, Butler PE. Breast reconstruction with a tissue engineering and regenerative medicine approach (systematic review). Annals of

Biomedical Engineering. 2020;**48**(1): 9-25

[82] Banyard DA, Bourgeois JM, Widgerow AD, Evans GRD. Regenerative biomaterials: A review. Plastic and Reconstructive Surgery. 2015;**135**(6):1740-1748

[83] O'Halloran N, Potter S, Kerin M, Lowery A. Recent advances and future directions in postmastectomy breast reconstruction. Clinical Breast Cancer. 2018;**18**(4):e571-e585

[84] Kearney AM, Yan Y, Bricker JT, Pincus JL, Alghoul MS. Acellular dermal matrix–associated contracture: A clinical and histologic analysis of patients undergoing prosthetic breast reconstruction. Plastic and Reconstructive Surgery. 2021;**148**(5): 968-977

[85] Banani MA, Rahmatullah M, Farhan N, Hancox Z, Yousaf S, Arabpour Z, et al. Adipose tissue-derived mesenchymal stem cells for breast tissue regeneration. Regenerative Medicine. 2021;**16**(01):47-70

[86] Cleversey C, Robinson M, Willerth SM. 3D printing breast tissue models: A review of past work and directions for future work. Micromachines (Basel). 2019;**10**(8):501

[87] Panayi AC, Orgill DP. Current use of biological scaffolds in plastic surgery. Plastic and Reconstructive Surgery. 2019;**143**(1):209-220

[88] Mu X, Zhang J, Jiang Y. 3D printing in breast reconstruction: From bench to bed. Frontiers in Surgery. 2021; **8**:641370

[89] Turner A, Abu-Ghname A, Davis MJ, Winocour SJ, Hanson SE, Chu CK. Fat grafting in breast reconstruction. In: Seminars in Plastic Surgery. Thieme Medical Publishers; 2020. pp. 17-23

[90] Oh C, Winocour SJ, Lemaine V. Latest trends in subpectoral breast reconstruction. In: Seminars in Plastic Surgery. Thieme Medical Publishers; 2019. pp. 224-228

[91] Simonacci F, Bertozzi N, Grieco MP, Grignaffini E, Raposio E. Autologous fat transplantation for breast reconstruction: A literature review. Annals of Medicine and Surgery. 2016; **12**:94-100

[92] Shurell E, Olcese C, Patil S, McCormick B, van Zee KJ, Pilewskie ML. Delay in radiotherapy is associated with an increased risk of disease recurrence in women with ductal carcinoma in situ. Cancer. 2018;**124**(1):46-54

[93] Clement Z, Egbeare D, Kollias J, Gill G, Whitfield R, Bingham J, et al. Safety and efficacy of immediate autologous breast reconstruction after mastectomy in patients undergoing neoadjuvant chemoradiotherapy for locally advanced breast cancer. Breast Disease. 2022;**41**(1):267-272

[94] Berbers J, van Baardwijk A, Houben R, Heuts E, Smidt M, Keymeulen K, et al. 'Reconstruction: Before or after postmastectomy radiotherapy? 'A systematic review of the literature. European Journal of Cancer. 2014;**50**(16):2752-2762

[95] Steele KH, Macmillan RD, Ball GR, Akerlund M, McCulley SJ. Multicentre study of patient-reported and clinical outcomes following immediate and delayed Autologous Breast Reconstruction And Radiotherapy (ABRAR study). Journal of Plastic, Reconstructive & Aesthetic Surgery. 2018;**71**(2):185-193

[96] Mehrara BJ, Santoro TD, Arcilla E, Watson JP, Shaw WW, da Lio AL. Complications after microvascular breast reconstruction: Experience with 1195 flaps. Plastic and Reconstructive Surgery. 2006;**118**(5):1100-1109

[97] Kronowitz SJ, Feledy JA, Hunt KK, Kuerer HM, Youssef A, Koutz CA, et al. Determining the optimal approach to breast reconstruction after partial mastectomy. Plastic and Reconstructive Surgery. 2006;**117**(1):1-11

[98] Reish RG, Lin A, Phillips NA, Winograd J, Liao EC, Cetrulo CL Jr, et al. Breast reconstruction outcomes after nipple-sparing mastectomy and radiation therapy. Plastic and Reconstructive Surgery. 2015;**135**(4): 959-966

[99] Matar DY, Wu M, Haug V, Orgill DP, Panayi AC. Surgical complications in immediate and delayed breast reconstruction: A systematic review and meta-analysis. Journal of Plastic, Reconstructive & Aesthetic Surgery. Nov 2022;**75**(11):4085-4095

[100] Angarita FA, Dossa F, Hermann N, McCready DR, Cil TD. Does timing of alloplastic breast reconstruction in older women impact immediate postoperative complications? An analysis of the American College of Surgeons National Surgical Quality Improvement Program (ACS NSQIP) database. The Breast. 2019;**48**:58-64

[101] Lam TC, Hsieh F, Boyages J. The effects of postmastectomy adjuvant radiotherapy on immediate two-stage prosthetic breast reconstruction: A systematic review. Plastic and Reconstructive Surgery. 2013;**132**(3): 511-518

[102] Tomita S, Matsunaga N, Fujita Y, de Kerckhove M, Fujii M, Honda Y, et al. Safety evaluation of immediate breast reconstruction for locally advanced breast cancer in Japanese patients. Journal of Plastic, Reconstructive & Aesthetic Surgery. Aug 2022;**75**(8): 2526-2534

[103] Weber WP, Shaw J, Pusic A, Wyld L, Morrow M, King T, et al. Oncoplastic breast consortium recommendations for mastectomy and whole breast reconstruction in the setting of post-mastectomy radiation therapy. The Breast. 2022;**63**:123-139

[104] Olawoyin OM, Mehta S, Chouairi F, Gabrick KS, Avraham T, Pusztai L, et al. Comparison of autologous breast reconstruction complications by type of neoadjuvant chemotherapy regimen. Plastic and Reconstructive Surgery. 2021;**148**(6):1186-1196

[105] Chang EI, Chang EI, Ito R, Zhang H, Nguyen AT, Skoracki RJ, et al. Challenging a traditional paradigm: 12-year experience with autologous free flap breast reconstruction for inflammatory breast cancer. Plastic and Reconstructive Surgery. 2015;**135**(2): 262e-269e

[106] Sun J, Liang H, Lin D, Han B, Zhang T, Gao J. Oncological safety of reconstruction with autologous fat grafting in breast cancer patients: A systematic review and meta-analysis. International Journal of Clinical Oncology. 2022;**2022**:1-7

[107] Pinell-White XA, Etra J, Newell M, Tuscano D, Shin K, Losken A. Radiographic implications of fat grafting to the reconstructed breast. The Breast Journal. 2015;**21**(5):520-525

Chapter 15

Breast Reconstructive Options

Benjamin Liliav and Luis Torres-Strauss

Abstract

Breast reconstructive options have evolved over the past six decades. Despite advancements in technology, improved therapeutic options, and genetic testing, women are still, unfortunately, faced with a myriad of deformities after treatments for breast cancer. In order to restore an esthetically pleasing breast mound, a careful evaluation of the patient must be taken into account. There are, generally, three components or factors that need to be considered while devising an excellent reconstructive option for a particular patient. These are: patient factors, surgeons' factors, and oncologic factors. It is only with a detailed understanding of each one of these factors that a sound solution is arrived at. In this chapter, we will explore the various modalities of breast reconstruction available to patients. We will also demonstrate specific considerations in order to optimize an excellent outcome for our breast cancer patients.

Keywords: breast reconstruction, breast cancer, implant based reconstruction, autologous reconstruction, lipofilling of breast, fat grafting breast, advances, and trends in reconstruction of the breast

1. Introduction

Breast cancer (BC) is the most common cancer of women in the United States and worldwide [1, 2]. The management of BC is in constant evolution. Multiple landmark studies published in the last several decades have led to a transition from a more radical surgical approach towards breast conserving surgery and less deforming mastectomies [3–7] (**Figure 1**). Similarly, the field of breast reconstruction (BR) has seen many changes in the form of new knowledge and technical advancements that have led to the development of modern reconstructive practices for restoration of a breast mound.

The surgical treatment of BC is best achieved in a multidisciplinary approach [8–10]. The patient typically requires the expertise of many medical and surgical specialists as part of their collaborative treatment plan. Adjuvant therapies in the form of chemotherapy, radiation therapy, hormonal therapy, biologic therapy, and psychologic therapies, may be required for optimal treatment of BC patients. For those undergoing a surgical treatment, reconstruction should be an integral part of the treatment plan as well. The goal of BR is to restore an esthetically pleasing breast mound. With many recent advancements in knowledge and surgical techniques, the ability to restore a cosmetically appealing breast utilizing BR has evolved into its modern practice.

The female breast is the most revered symbol of femininity. From physiological stand point, the breasts main function is lactation. From an anatomical perspective,

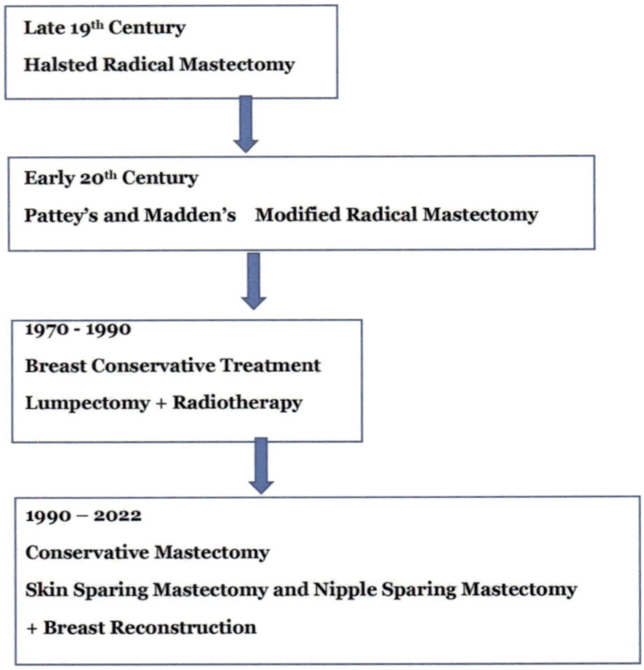

Figure 1.
Evolution of breast cancer surgery.

they serve as a crucial part of the female body image and sexuality [11]. Breast oncologic surgery for the treatment of BC may lead to anatomic deformities with the consequence of adverse impact on the patient's quality of life [12]. Many studies have shown the psychologic and therapeutic benefits in women who undergo BR [13]. The breast restoration experience has been shown not only to reinstate the esthetically pleasing breast but also to improve the personal body image in these women [14].

When a BC patient undergoes a surgical treatment for a tumor, it may result in breast deformities or the complete acquired absence of a breast.

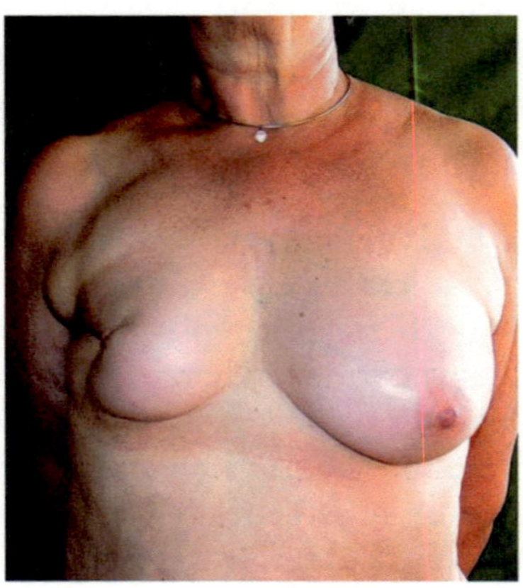

Figure 2.
48 year old female after lumpectomy and radiation to her right breast. Volume distortion and contour abnormality is clearly visible in the right breast compared with left.

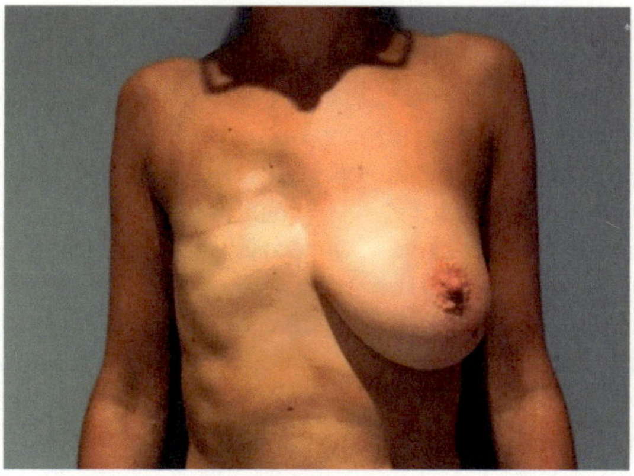

Figure 3.
32 year old female after right mastectomy with total acquired breast absence.

With breast conserving therapy, which entails lumpectomy and radiation, several breast contour deformities and volume distortion may result from tumor excision and radiation treatment (**Figure 2**) [15, 16].

In patients undergoing mastectomy either as a Skin Sparing Mastectomy (SSM) or a Nipple Sparing Mastectomy (NSM), the result is a patient with acquired breast absence (**Figure 3**). In order to offset these deformities, and optimize the surgical outcome, the patient should be informed of reconstructive options prior to undergoing the lumpectomy or mastectomy procedures. Therefore, it is absolutely imperative to involve the reconstructive plastic surgeon as part of the multidisciplinary team as soon as the diagnosis for BC is made. This will allow the patient to have access to and be carefully evaluated by the reconstructive plastic surgeon and help determine what breast restoration options are available to the patient early in the treatment process.

2. Options for breast cancer surgery

- Conservative treatment (lumpectomy +radiation)
  In some cases, Oncoplastic surgery.
- Mastectomy
  Modified radical, Skin Sparing, Nipple Sparing
  1. With Reconstruction
     a. Autologous Tissue
     b. Implant based reconstruction
     c. Fat grafting
  2. Without Reconstruction
- Contralateral Breast surgery

3. Considerations in breast reconstruction

There are three different factors that must be considered while choosing a BR option. These are patient related factors, Oncologic factors, and surgeon related factors. The plan must be individualized to each patient based on these factors. Furthermore, the decision process of reconstructive procedure must entail a collaborative approach between the plastic surgeon and the affected patient [17]. More specifically, the reconstructive plastic surgeon presents the available options based on the above mentioned factors, while the patient states her desires to finally arrive at the optimal breast reconstructive plan.

Patient related factors are: the age of the patient, the patient's desires, overall health and comorbidities, previous breast or other body surgeries, smoking history, and patient anatomy. Oncologic factors involve BC history, history of radiation therapy, history of breast biopsies, tumor biological features, and the potential need for adjuvant chemotherapy, radiation therapy, biological and hormonal therapy. Surgeon related factors include the availability of a plastic surgeon to perform a particular reconstruction, and optimal facility with appropriate capabilities and ancillary staff where the surgery will be performed.

4. Who is a candidate for BR after BC surgery?

Most women diagnosed with BC are candidates for BR which is viewed as part of the healing process. Every patient, regardless of disease stage, socioeconomic status, or demographics, must be informed about options and techniques available to them. Historically, there was a concern that BR may mask locoregional recurrence or that it may compromise adjuvant treatments [18]. However, the available evidence suggest that BR does not adversely affect disease-free or overall survival and there is no significant delay in recurrent disease presentation [19]. Currently, with improved social media and internet access, there is an increase in frequency of patients who are desiring breast reconstruction after mastectomy [20].

The multidisciplinary team should review important parameters in order to obtain a complete evaluation of any particular patient (**Figure 4**).

There is a particular group of patients who is considered high risk based on genetic mutations. Less than 15%of all BC are associated with germline mutations [21]. The majority of hereditary breast tumors are due to mutations in BrCa1 and/or

Breast Reconstruction Patient's Criteria

- Patients age
- Body Mass Index (BMI)
- Breast Anatomy
- Patients preferences
- Overall Health and comorbidities
- Previous surgeries
- Smoking
- Stage of BC
- First occurrence vs recurrent
- Use of adjuvant therapy (chemotherapy, radiation, and hormonal therapy)
- Immediate vs delayed reconstruction
- Single or two-stage reconstruction
- Uni or bilateral surgery and reconstruction
- Facility capability of supporting microsurgery

Figure 4.
Breast reconstruction patient's criteria.

BrCa2 genes, these patients often have bilateral and multicentric disease, early-onset, and more likely to be Triple Negative (ER-, PR-, HER2-) [22, 23]. One of the most effective strategies in treating these women is the prophylactic mastectomy better defined as Risk Reduction mastectomy (RRM). This technique provided the greatest reduction in risk of BC development (around 90%) and also diminishes the anxiety and fear in these affected women [24]. As a result of that, this subset of patients can benefit from prophylactic mastectomy, and require breast reconstruction of their affected breast as well as a restoration procedure for their contralateral breast. It should be noted that contralateral RRM does not improve survival in patients without deleterious genetic mutations or lobular histology [25]. In the USA, a growing rate of bilateral mastectomy for unilateral BC is being observed. Availability of immediate BR, young age, pathogenic BrCa mutations, significant family history, and Triple Negative disease play a significant role in choosing this type of surgery. NSM plus immediate BR is nowadays considered the gold standard in this group of women [26].

5. No reconstruction

Some patients prefer not to have BR and opt for a breast prosthesis instead. The advantage of this device is not taxing the body with additional surgery other than the required oncologic procedure. The disadvantages are significant discomfort, skin irritation and rashes, and inability to wear a bathing suit or clothing comfortably. This option is reasonable for an elderly patient who is not concerned about cosmesis or a patient with many comorbidities who is not a candidate for BR.

6. Delayed reconstruction

A delayed BR is breast restoration performed at a later date as an independent separate procedure by the plastic surgeon. The patient initially undergoes the oncologic procedure with a mastectomy or breast conserving therapy. Subsequently, the patient pursues Breast reconstruction based on a collaborative approach with the plastic surgeon. This reconstructive option is ideal if there is no availability of plastic surgeon at the facility or if negative margins could not be achieved during the oncologic procedure. Once the patient is cleared from an oncologic standpoint, the BR can be pursued at a later date. Advantages include allowing time to identify a board certified plastic surgeon who will perform the reconstruction at a nearby facility as well as appropriate allotted time for oncologic treatment in terms of achieving final negative margins. The disadvantage of this approach is that by waiting, the patient endures the negative psychologic implications of not having a breast or having a deformed breast until the reconstruction is performed. In addition, with delayed reconstruction there is scarring and fibrosis that forms as part of the healing process that may impact the type of reconstruction that can be performed at a later date [27, 28].

7. Implant based reconstruction (IBR)

IBR entails using a breast implant (silicone or saline) to create a breast mound after mastectomy. The advantages of IBR are that this procedure is relatively simple, expedient, and has short recovery time. The disadvantages are implant related complications such as implant rupture, exposure, extrusion, and capsular contractures [29]. IBR can be performed in a single or two stage technique. In a single stage IBR, the plastic surgeon places the breast implant to reconstruct the breast mound at the same operation immediately after mastectomy [30]. Alternatively, IBR can be performed in two stages. This is particularly useful in cases where extra skin needs to be recruited. In this approach, a tissue expander is placed first at the time of mastectomy. The device is expanded over time on a weekly basis in the medical office. Several months later, the second stage of the procedure is performed where the tissue expander is removed and replaced with a permanent breast implant [31].

Irrespective of single or two stage implant reconstruction technique, anatomically, these devices (expander and/or implant) can be placed either above or below the pectoralis muscle. In the early period of breast reconstruction, pre-pectoral (above the pectoralis muscle) implant placement was abandoned due to high rates of capsular contracture, implant extrusion and poor esthetic results. Subsequently, the shift to subpectoral plane (under the pectoralis muscle) offered an increased coverage of the implant and less of the above implant related complications However, over the years it became apparent that submuscular implant placement is associated with chronic muscle related pain, muscle spasms, animation deformity, and reduced physical mobility. With optimization of mastectomy technique, advances in radiotherapy, use of alloplastic devices, fat grafting, and new implant designs, the prepectoral approach has undergone a revival and is now performed in many centers around the world [32].

With certain surgical advancements, oncologic surgeons are transitioning to SSM and NSM. Technological breakthrough has contributed to the availability of mesh (Human/animal/synthetic) for reconstructive support [33]. Improvements in the breast implant device characteristics have led to improved outcomes for patients undergoing IBR as well. Furthermore, due to these advances in mastectomy techniques, and the recent increase in bilateral mastectomies performed, IBR is the most common approach currently used for breast reconstruction. According to The American Society of Plastic Surgeons 2018 publication, 40% of women who underwent mastectomy had reconstruction and the most common practice in the US was immediate reconstruction (75% of the cases) of these 81% corresponded to Implant based (two-stage 68%, one stage 13% (**Figures 5** and **6**) [34].

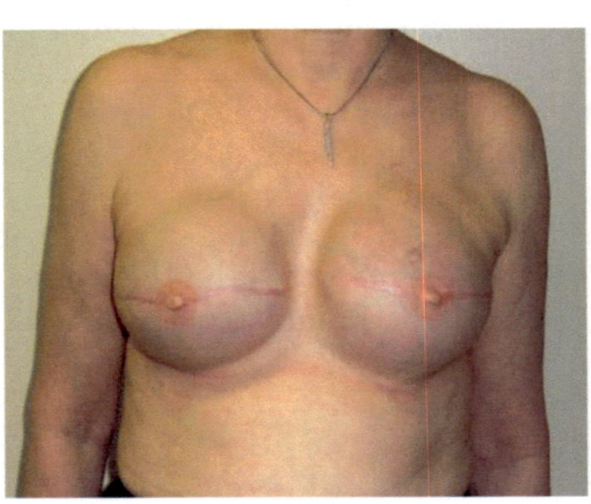

Figure 5.
36 year old female with history of bilateral SSM and immediate subpectoral implant based BR. Of note she also had bilateral nipple reconstruction.

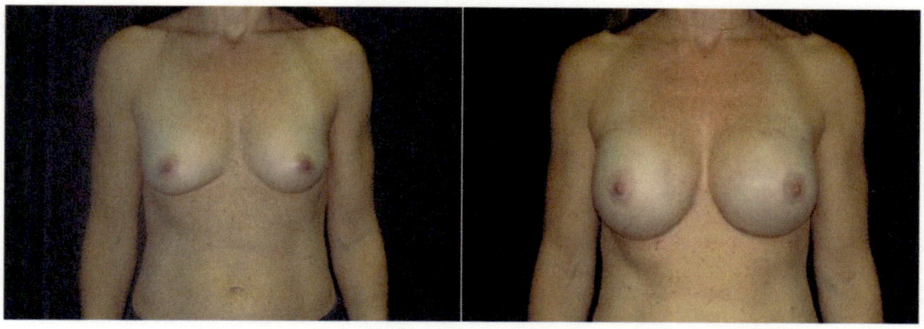

Figure 6.
28 year old female with history of BRCA gene mutation. Left: demonstrates her pre surgery (pre mastectomy). Right: patient 6 months after Bilateral prophylactic NSM with immediate prepectoral implant based BR.

8. Autologous breast reconstruction (AR)

The premise in AR is utilizing tissue such as skin, fat, and sometimes muscle from another place on the patient's body in order to create a breast mound. AR can be performed in immediate or delayed fashion as well [35]. Many different types of flaps have been described in the literature for restoration of breast mound using patients

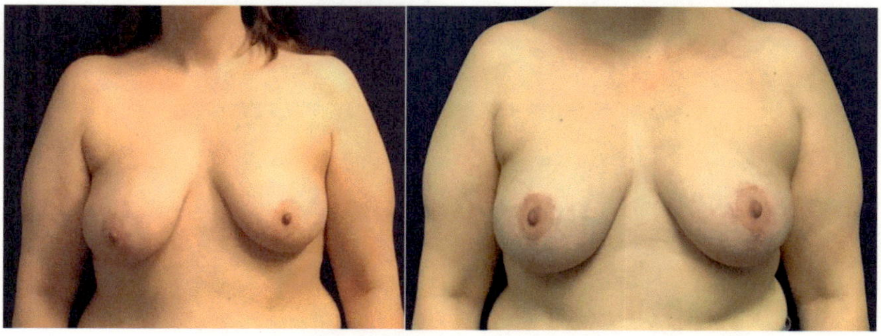

Figure 7.
Top: 39 year female diagnosed with left breast cancer. Bottom: after Left NSM and reconstruction with abdominal based flap.

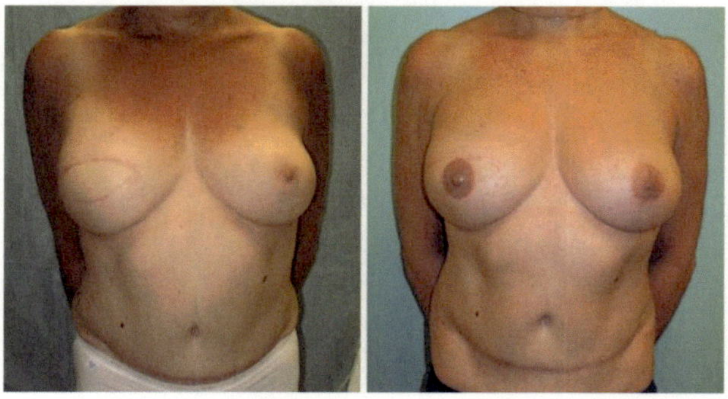

Figure 8.
49 year old female with history of right breast cancer. Patient underwent autologous reconstruction with abdominal based flap. Left: right breast reconstruction with DIEP (deep inferior epigastric perforator) flap. Right: same patient after nipple reconstruction.

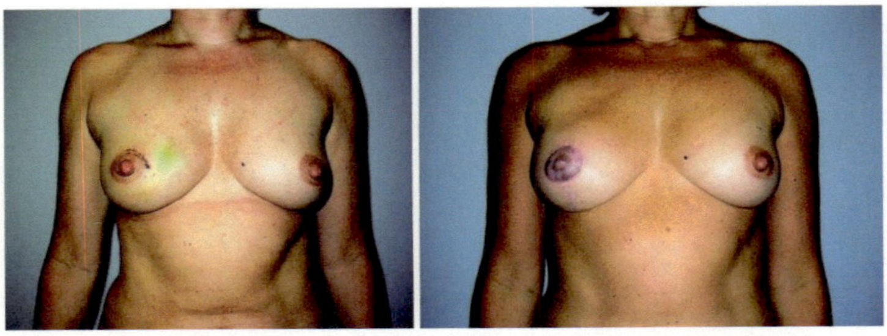

Figure 9.
Left: 38 years old female diagnosed with invasive right breast cancer. Right: same patient after right NSM and reconstruction with TUG (transverse upper gracilis) flap.

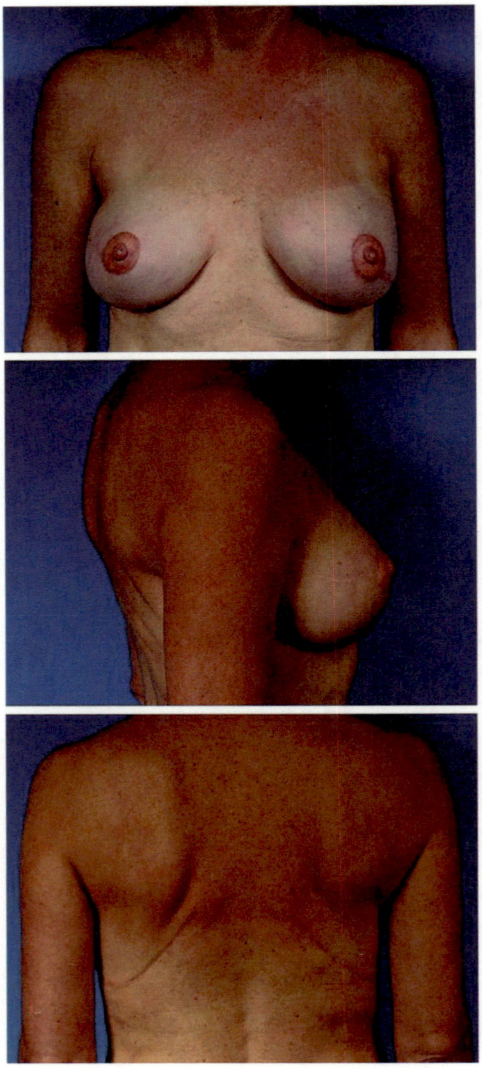

Figure 10.
Patient with history of bilateral breast cancer, right invasive ductal and left lobular in situ. She is shown after bilateral SSM and immediate reconstruction with bilateral LD (latissimus Dorsi) flaps. Delayed tattooing nipple reconstruction.

own body tissues [36]. Some are abdominal based flaps (TRAM, DIEP, SIEA), others are gluteal based flaps (SGAP, IGAP), there are thigh based flaps (PAP, TUG) and back based flaps (LD, TDAP) [37]. Most of these flaps require a microsurgeon who is well versed in microsurgical techniques, the availability of a microscope, a well-trained surgical team in microsurgery, and a facility that can support these types of complex and delicate operations. The advantages of BR using these flaps are natural appearing results, esthetically pleasing outcome, and improved patient satisfaction [38]. The disadvantages are the need for a skilled microsurgeon, long procedure time, longer recovery period, extra scarring in the donor sites, and increased pain. **Figures 7–10** show examples of Autologous Breast reconstruction.

9. BR with lipofilling

BR could be achieved by lipofilling (fat transfer) after mastectomy. This technique involves removing fat from certain areas in the body by way of liposuction, processing the fat cells, and transferring them to the area of absent breast. It is important to note that there is a limitation of how much fat can be injected in order for the fat cells to survive and often times this requires several sessions of fat grafting in order to obtain the desired result. Patients who undergo breast conserving therapy with lumpectomy resulting in a contour deformity or volume deficiency after excision, may benefit from fat transfer procedure in order to restore the loss of volume in the treated breast [39]. Of note, BR with lipofilling has been shown to be ontologically safe [40]. Advantages of lipofilling for breast reconstruction

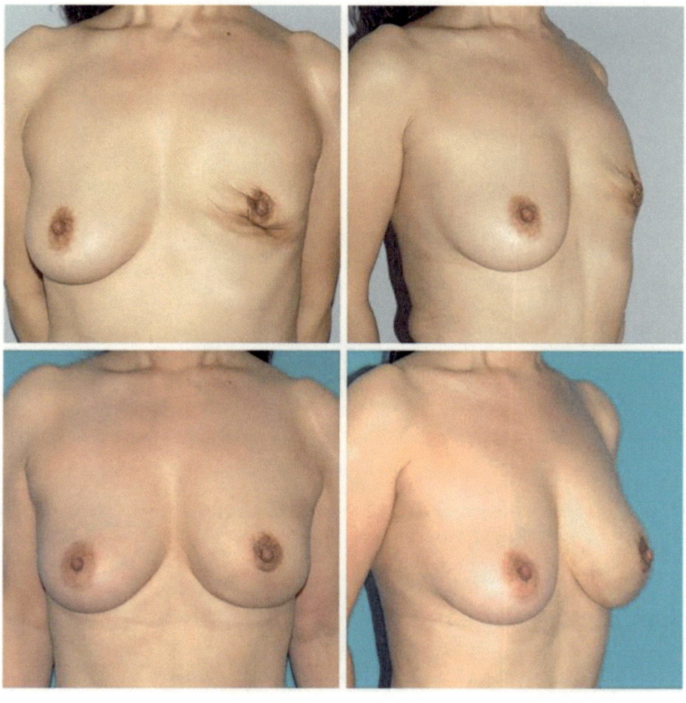

Figure 11.
BR with lipofilling. Left: Patient with history of NSM for left BC resulting in contour deformity. Right: patient after Reconstruction with 4 sessions of lipofilling and scar release.

include the creation of a breast with a natural consistency, minimal scarring, could be use in patients with comorbidities, relatively simple procedure, and low costs [41]. The main limiting factor of this technique is that fat transfer uptake may require multiple fat grafting sessions [42]. This procedure is better offered to patients with small brassiere cup. Some teams report the use of a skin expansion with expander or an expansion device like BRAVA system [43]. Although BR with lipofilling is a relatively new technique, it is gaining in popularity in the United States and worldwide (**Figure 11**) [44].

10. Oncoplastic breast reconstruction

In certain BC patients, particularly if they have larger breast size, it is oftentimes possible for them to have the excision of the tumor and have the plastic surgeon perform local breast tissue rearrangement by either lifting the breast or reducing the total size of the breast at the same time that the tumor is being removed. This technique is ideal for a patient with large ptotic breasts who desires breast reduction or lift at the same time of oncologic excision surgery. The advantages are that the tumor is removed with very wide margins and once the tissues are rearranged by way of lifting or reduction, the new breast mound appears even more esthetically pleasing then prior to the patient undergoing surgery. The disadvantages are that the contralateral breast which is not affected from oncologic standpoint is undergoing a surgical procedure as well. Also, many patients are not candidates for this technique especially if their breasts are too small or if the tumor is not in a favorable location (**Figure 12**) [45, 46].

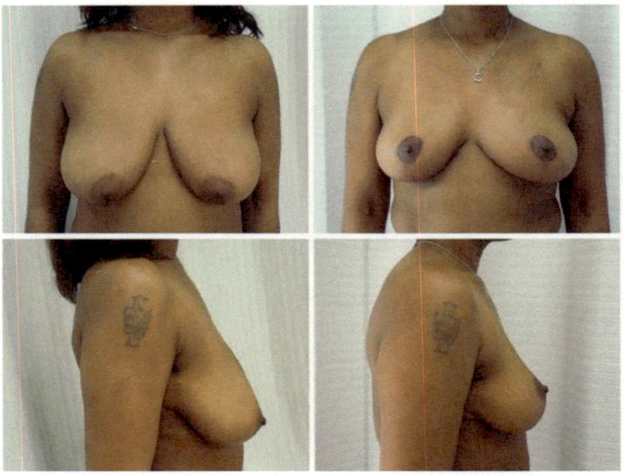

Figure 12.
46 year old female diagnosed with left invasive breast cancer. Left: preoperative photos. Right: patient after Oncoplastic Surgery with excision of left breast tumor with concurrent bilateral breast reduction.

11. Approach to the opposite breast

Many BC patients who undergo surgical treatment with or without reconstruction oftentimes require treatment to their contralateral breast. The main reason is for symmterization of both breasts and to improve the esthetic outlook. Depending on what treatment is indicated, the contralateral breast may require breast augmentation with implant, breast reduction, or breast lift. When speaking with the BC patients, it is important to make sure they are aware that reconstruction is a process. We must clearly inform the patient not only about the reconstructive options but also symmetrizing procedures that may be needed either at the same time as BR or later on as a separate procedure.

12. Breast implant associated illness

Although rare, it must be mentioned that there are several cases of Breast Implant illness reported in the literature. As of April 1, 2022 The Food and Drug Administration has received a total of 1130 US and global medical device reports of breast implant-associated anaplastic large cell lymphoma (BIA-ALCL) [47]. These cases, must be confirmed by pathology/cytology test or Anaplastic Lymphoma Kinase and CD30 biomarkers. More recently, Sept, 2022, the FDA released a new safety communication about Squamous cell carcinoma and various lymphomas in the capsule around breast implants. The current data is limited but evolving. More studies are required to ascertain the magnitude of these findings. Nonetheless, clinical awareness is paramount [48].

13. The impact of post mastectomy radiation therapy on breast reconstruction

Radiation Therapy (RT) is delivered to those patients who are at high risk for developing local recurrence. Indications for radiation therapy include patients undergoing breast conservative surgery as well as patients who undergo mastectomy based on the stage of the tumor and the extent of lymph node metastasis [49]. The need for radiation therapy may not be known until the final pathologic classification of the tumor is completed. Therefore, the reconstructive surgical technique, whether implant based or autologous, should remain the same even in patient who will require post mastectomy radiation therapy. Despite reported data of potential increase in surgical and wound related complications in IBR and to a lesser extent Autologous reconstruction, current literature suggests that there are no absolute contraindications for implant based reconstructions in the setting of post mastectomy radiation therapy [50].

14. Nipple areola reconstruction

Nipple areolar reconstruction (NAR) is the final stage of the breast reconstructive process. The individual who requires NAR is a patient that underwent SSM where the nipple areolar complex is excised as part of the oncologic procedure. In addition, any patient who undergoes NSM, but the nipple areolar complex was compromised due to poor vascularity is a candidate for NAR as well. NAR can be performed as an outpatient procedure under local anesthetic and yields superb results for the patients. Many different techniques are described in the literature for NAR [51]. The authors favorite technique is single stage NAR and tattooing (**Figure 13**) [52].

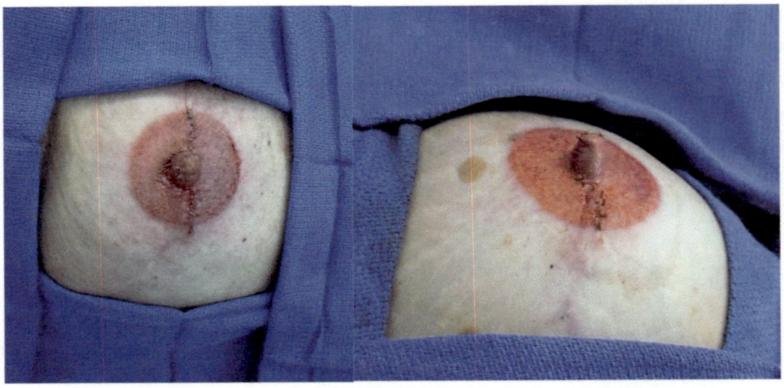

Figure 13.
Left: 35 year old female after nipple areolar complex Reconstruction and tattooing in a single stage technique. Right: same patient with side photo showing adequate projection of nipple.

Conflict of interest

The authors declare no conflict of interest.

Author details

Benjamin Liliav[1]* and Luis Torres-Strauss[2]

1 South Miami Hospital, Larkin Hospital, Jackson Memorial Hospital, Miami, FL, USA

2 Clinica El Vinedo and Red Cross Hospital, Valencia, Venezuela

*Address all correspondence to: associatesinplasticsurgery20@gmail.com

References

[1] American Cancer Society, CA: A Cancer Journal for Clinicians. The Facts and Figures 2022

[2] World Health Organization. Breast Cancer Fact Sheets. 2021

[3] Fisher B, Redmond C, Poisson R, Margolese R, Wolmark N, Wickerman L, et al. Eight-year results of a randomized clinical trial comparing total mastectomy and lumpectomy with or without irradiation in the treatment of breast cancer. The New England Journal of Medicine. 1989;**320**:822-828. DOI: 10.1056/NEJM198903303201302

[4] Veronesi U, Salvadori B, Luini A, Banfi A, Del Vecchio M, Saccozzi R, et al. Conservative treatment of early breast cáncer. Long-term resuls of 1232 cases treated with qudrantectomy, axillary dissection and radiotherapy. Annals of Surgery. 1990;**211**:250-259

[5] Lichter AS, Lippman ME, Danforth DN, et al. Mastectomy versus brest-conserving therapy in the treatment of stage I and II carcinoma of the breast: A randomized trial at the National Cancer Institute. Journal of Clinical Oncology. 1992;**10**:976-983. DOI: 10.1200/JCO.1992.10.6.976

[6] Fisher B, Anderson S, Bryant J, Margolese RG, Deutsch M, Fisher ER, et al. Twenty-year follow-up f a randomized trial comparing total mastectomy, lumpectomy ad lumpectomy plus irradiation for the treatment of invasive breast cancer. The New England Journal of Medicine. 2002;**347**:1233-1241. DOI: 10.1056/NEJMoa022152

[7] Veronesi U, Cascinelli N, Mariani L, Greco M, Saccozzi R, Luini A, et al. Twenty-year follow-up off a randomized study comparing breast-conserving surgery with radical mastectomy for early breast cancer. The New England Journal of Medicine. 2002;**92**:1143-1150. DOI: 10.1056/NEJMoa0220989

[8] Cevik J, Hunter-Smith D, Rozen W. Current Advances in breast reconstruction. Journal of Clinical Medicine. 2022;**11**(12):3328. DOI: 10.3390/jcm11123328

[9] Pan E-SB, Sosin M, Carey JN, Nahabedian MY, Km P. Breast Reconstruction and adjuvant therapy: A systematic review of surgical outcomes. Surgical Oncology. 2015;**112**(5):458-464

[10] Kaidar-Person O, Offersen B, Boersma L, Ruysscher D, Tramm T, Kuhn T, et al. A multisciplinary view of mastectomy and breast reconstruction: Understanding the challenges. Breast. Apr 2021;**56**:42-52. DOI: 10.1016/jbreast.2021.02.004

[11] Shashanka M. Breast Cancer Comprehensive Management. 2022. Chapter 22; p.465-495 DOI: 10.1007/978-981-16-4546-4

[12] Al-Hilli Z, Wilkerson A. Breast surgery: Management of postoperative complications following operations for breast cancer. Surgical Clinics North America. 2021;**101**(5):845-863. DOI: 10.1016/j.suc.2021.06.014

[13] Planchal H, Matros E. Current trends in post-mastectomy breast reconstruction. Plastic and Reconstructive Surgery. 2017;**140**(5):7S-13S. DOI: 10.1097/PRS.0000000000003941

[14] Zehra S, Doyle F, Barry M, Walsh S, Kell MR. Health-related quality of life following breast reconstruction compared to total mastectomy and breast-conserving surgery among breast cancer survivors: A systematic review and meta-analysis. Breast Cancer. 2020;**27**(4):534-566. DOI: 10.1007/s12282-020-01076-1

[15] Dahlback C, Ringberg A, Manjer J. Aesthetic outcome following breast-conserving surgery assessed by three evaluation modalities in relation to health-related quality of life. The British Journal of Surgery. 2019;**106**(1):90-99. DOI: 10.1002/bjs.10963

[16] Deutinger M, Tairych G, Resch A, Biber E. Contour defects after breast preserving therapy of breast carcinoma. Primary and secondary possibilities of correction. Strahlentherapie und Onkologie. 1999;**175**(11):577-582. DOI: 10.1007/s000660050044

[17] Li X et al. Shared decision-making in breast reconstruction for breast cancer patients: A scoping review. Patient Preference and Adherence. 2021;**15**:2763-2781. DOI: 10.2047/PPA.S335080

[18] Galimberti V, Vicini E, Veronesi P. Nipple-sparing mastectomy: Review of aims, oncological safe and contraindications. Breast. 2017;**34**(Suppl. 1):S82-S84. DOI: 10.1016/jbreast.2017.06.034

[19] Platt J et al. Does breast reconstruction after mastectomy for breast cancer affect overall survival? Long-term follow-up of a retrospective population-based cohort. Plastic and Reconstructive Surgery. 2015;**135**(3):468e-476e. DOI: 10.1097/PRS.0000000000001054

[20] Panchal H, Matros E. Advances in breast reconstruction. Plastic and Reconstructive Surgery. 2017;**140**(5S):7S-13S. DOI: 10.1097/PRS.0000000000003941

[21] Wei G, Kumar A, Lee MC, Wang X. Influential factors on risk-reduction mastectomy in a high-risk breast cancer population with genetic predispositions. Clinical Breast Cancer. 2021;**21**(4):e427-e433. DOI: 10.1016/j.clbc.2021.01.008

[22] Yip CH, Newman LA. Guideline for management of hereditary breast cancer. American society of clinical oncology, American society for radiation oncology, and society of surgical oncology. JAMA Surgery. 2021;**156**:284-285. DOI: 10.1001/jamasurg.2020.6254

[23] Yoshida R. Hereditary breast and ovarian cancer (HBOC): Review of its molecular characteristics, screening, treatment, and prognosis. Breast Cancer. 2021;**28**(6):1167-1180. DOI: 10.1007/s12282-020-01148-2

[24] Tung NM, Boughey JC, Pierce LJ, Robson ME, Bedrosian I. Management of hereditary breast cancer: American society of clinical oncology, American society for radiation oncology, and society of surgical oncology guideline. Journal of Clinical Oncology. 2020;**38**:2080-2106. DOI: 10.1200/JCO.20.00299

[25] Eisemann B, Spiegel A. Risk-reducing mastectomy and breast reconstruction: Indications and evidence for current management strategies. Review Clinical Plastic Surgery. 2018;**45**(1):129-136. DOI: 10.1016/j.cps.2017.08.013

[26] Headon H, Kasem A, Mokbel K. The oncological safety of nipple-sparing mastectomy: A systematic review of the literature with a pooled analysis of 12,358 procedure. Archives of Plastic Surgery.

2016;**43**(4):328-338. DOI: 10.5999/aps.2016.43.4.328

[27] Shammas RL, Cason RW, Sergesketter AR, Glener AD. Broadwater a comparison of surgical complications in patients undergoing delayed versus staged tissue-expander and free-flap breast reconstruction. Plastic and Reconstructive Surgery. 2021;**148**(3):501-509. DOI: 10.1097/PRS.0000000000008208

[28] Matar DY, Wu M, Haug V, Orgill DP, Panayi AC. Surgical complications in immediate and delayed breast reconstruction: A systematic review and meta-analysis. Journal of Plastic, Reconstructive & Aesthetic Surgery. 2022;**75**(11):4085-4095. DOI: 10.1016/j.bjps.2022.08.029

[29] Kumbla PA, Ananthasekar S, Denney BD. Two-stage, prepectoral breast reconstruction: Standardized technique and outcomes. Analysis during first stage to reduce complications and ensure reliability. Annals of Plastic Surgery. 2021;**86**(6S Suppl 5):S482-S486. DOI: 10.1097/SAP.0000000000002700

[30] Colwell AS, Taylor EM. Recent Advances in Implant-Based Breast Reconstruction. Plastic and Reconstructive Surgery. 2020;**145**(2):421e-432e. DOI: 10.1097/PRS.0000000000006510

[31] Caputo GG, Vigato E, Rampino Cordaro E, Parodi PC, Governa M. Comparative study of patient outcomes between direct to implant and two-stage implant-based breast reconstruction after mastectomy. Journal of Plastic, Reconstructive & Aesthetic Surgery. 2021;**74**(10):2573-2579. DOI: 10.1016/j.bjps.2021.03.058

[32] Weinzierl A, Schmauss D, Brucato D, Harder Y. Implant-based breast reconstruction after mastectomy, from the subpectoral to the prepectoral approach: An evidence-based change of mind Journal of Clinical Medicine 2022;**11**(11):3079. DOI: 10.3390/jcm11113079

[33] Rolph R, Farhadi J. The use of meshes and matrices in breast reconstruction. British Journal of Hospital Medicine (London, England). Aug 2018;**79**(8):454-459. DOI: 10.12968/hmed.2018.79.8.454

[34] American Society of Plastic Surgeon. Supplement 2018. Breast reconstruction

[35] Saldanha I, Broyles J, Adam G, Cao W, Bhuma M, Mehta S, et al. Autologous breast reconstruction after mastectomy for breast cancer: A systematic review. Plastic and Reconstructive Surgery. Global Open. 2022;**10**(3):e4181. DOI: 10.1097/GOX.0000000000001481

[36] Costanzo D, Klinger M, Lisa A, Maione L, Battistini A, Vinci V. The evolution of autologous breast reconstruction. The Breast Journal. 2020;**26**(11):2223-2225. DOI: 10.1111/tbj.14025

[37] Chang EI. Latest advancements in autologous breast reconstruction. Plastic and Reconstructive Surgery. 2021;**147**(1):111e-122e. DOI: 10.1097/PRS.0000000000007480

[38] Toyserkani NM, Jørgensen MG, Tabatabaeifar S, Damsgaard T, Sørensen JA. Autologous versus implant-based breast reconstruction: A systematic review and meta-analysis of Breast-Q patient-reported outcomes. Journal of Plastic, Reconstructive & Aesthetic Surgery. 2020;**73**(2):278-285. DOI: 10.1016/j.bjps.2019.09.040

[39] Piffer A, Aubry G, Cannistra C, Popescu N, Nikpayam M, Koskas M, et al. Breast reconstruction by exclusive

lipofilling after total mastectomy for breast cancer: Description of the technique and evaluation of quality of life. Journal of Personalized Medicine. Feb 2022;**12**(2):153. DOI: 10.3390/jpm12020153

[40] Chung J, Kim K, Jung S, Park S, Yoon E. Analysis of oncological safety of autologous fat grafting after immediate breast reconstruction. Gland Surgery. 2021;**10**(2):584-594. DOI: 10.21037/gs-20-645

[41] Turner A, Abu-Ghname A, Davis MJ, Winocour SJ, Hanson SE, Chu CK. Fat grafting in breast reconstruction. Seminars in Plastic Surgery. 2020;**34**: 17-23. DOI: 10.1055/s-0039-1700959

[42] Kellou K, Lequesne J, Georgescu D, De Gournay E, Breard H, et al. Limitations of breast reconstruction using exclusive lipofilling: A retrosoective study over 10 years. Gynecologie, Obstetrique, Fertilite & Senologie. 2019;**47**:347-351. DOI: 10.1016/j.gofs.2019.02.007

[43] Mestak O et al. Breast reconstruction after bilateral mastectomy using the BRAVA expansion system and fat grafting. Plastic and Reconstructive Surgery Global Open. Nov 2013;**1**(8);e71. DOI: 10.1097/GOX.0000000000000022

[44] Alessandri Bonetti M, Carbonaro R, Borelli F, Amendola F, Cottone G, Mazzocconi L, et al. Outcomes in hybrid breast reconstruction: A systematic review. Medicina (Kaunas, Lithuania). 2022;**58**(9):1232. DOI: 10.3390/medicina58091232

[45] Kaufman CS. Increasing role of oncoplastic surgery for breast cancer. Current Oncology Reports. 2019;**21**(12):111. DOI: 10.1007/s11912-019-0860-9

[46] Salibian AA, Olson B, Shauly O, Patel KM. Oncoplastic breast reconstruction: Principles, current techniques, and future directions. Journal of Surgical Oncology. 2022;**126**(3):450-459. DOI: 10.1002/jso.26897

[47] The US Food and Drug Administration. Medical Device Reports of Breast Implant-Associated Anaplastic Large Cell Lymphoma. 2022. Available from: www.fda.gov

[48] The US Food and Drug Administration Breast Implants: Reports of Squamous Cell Carcinoma and Various Lymphomas in Capsule Around Implants: FDA Safety Communication. 2022. Available from: www.fda.gov

[49] McCormick B. Breast journal 2020 special issue: Post-mastectomy radiation: Tracking changes in the standard of care over 25 years. The Breast Journal. 2020;**26**(1):55-58. DOI: 10.1111/tbj.13726

[50] Weber P et al. Oncoplastic breast consortium recommendations for mastectomy and whole breast reconstruction in the setting of post-mastectomy radiation therapy. The Breast. DOI: 10.1016/j.breast.2022.03.008

[51] Paolini G, Firmani G, Briganti F, Sorotos M, Santanelli di Pompeo F. Guiding nipple-areola complex reconstruction: Literature review and proposal of a new decision-making algorithm. Plastic Surgery. 2021;**45**(3):933-945. DOI: 10.1007/s00266-020-02047-9

[52] Liliav B et al. Single-stage nipple-areolar complex reconstruction technique, outcomes and patient satisfaction. Annals of Plastic Surgery. Nov 2014;**73**(5):492-497. DOI: 10.1097/ SAP.0b013e318276dac0

Chapter 16

Oncoplastic Breast Conservation: A Standard of Care in Modern Breast Cancer Surgical Management

Ana Car Peterko

Abstract

Within the multimodal treatment, the extent of surgery for early-stage breast cancer treatment may be safely de-escalated. This strategy is associated with less morbidity, therefore significant improvements in quality of life (QoL). Nevertheless, conventional, ablative-only breast conservative surgery (BCS) has several limitations considering breast aesthetics and may impact QoL just opposite than anticipated. The concept of oncoplastic breast conservation emerged at the end of the last century intending to overcome these limitations. Although the primary goal remains oncological safe cancer resection, the enhanced aesthetic outcomes, achieved with this approach, significantly contribute to higher patient satisfaction. The author believes that mastectomy should no longer be offered as an equivalent treatment option for early-stage breast cancer patients with low-volume breast disease, irrespective of the availability of postmastectomy breast reconstruction. Moreover, with the opportunities of oncoplastic breast conservative surgery, the technical feasibility of breast conservation should not represent an issue even in a higher stage of the disease. Clinical decision on the type of oncoplastic procedure is mainly based upon the anticipated percentage of breast volume loss and the residual breast volume, as well as the availability of additional donor sites, patients' preference, and surgeons' skills.

Keywords: breast cancer, surgery, mastectomy, breast conservation, oncoplastic, quality of life

1. Introduction

Breast cancer was the most common malignant disease in the general population worldwide, contributing 12.5% of the total number of new cases and 25.8% of new cases in females diagnosed in 2020 [1]. The average woman's lifetime risk of breast cancer diagnosis is as high as 12–13%, that is, statistically, one in every eight women will be diagnosed with breast cancer during her life [2].

Due to population screening programmes and increased breast awareness in the developed world, breast cancer is nowadays detected predominantly (80%) in the preclinical and early stages of the disease. With the multidisciplinary management and the modern multimodal treatments, in this subgroup of patients, the oncological outcomes are excellent, with a 5-year overall survival (OS) rate reaching over 95%. Moreover, the cumulative 10-year OS rate of 70–80% has been reported as well [3].

In addition to conventional oncologic outcomes, quality of life (QoL) has emerged as an important outcome measure and has been recently established in breast cancer management evaluation. The world's most prevalent cancer, with 2.3 million newly diagnosed patients yearly and 7.8 million new breast cancer survivors every 5 years [4], clearly justifies the QoL evaluation in all breast cancer management trials.

The ultimate goals of modern breast cancer surgery are optimal local and regional control of the disease, associated with minimal morbidity and enhanced aesthetic outcomes.

2. Surgical management of early-stage breast cancer

Until the seventies, mutilating procedures in the breast and axilla, intended for disease eradication, were the only available surgical options in breast cancer treatment, irrespective of the stage of the disease. Better insights into breast cancer biology, as well as a better understanding of the natural course of the disease, have contributed to substantial changes in surgical management over the last five decades. Clinical trials, initiated by Veronesi and Fisher [5–7], have demonstrated that breast conservative surgery, accompanied by adjuvant breast irradiation, is not an inferior option for the early-stage (T1-T2) breast cancer treatment. Moreover, the survival outcomes in several, more recent, population-based studies [8–13] favour a conservative approach (**Table 1**).

As no benefit has not ever been associated with the more extensive procedures, breast surgery has been de-escalated to the more conservative options. Several synonyms for breast conservative surgery (BCS) are present in the literature: partial mastectomy, quadrantectomy, segmentectomy and lumpectomy. Although there are slight differences among the original definitions, nowadays the term represents

Reference	Number of patients included	Years of follow up	Endpoint(s)	Results
Milan trial [5, 6]	701	20	OS (Mx vs. BCS)	41% vs. 42%
NSABP B-06 [7]	1843	20	OS (Mx vs. BCS)	47% vs. 46%
Norwegian population register [8, 9]	13,015	10	BCSS (Mx vs. BCS) OS (Mx vs. BCS)	82% vs. 93% 64% vs. 86%
Indian hospital-based registers [10]	7609	5	OS (Mx vs. BCS) Stage I Stage II Stage III	99% vs. 91% 86% vs. 94% 69% vs. 87%
SEER [11]	132,149	10	BCSS (Mx vs. BCS)	90% vs. 94%
Danish population register [12]	58,331	10	OS (Mx vs. BCS) vs. BCS and Mx	57% vs. 82% vs. 74%
Dutch population register [13]	129,692	6 12	OS (Mx vs. BCS) OS (Mx vs. BCS)	80% vs. 91% 72% vs. 52%

Table 1.
Overall survival (OS) and/or breast cancer specific survival (BCSS) in relation to surgical treatment: Mastectomy (Mx) vs. breast conservative surgery (BCS).

a breast tumour resection with appropriate histological margins, that is, 'no ink on tumour' for invasive breast cancer and a minimum of 2 mm of benign breast tissue surrounding the *in situ* disease [14, 15]. The goal of this treatment de-escalation strategy is QoL improvement, related to breast preservation. Nevertheless, the conventional, ablative-only approach in BCS has several limitations considering breast shape and symmetry, that is, breast aesthetics, and may impact QoL just opposite than anticipated [16].

The breast resection volume and the lesion location within the breast are major determinants of the aesthetic outcome following conventional BCS. Even in the early stage of the disease (T1-T2), a 30% risk of breast deformity is reported in the literature. Resection volume over 15–20% of breast volume in outer quadrants and over 10% in medial or central quadrants, without partial breast reconstruction, may already result in some degree of breast deformity [17, 18]. In addition, natural (preoperative) breast shape, degree of ptosis and breast glandular density impact the aesthetic outcome as well. According to available literature data [19], four degrees of breast deformity have been reported following BCS, from a mild NAC retraction to the severe distortion of the entire breast.

The oncoplastic approach emerged at the end of the last century with intention of overcoming the limitations of conventional BCS. Following oncoplastic procedures, breast shape and symmetry remain preserved, although the breast volume may be reduced. Moreover, breast aesthetics can be improved with this type of cancer surgery.

The term 'oncoplastic' was first mentioned by German surgeon Audretsch in 1993 [20]. Merged from the Greek words 'onco' (tumour) and 'plastic' (shaping), it signifies reshaping the breast after the tumour resection. Although the primary goal remains oncological safe cancer resection, the enhanced aesthetic outcomes, achieved within this approach, contribute to the improvements of the QoL among the survivors. The concept was therefore easily accepted worldwide and is further developing into a new surgical discipline.

Superior aesthetic outcomes are not the only advantage of the oncoplastic approach. In a meta-analysis of 8659 patients from 61 studies [16], specimen weight, re-excision rate, local recurrence rate and patient satisfaction were compared between conventional and oncoplastic BCS. All analysed endpoints favour the oncoplastic approach, indicating that higher rates of BCS with lower re-excision rates can be achieved in addition to lower local recurrence rates and higher patient satisfaction. It is interesting to consider that the same endpoints are proposed by the EUSOMA working group [21] for quality indicators (QIs) in the early-stage breast cancer surgical management evaluation. Accordingly, higher rates of breast conservation for low volume *in situ* and invasive breast disease, as well as lower rates of re-excision following BCS, suggest a higher quality of surgical management. In other words, the mastectomy rate of over 30%, in this subgroup of patients, indicates the poor quality of surgical management. Additional arguments that further support the latest observation are available in the scientific literature as well. Potter reports significantly higher rates of complications, re-operations and re-admissions to hospital in the oncoplastic mastectomy group as compared to oncoplastic breast conservation, in patients with tumour size less than 3 cm [22]. In Chands' QoL analysis, all aspects of the validated questionnaire (breast appearance, physical, emotional and sexual well-being) were better in the oncoplastic BCS group, when compared to any type of postmastectomy reconstruction [23]. Finally, in the Dutch cost-utility study, oncoplastic BCS is reported as more cost-effective than mastectomy followed by implant-based or autologous breast reconstruction [24].

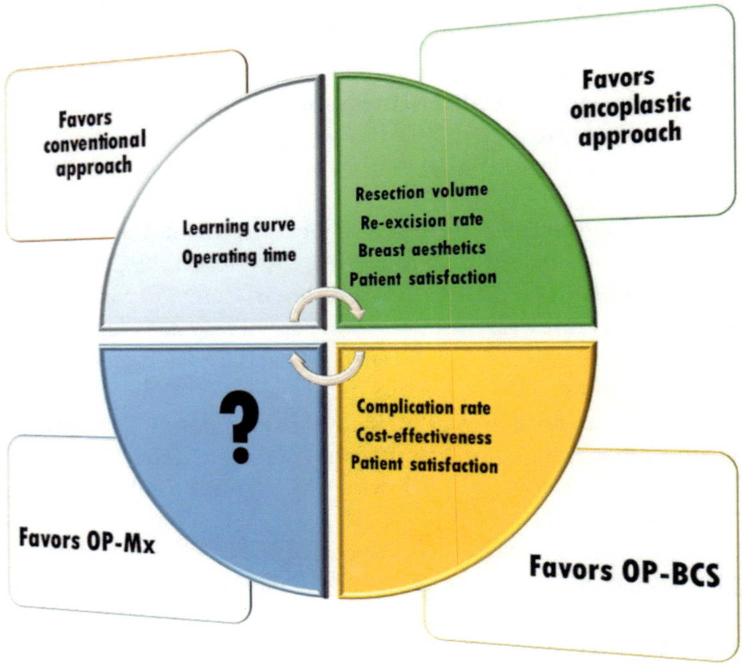

Figure 1.
Surgical options in early-stage breast cancer treatment. OP-BCS = oncoplastic breast conservative surgery, OP-Mx = oncoplastic mastectomy.

Considering all the above-mentioned arguments favouring oncoplastic BCS, the author believes that mastectomy should no longer be offered as a comparable treatment option for a low-volume breast disease unless there is a strong oncologic contraindication for breast conservation (**Figure 1**).

With all available oncoplastic techniques, the technical feasibility of surgery should not represent an issue in this stage of the disease. Moreover, the oncoplastic approach offers the opportunity for breast preservation even in selected patients with locally advanced disease [25].

3. Surgical management of locally advanced breast cancer (LABC)

Irrespective of screening programmes, 15% of all breast cancer is still diagnosed with the locally advanced stage of the disease (T3-4 and/or N2-3). However, the reported 5-year OS is still 70–80%. Therefore, QoL, as an important outcome measure in the management evaluation, cannot be ignored either in this group of patients.

In the modern multimodal approach, neoadjuvant systemic treatment is the first-line option for these patients. According to all relevant treatment recommendation guidelines, neoadjuvant chemotherapy (NAC) should be offered to all aggressive breast cancer phenotypes (TNBC and HER2 enriched) with a tumour size of over 2 cm or/and axillary lymph node involvement. From the surgical point of view, the major benefit of this approach is tumour downsizing, allowing a higher rate of conservative procedures in the breast and axilla. However, the high rate of treatment response following NAC is still not accompanied by the equivalent increase in BCS in everyday clinical practice; that is, the surgical overtreatment is consistently reported in the literature [26, 27].

According to evidence-based practice guidelines, as well as expert consensus guidelines, response-adjusted surgery is the recommended option following NAC; that is, only the residual disease in the breast should be removed following treatment response. For the non-responders, those with a poor response or with scattered patterns of response, the oncoplastic approach has broadened the possibilities for breast conservation. However, care should be taken in those patients with the multifocal residual pattern, lymphatic vascular invasion, residual T size over 2 cm, and extensive nodal involvement following NAC, as a higher risk of local and regional recurrence was reported for the subgroup of patients with multiple above-mentioned factors detected [28].

Nevertheless, extensive *in situ* disease, as well as extensive invasive breast cancer (T3), no longer represents an absolute contraindication for breast conservation. The results reported by Silverstein and Libson [25, 29] indicate that extreme oncoplastic breast conservation is an oncological safe approach for patients with high-volume breast disease. In addition, it allows safe and aesthetically pleasing breast preservation in patients with multifocal and multicentric diseases [30–33]. However, the decision on the type of surgical procedure for the LABC patient should be always made in a multidisciplinary fashion, considering all aspects of multimodal treatment, rather than the technical feasibility of surgery exclusively.

4. Relative contraindications for breast-conserving surgery

Although good aesthetic results and a large volume of resection can be achieved with oncoplastic BCS, mastectomy may still be required in patients with the multicentric disease when appropriate resection cannot be achieved in a single resection volume, especially for those patients with a higher risk of local relapse, in whom irradiation boost to tumour bed might be required for optimal oncologic outcomes.

Hereditary breast cancer with a proven high-risk genetic mutation, as well as strong family history without a proven high-risk mutation, but with a calculated lifetime risk of contralateral breast cancer of over 30%, may also represent a relative contraindication for BSC. For these patients, a bilateral mastectomy may be recommended, although the evidence of survival benefit is reported only after a long-term follow-up (>15 years) [34, 35]. In addition to young age, patients diagnosed with less aggressive tumour subtypes might as well benefit from the radical bilateral procedure [36]. When considering the risk of local relapse in patients with proven high-risk mutations, the results of scientific reports are unclear. Although there are literature data favouring mastectomy, other studies did not confirm any benefit for local control management in these patients [37].

Another issue requiring clarification in surgical management decision-making is ipsilateral breast recurrence following previous BCS and whole breast irradiation. Although better oncological outcomes following radical procedures have not been confirmed by the results of any randomised control trials, mastectomy is the most often recommended clinical practice for this condition. Nevertheless, several non-randomised clinical trials have reported non-inferiority of BCS for the selected subgroup of patients, even for those cases in which re-irradiation was omitted [38, 39].

In conclusion, when deciding on the type of breast surgery for LABC, multicentric, hereditary and familial breast cancer, as well as for ipsilateral recurrence, the author recommends a multidisciplinary and highly personalised approach to every case. The scientific evidence is not yet strong enough to support standardisation for optimal management in these patients. Randomised clinical trials are needed for a better understanding of these cases, although the low frequency of the condition and ethical issues involved represent obstacles to the appropriate study design.

5. Absolute contraindications for breast-conserving surgery

Only a few situations represent the absolute contraindication to BCS: inflammatory breast cancer, irrespective of NAC treatment response, inability to obtain adequate resection margins due to diffuse breast disease, and inability to deliver adjuvant breast irradiation (lack of required facilities or patient comorbidities that prevent safe irradiation delivery). Although rare nowadays, in these cases mastectomy is considered mandatory, with or without immediate or delayed breast reconstruction.

Patients' desire for radical surgery is another issue that requires consideration. It is often driven by patients' knowledge gaps and subsequent fear of disease recurrence. The surgeon's role in modifying patients' decisions is tremendous. Most of the patients can be reassured easily with the appropriate information concerning both procedures, as well as their impact on oncologic outcomes and QoL [22, 23]. A decision for mastectomy should never reflect the surgeon's desire to avoid complex oncoplastic surgery. The optimal treatment strategy must be offered to every patient and ignorance may not be an excuse for suboptimal management.

Relative and absolute contraindications for BCS are summarised in **Table 2**.

Relative contraindications for BCS	Absolute contraindications for BCS
Locally advanced breast cancer	
Multicentric disease	Inflammatory breast cancer
Hereditary breast cancer	Diffuse breast disease
Familial breast cancer	Adjuvant breast irradiation cannot be delivered
Ipsilateral breast cancer recurrence	
Patient opting for mastectomy?	

Table 2.
Relative and absolute contraindications for breast conserving surgery in breast cancer management.

6. Oncoplastic techniques in breast conservative surgery

For academic purposes, the techniques of partial breast reconstruction following tumour resection can be divided into two major groups: breast volume displacement and breast volume replacement (**Figure 2**). The basic difference is in the donor area utilised for partial breast reconstruction. The resected volume can be substituted by displacement of the remaining breast parenchyma, or replaced with fat tissue harvested adjacent to the breast.

Volume displacement techniques may further be categorised into level I (simple breast tissue advancement) and level II procedures (breast tissue rearrangement); however, due to variable definitions in the literature, certain techniques can be

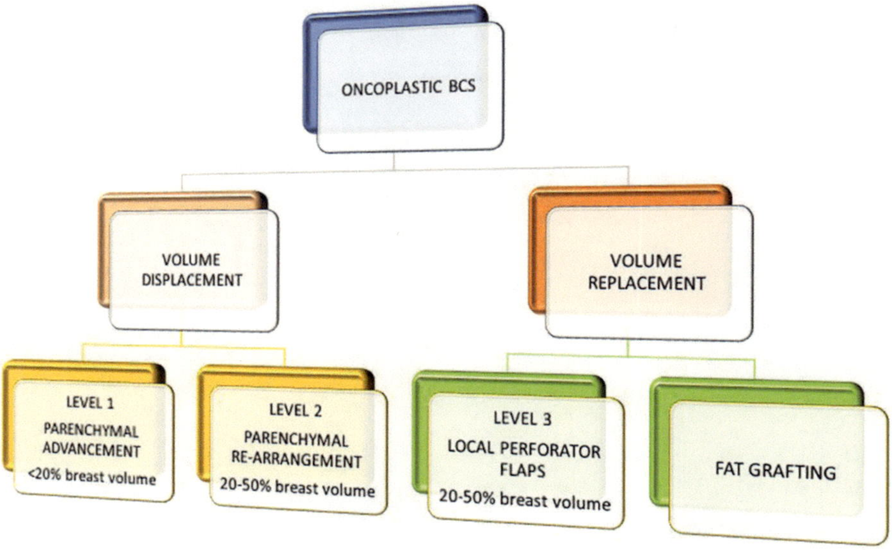

Figure 2.
Oncoplastic techniques in breast conserving surgery.

categorised in both groups. Although basic concepts originate from reconstructive surgery (advancement flaps) and aesthetic breast surgery (mastopexy and breast reduction), the adopted procedures were significantly modified and enriched with new techniques, designed for cancer surgery. Different oncoplastic breast surgery atlas recommendations, proposed by different authors, suggest a lack of standardisation in the field. Nevertheless, a multitude of techniques enables a personalised surgical approach for each patient.

Volume replacement techniques, local perforator flaps (level III) and fat grafting, both adopted from reconstructive surgery, have recently emerged as popular alternatives in partial breast reconstruction.

Clinical decision on the type of oncoplastic procedure is mainly based upon the anticipated percentage of breast volume loss and the residual breast volume [40], as well as the availability of additional donor sites, patients' preference and surgeons' skills.

Profound knowledge of breast anatomy is required for optimal performance for both ablative and reconstructive parts of all breast oncoplastic procedures. Compliance with the proposed oncoplastic planes of dissection, as well as respecting the breast as an aesthetic unit (shape, nipple position and symmetry with the contralateral breast), in addition to oncological safe tumour resection, is mandatory for the successful outcome of the oncoplastic surgery. Otherwise, it may result in higher complication rates (bleeding, skin and NAC necrosis, fat necrosis, infection), higher re-excision rates, and higher rates of local recurrence and disease progression. However, detailed breast anatomy and a description of surgical techniques are both beyond the scope of this chapter.

6.1 Level 1 volume displacement (parenchymal advancement)

Every oncoplastic breast surgery starts with skin incision planning. If the skin overlying the tumour is closed or involved, the skin incision is determined by the

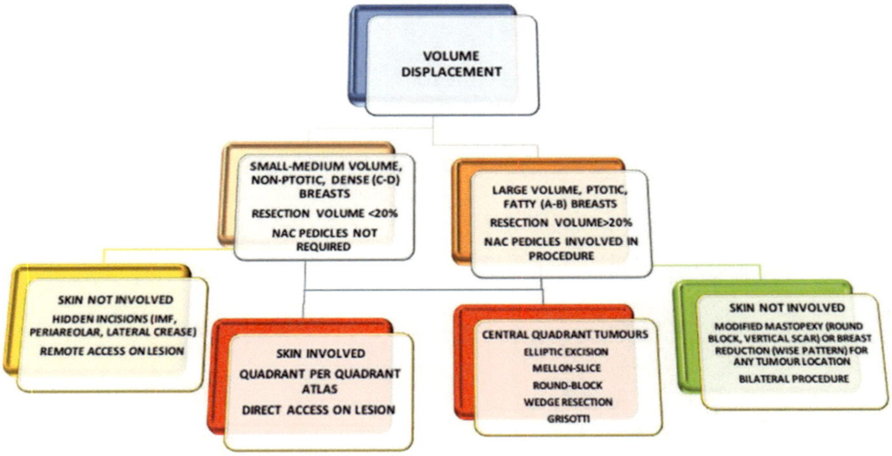

Figure 3.
Oncoplastic volume displacement level 1 and level 2.

tumour position. However, whenever oncology is safe, the preferred approach is the skin incision hidden in the inframammary fold (IMF), peri-areolar region or lateral mammary fold, accompanied by retro-glandular or subcutaneous access to the breast lesion and oncoplastic lumpectomy.

From the surgical perspective, oncoplastic level 1 procedures are technically the least demanding with a fast learning curve and wide applicability. It represents the optimal surgical approach for the majority of early-stage breast cancer patients. The best results are achieved for resections not exceeding 20% of the breast volume, ideally, in small- to medium-size, non-ptotic, firm, dense (BIRADS C-D) breasts. The basic concept of level 1 partial breast reconstruction relays upon single- or dual-layer mobilisation of the breast parenchyma surrounding the resected area and its closure by simple parenchymal advancement.

Nipple and areola complex (NAC) repositioning into a new breast centre may be required following extensive parenchymal advancement. However, if NAC pedicles and significant tissue rearrangement are involved, it would be more appropriate to categorise it as a level 2 procedure (**Figure 3**).

6.2 Level 2 volume displacement (parenchymal rearrangement)

Except for the NAC pedicle formation, significantly extensive breast tissue rearrangement is involved in level 2 procedures. Consequently, the procedures are more complex, as compared to level 1, and a longer learning curve is required. A resection volume of over 20% of breast volume is an indication for the level 2 procedure. However, only selected patients, with ptotic, medium or large volume, fatty (BIRADS A-B) breasts are appropriate candidates for level 2 oncoplastic breast conservation.

Although mastopexy and reduction mammoplasty represent the origins of the level 2 procedures, the techniques have been significantly modified for cancer surgery. If the skin is not involved, the type of the skin incision (round block, vertical scar, inverted T) is determined by surgeons' preference, breast volume and the degree of breast ptosis. Subcutaneous lumpectomy for any tumour location can be performed

DOI: http://dx.doi.org/10.5772/intechopen.108944

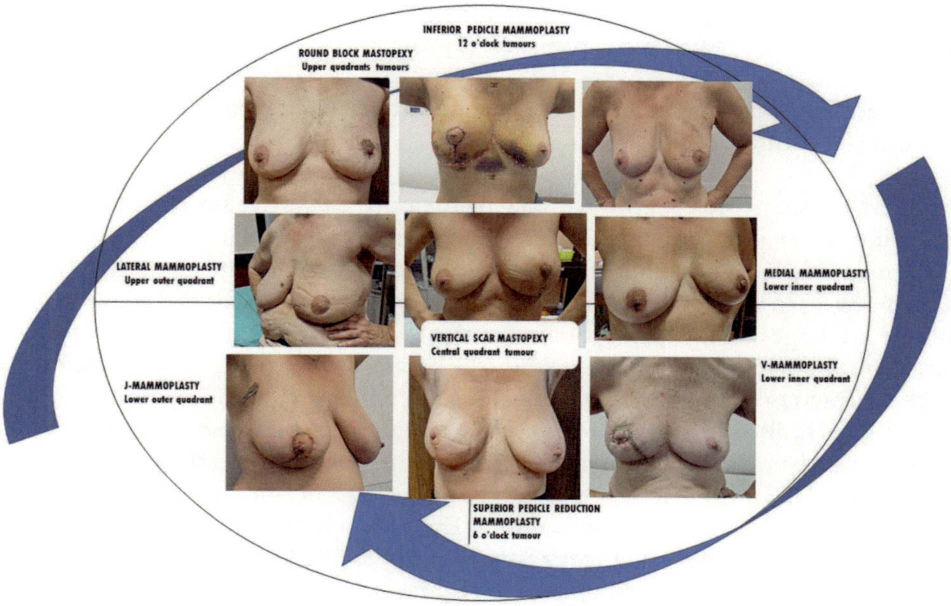

Figure 4.
Quadrant per quadrant atlas of oncoplastic volume displacement techniques.

through any of the above-proposed types of skin incision. However, the choice of NAC pedicle, parenchymal resection and rearrangement are influenced by the tumour location within the breast [19]. Nevertheless, if the overlying breast skin is involved, the tumour location determines the skin incision and the technique modification accordingly. For these situations, a quadrant-per-quadrant atlas of oncoplastic procedures has been proposed [41] as follows: lateral mammoplasty for the upper outer quadrant, J/L mammoplasty for the lower outer quadrant, V mammoplasty for the lower inner quadrant, batwing mastopexy for the upper inner quadrant, and superior/inferior pedicle mammoplasty for 12 and 6 o clock tumours (**Figure 4**).

For small-volume tumours in the small-to-medium volume, firm (dense), non-ptotic breasts, good results can be achieved in a single oncoplastic procedure. However, if a larger resection volume is required or the procedure is performed in hypertrophic, fatty and/or severe ptotic breasts, symmetry can only be achieved with an additional surgical procedure in the contralateral healthy breast. Following level 2 oncoplastic surgery, a symmetrisation procedure for the contralateral breast is usually required. Aesthetically pleasing results (good symmetry) can be accomplished with an equal procedure in the healthy breast at the time of cancer surgery or following adjuvant oncologic treatment(s) and an additional 6–12-month period required for breast stabilisation.

6.3 Oncoplastic breast conservation for central quadrant tumours

For central quadrant tumours, several procedures have been proposed: elliptic horizontal/vertical excision of the central portion of the breast, melon slice, round block and wedge resection. The choice of the optimal procedure depends on the breast volume and shape, as well as the breast volume required for oncological safe resection. The goal is to maintain the maximum projection site in the centre of the breast.

The proposed methods for NAC reconstruction are local skin flaps, contralateral NAC (grafting), NAC tattooing and external NAC prosthesis.

6.4 Level 3: volume replacement (local perforator flaps in partial breast reconstruction)

Another reconstructive option following breast conservative surgery is volume replacement (level 3 oncoplastic breast conservative surgery). The technique is the ideal choice if a large resection volume is required in a small volume breast and a patient desires to avoid mastectomy. It is also a good alternative for a large resection volume in a large volume breast, but in a patient wishing to avoid additional procedures for symmetry in a contralateral healthy breast. Moreover, it is a useful option for the correction of deformity following unsuccessful previous BCS.

The flaps utilised in partial breast reconstruction can be harvested as random or perforator-based flaps. The irrigation of the flap is based on nearby perforator arteries: medial, anterior, and lateral intercostal arteries perforators (MICAP, AICAP, LICAP), lateral thoracic artery perforators (LTAP) and thoracodorsal artery perforators (TDAP). These adipo-cutaneous flaps may be designed in the epigastric area, just below to IMF or in the lateral thoracic region, connected to a lateral mammary crease, and therefore can be easily inserted in a breast defect following tumour resection (**Figure 5**). However, additional scars, donor site morbidity and a higher risk of complications associated with these techniques mandate additional surgical training, as well as appropriate patient selection. A detailed description of the techniques is available widely across the literature [42–46] and is beyond the scope of this chapter.

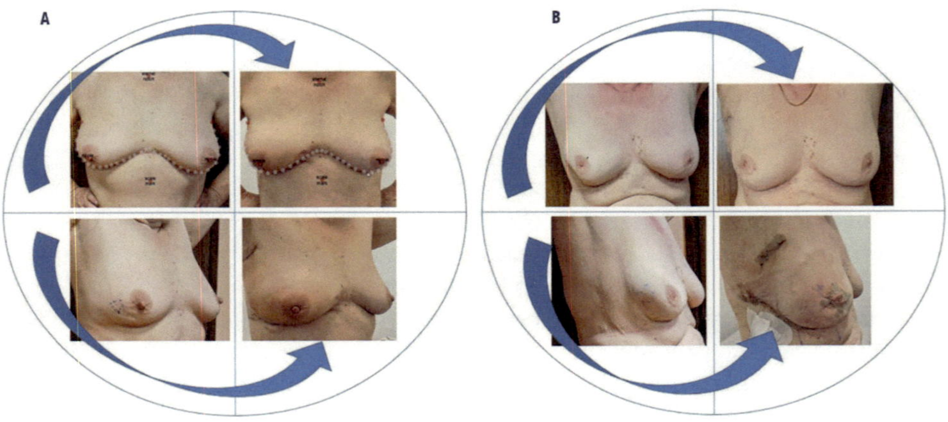

Figure 5.
Local perforator flaps for partial breast reconstruction harvested in a) epigastric region and b) lateral thoracic region.

7. Conclusion

Modern breast cancer surgical management should consider QoL as an equally important treatment outcome as the traditional oncological endpoints. Implementation of an oncoplastic breast conservative approach has significantly improved the QoL as compared to conventional BCS in early-stage breast cancer patients. Moreover, oncoplastic BCS has become a treatment option even for patients diagnosed in the locally advanced stage of the disease and irrespective of the tumour response to NAC. As compared to oncoplastic mastectomy, it does not affect the oncological outcomes; however, fewer complications, better QoL and fewer expenses for the healthcare system have been reported for the oncoplastic BCS.

Oncoplastic breast surgery has emerged as a new concept, and it is developing into a new surgical discipline. Basic surgical training in general or plastic surgery is no longer an optimal level of education for the surgeons involved in breast cancer management. Additional theoretical and practical knowledge is highly recommended. In addition, for optimal margin assessment, appropriate irradiation dose delivery and patient follow-up after an oncoplastic procedure, all breast specialists within the modern oncoplastic breast multidisciplinary team should become familiar with the oncoplastic techniques as well.

Conflict of interest

The author declares no conflict of interest.

Author details

Ana Car Peterko
Department of General Surgery and Surgical Oncology, Clinical Hospital Centre Rijeka, Rijeka, Croatia

*Address all correspondence to: anacarpeterko@gmail.com

References

[1] World Cancer Research Fund International. Breast Cancer Statistics. World Cancer Research Fund International; 2020. Available from: https://www.wcrf.org/cancer-trends/worldwide-cancer-data/

[2] National Cancer Institute. Surveillance, Epidemiology, and End Results Program Stat Fact Sheets: Female Breast Cancer. National Cancer Institute; 2019. Available from: https://seer.cancer.gov/statfacts/html/breast.html

[3] Allemani C, Minicozzi P, Berrino F, Bastiaannet E, Gavin A, Galceran J, et al. Predictions of survival up to 10 years after diagnosis for European women with breast cancer in 2000-2002. International Journal of Cancer. 2013;**132**(10):2404-2412. DOI: 10.1002/ijc.27895

[4] World Health Organization. Breast Cancer. World Health Organization; 2021. Available from: https://www.who.int/news-room/fact-sheets/detail/breast-cancer

[5] Veronesi U, Cascinelli N, Mariani L, Greco M, Saccozzi R, Luini A, et al. Twenty-year follow-up of a randomized study comparing breast-conserving surgery with radical mastectomy for early breast cancer. The New England Journal of Medicine. 2002;**347**(16):1227-1232. DOI: 10.1056/NEJMoa020989

[6] Veronesi U, Luini A, Galimberti V, Zurrida S. Conservation approaches for the management of stage I/II carcinoma of the breast: Milan cancer institute trials. World Journal of Surgery. 1994;**18**(1):70-75. DOI: 10.1007/BF00348194

[7] Fisher B, Anderson S, Bryant J, Margolese RG, Deutsch M, Fisher ER, et al. Twenty-year follow-up of a randomized trial comparing total mastectomy, lumpectomy, and lumpectomy plus irradiation for the treatment of invasive breast cancer. The New England Journal of Medicine. 2002;**347**(16):1233-1241. DOI: 10.1056/NEJMoa022152

[8] Hartmann-Johnsen OJ, Karesen R, Schlichting E, Nygard JF. Better survival after breast-conserving therapy compared to mastectomy when axillary node status is positive in early-stage breast cancer: A registry-based follow-up study of 6387 Norwegian women participating in screening, primarily operated between 1998 and 2009. World Journal of Surgical Oncology. 2017;**15**(1):118. DOI: 10.1186/s12957-017-1184-6

[9] Hartmann-Johnsen OJ, Kåresen R, Schlichting E, Nygård JF. Survival is better after breast conserving therapy than mastectomy for early stage breast cancer: A registry-based follow-up study of Norwegian women primary operated between 1998 and 2008. Annals of Surgical Oncology. 2015;**22**(12):3836-3845. DOI: 10.1245/s10434-015-4441-3

[10] Nandakumar A, Rath GK, Kataki AC, Bapsy PP, Gupta PC, Gangadharan P, et al. Decreased survival with mastectomy Vis-à-Vis breast-conserving surgery in stage II and III breast cancers: A comparative treatment effectiveness study. J Glob Oncol. 2016;**3**(4):304-313. DOI: 10.1200/JGO.2016.004614

[11] Agarwal S, Pappas L, Neumayer L, Kokeny K, Agarwal J. Effect of breast conservation therapy vs mastectomy on disease-specific survival for early-stage breast cancer. JAMA Surgery. 2014;**149**(3):267-274. DOI: 10.1001/jamasurg.2013.3049

[12] Christiansen P, Carstensen SL, Ejlertsen B, Kroman N, Offersen B, Bodilsen A, et al. Breast conserving surgery versus mastectomy: Overall and relative survival-a population based study by the Danish breast cancer cooperative group (DBCG). Acta Oncologica. 2018;**57**(1):19-25. DOI: 10.1080/0284186X.2017.1403042

[13] Lagendijk M, van Maaren MC, Saadatmand S, Strobbe LJA, Poortmans PMP, Koppert LB, et al. Breast conserving therapy and mastectomy revisited: Breast cancer-specific survival and the influence of prognostic factors in 129,692 patients. International Journal of Cancer. 2018;**142**(1):165-175. DOI: 10.1002/ijc.31034

[14] Moran MS, Schnitt SJ, Giuliano AE, Harris JR, Khan SA, Horton J, et al. Society of Surgical Oncology-American Society for Radiation Oncology consensus guideline on margins for breast-conserving surgery with whole-breast irradiation in stages I and II invasive breast cancer. International Journal of Radiation Oncology, Biology, Physics. 2014;**88**(3):553-564. DOI: 10.1016/j.ijrobp.2013.11.012

[15] Morrow M, Van Zee KJ, Solin LJ, Houssami N, Chavez-MacGregor M, Harris JR, et al. Society of Surgical Oncology-American Society for Radiation Oncology-American Society of Clinical Oncology consensus guideline on margins for breast-conserving surgery with whole-breast irradiation in ductal carcinoma In situ. Annals of Surgical Oncology. 2016;**23**(12):3801-3810. DOI: 10.1245/s10434-016-5449-z

[16] Losken A, Dugal CS, Styblo TM, Carlson GW. A meta-analysis comparing breast conservation therapy alone to the oncoplastic technique. Annals of Plastic Surgery. 2014;**72**(2):145-149. DOI: 10.1097/SAP.0b013e3182605598

[17] Cochrane RA, Valasiadou P, Wilson AR, Al-Ghazal SK, Macmillan RD. Cosmesis and satisfaction after breast-conserving surgery correlates with the percentage of breast volume excised. The British Journal of Surgery. 2003;**90**(12):1505-1509. DOI: 10.1002/bjs.4344

[18] Pukancsik D, Kelemen P, Újhelyi M, Kovács E, Udvarhelyi N, Mészáros N, et al. Objective decision making between conventional and oncoplastic breast-conserving surgery or mastectomy: An aesthetic and functional prospective cohort study. European Journal of Surgical Oncology. 2017;**43**(2):303-310. DOI: 10.1016/j.ejso.2016.11.010

[19] Losken A, Hamdi M. Partial Breast Reconstruction-Techniques in Oncoplastic Surgery. 2nd ed. New York: Thieme; 2017

[20] Audretsch W, Rezai M, Kolotas C, et al. Onco-plastic surgery: "Target" Volume Reduction (BCT-mastopexy), Lumpectomy, Reconstruction (BCT-Reconstruction), and Flap-supported Operability in Breast Cancer. Proceedings of 2nd European Congress on Senology, Vienna, Austria, Bologna. October 1994;**2**(6):139-157

[21] Biganzoli L, Marotti L, Hart CD, Cataliotti L, Cutuli B, Kühn T, et al. Quality indicators in breast cancer care: An update from the EUSOMA working group. European Journal of Cancer. 2017;**86**:59-81. DOI: 10.1016/j.ejca.2017.08.017

[22] Potter S, Trickey A, Rattay T, O'Connell RL, Dave R, Baker E, et al. Therapeutic mammaplasty is a safe and effective alternative to mastectomy with or without immediate breast reconstruction. BJS. 2020;**107**(7):832-844. DOI: 10.1002/bjs.11468

[23] Chand ND, Browne V, Paramanathan N, Peiris LJ,

Laws SA, Rainsbury RM. Patient-Reported Outcomes Are Better after Oncoplastic Breast Conservation than after Mastectomy and Autologous Reconstruction.Plast Reconstr Surg Glob Open. 24 Jul 2017;**5**(7):e1419. DOI: 10.1097/GOX.0000000000001419. PMID: 28831358; PMCID: PMC5548581

[24] Kouwenberg CAE, Mureau MAM, Kranenburg LW, Rakhorst H, de Leeuw D, Klem TMAL, et al. Cost-utility analysis of four common surgical treatment pathways for breast cancer. European Journal of Surgical Oncology. 2021;**47**(6):1299-1308. DOI: 10.1016/j.ejso.2020.11.130

[25] Silverstein MJ. Radical mastectomy to radical conservation (extreme Oncoplasty): A revolutionary change. Journal of the American College of Surgeons. 2016;**222**(1):1-9. DOI: 10.1016/j.jamcollsurg.2015.10.007

[26] McGuire K, Santillan A, Kaur P, Meade T, Parbhoo J, Mathias M, et al. Are mastectomies on the rise? A 13-year trend analysis of the selection of mastectomy versus breast conservation therapy in 5865 patients. Annals of Surgical Oncology. 2009;**16**:2682-2690

[27] Pollom EL, Qian Y, Chin AL, Dirbas FM, Asch SM, Kurian AW, et al. Rising rates of bilateral mastectomy with reconstruction following neoadjuvant chemotherapy. International Journal of Cancer. 2018;**143**(12):3262-3272. DOI: 10.1002/ijc.31747

[28] Chen AM, Meric-Bernstam F, Hunt KK, Thames HD, Outlaw ED, Strom EA, et al. Breast conservation after neoadjuvant chemotherapy. Cancer. 2005;**103**(4):689-695. DOI: 10.1002/cncr.20815

[29] Libson S, Koshenkov V, Rodgers S, Hurley J, Avisar E. Breast conservation after neoadjuvant therapy for tumors ≥5 cm: A prospective cohort study. International Journal of Surgery Open. 2015;**1**:10-13. DOI: 10.1016/j.ijso.2015.12.001

[30] Lynch SP, Lei X, Hsu L, Meric-Bernstam F, Buchholz TA, Zhang H, et al. Breast cancer multifocality and multicentricity and locoregional recurrence. The Oncologist. 2013;**18**(11):1167-1173. DOI: 10.1634/theoncologist.2013-0167

[31] Houvenaeghel G, Tallet A, Jalaguier-Coudray A, Cohen M, Bannier M, Jauffret-Fara C, et al. Is breast conservative surgery a reasonable option in multifocal or multicentric tumors? World J Clin Oncol. 2016;**7**(2):234-242. DOI: 10.5306/wjco.v7.i2.234

[32] Neri A, Marrelli D, Megha T, et al. Clinical significance of multifocal and multicentric breast cancers and choice of surgical treatment: A retrospective study on a series of 1158 cases. BMC Surgery. 2015;**15**:1. DOI: 10.1186/1471-2482-15-1

[33] Vera-Badillo FE, Napoleone M, Ocana A, Templeton AJ, Seruga B, Al-Mubarak M, et al. Effect of multifocality and multicentricity on outcome in early stage breast cancer: A systematic review and meta-analysis. Breast Cancer Research and Treatment. 2014;**146**(2):235-244. DOI: 10.1007/s10549-014-3018-3

[34] Basu NN, Ross GL, Evans DG, Barr L. The Manchester guidelines for contralateral risk-reducing mastectomy. World Journal of Surgical Oncology. 2015;**13**:237. DOI: 10.1186/s12957-015-0638-y

[35] Valachis A, Nearchou AD, Lind P. Surgical management of breast cancer in BRCA-mutation carriers: A systematic review and meta analysis. Breast Cancer Research and Treatment. 2014;**144**:44

[36] Huang E, Buchholz TA, Meric F, Krishnamurthy S, Mirza NQ, Ames FC, et al. Classifying local disease recurrences after breast conservation therapy based on location and histology: New primary tumors have more favorable outcomes than true local disease recurrences. Cancer. 2002;**95**(10):2059-2067

[37] Pierce LJ, Phillips K-A, Griffith KA, Buys S, Gaffney DK, Moran MS, et al. Local therapy in BRCA1 and BRCA2 mutation carriers with operable breast cancer: Comparison of breast conservation and mastectomy. Breast Cancer Research and Treatment. 2010;**121**(2):389-398

[38] Gentilini O, Botteri E, Veronesi P, Sangalli C, Del Castillo A, Ballardini B, et al. Repeating conservative surgery after ipsilateral breast tumor reappearance: Criteria for selecting the best candidates. Annals of Surgical Oncology. 2012;**19**(12):3771-3776. DOI: 10.1245/s10434-012-2404-5

[39] Yoshida A, Takahashi O, Okumura Y, Arima N, Nakatsukasa K, Tanabe M, et al. Prognosis after mastectomy versus repeat lumpectomy in patients with ipsilateral breast cancer recurrence: A propensity score analysis. European Journal of Surgical Oncology. 2016;**42**(4):474-480. DOI: 10.1016/j.ejso.2016.01.011

[40] Macmillan RD, McCulley SJ. Oncoplastic breast surgery: What, when and for whom? Curr Breast Cancer Rep. 2016;**8**:112-117. DOI: 10.1007/s12609-016-0212-9

[41] Clough KB, Kaufman GJ, Nos C, Buccimazza I, Sarfati IM. Improving breast cancer surgery: A classification and quadrant per quadrant atlas for oncoplastic surgery. Annals of Surgical Oncology. 2010;**17**(5):1375-1391. DOI: 10.1245/s10434-009-0792-y

[42] Hamdi M, De Frene B. Pedicled perforator flaps in breast reconstruction. Seminars in Plastic Surgery. 2006;**20**(2):73-78. DOI: 10.1055/s-2006-941713

[43] Mangialardi ML, Baldelli I, Salgarello M, Raposio E. Breast reconstruction using the lateral thoracic, thoracodorsal, and intercostal arteries perforator flaps. Plastic and Reconstructive Surgery. Global Open. 2021;**9**(1):e3334. DOI: 10.1097/GOX.0000000000003334

[44] Yang JD, Ryu DW, Lee JW, Choi KY, Chung HY, Cho BC, et al. Usefulness of a lateral thoracodorsal flap after breast conserving surgery in laterally located breast cancer. Archives of Plastic Surgery. 2013;**40**(4):367-373. DOI: 10.5999/aps.2013.40.4.367

[45] Acea Nebril B, Builes Ramírez S, García Novoa A, Varela LC. Rotational flaps in oncologic breast surgery. Anatomical and technical considerations. Cirugía Española. 2016;**94**(7):372-378. DOI: 10.1016/j.ciresp.2016.03.004

[46] Schaverien MV, Kuerer HM, Caudle AS, Smith BD, Hwang RF, Robb GL. Outcomes of volume replacement Oncoplastic breast-conserving surgery using Chest Wall perforator flaps: Comparison with volume displacement Oncoplastic surgery and Total breast reconstruction. Plastic and Reconstructive Surgery. 2020;**146**(1):14-27. DOI: 10.1097/PRS.0000000000006911

Chapter 17

Physiotherapeutic Management in Breast Cancer Patients

Margit Eidenberger

Abstract

Breast cancer treatment can lead to various physic and psychic long-term morbidities, such as restricted shoulder joint range of motion, lymphedema, impaired muscle strength, or cancer-related fatigue. Physiotherapy is a body-oriented approach to tackle these different complaints. This chapter starts with possible prehabilitation approaches until therapy or surgery. It continues with early post-op mobilization and shoulder-arm exercises during the early stages and additionally breathing exercises. In the following rehabilitation period and after hospital discharge, the focus lies on shoulder joint range of motion, muscle strengthening, and body posture to regain normal activities of daily life. This is supported by easy learnable exercises and therapy measures. Lymphedema prevention and treatment are discussed as well as sports therapy, which is divided into endurance and strength training. Therefore, an active lifestyle is encouraged by also considering necessary precautions while training during chemotherapy cycles. Common symptoms and problems, such as cancer-related fatigue and chemotherapy-induced polyneuropathy, are tackled with techniques, such as yoga or balance training. Scar therapy and radiation-induced lung injury are delineated followed by massage therapy proposals and specified exercises to enhance oxygen uptake.

Keywords: prehabilitation, rehabilitation, shoulder joint mobility, lymphedema, endurance training, strength training, relaxation

1. Introduction

Breast cancer is the most common cancer type in women. The latest improvements in early detection and therapy have led to a 10-year overall survival rate of up to 78% [1] in central Europe. At the time of diagnosis, most women are between 55 and 69 years old [2], but also younger women are increasingly affected, every one of these interested in an ongoing high quality of life after completing therapy. This has necessarily brought attention to the treatment of morbidities following the diagnosis and/or side effects of modern breast cancer treatment [3]. Women not only resume their working position but also want to return to sports after breast cancer treatment and/or reconstructive breast surgery and therefore need support, advice, and medical expertise.

Physiotherapy is a body- and patient-oriented approach for tackling different complaints of breast cancer patients after surgery (breast-conserving surgery BCS, mastectomy, and/or breast reconstruction), radiation therapy (RT), chemotherapy

(CT), or hormone therapy. It aims at shoulder joint immobility, pain, scar complaints, or lymphedema with means of "hands-on techniques." Patients are furthermore educated to perform customized exercises, that is, "hands-off exercises" to regain their mobility and strength [4] and in doing so act as their own therapist.

The physiotherapeutic process starts with a thorough patient anamnesis, inspection and palpation, and further assessments to figure out the reason for the patient's problem. Afterward, the physiotherapist suggests a suitable treatment approach according to her/his expertise, medical research evidence, and the patient's values and preferences. Patient adherence to therapy is crucial for ongoing success.

This chapter gives an overview of different physiotherapeutic approaches, therefore guiding breast cancer patients through different stages of cancer treatment and afterward. Various common complaints and deficits are depicted followed by evidence-based exercise and therapy suggestions. It describes physiotherapy as an important part of the whole therapy concept contributing to a patient's better quality of life. Even in case of cancer-recurrence or metastasis, and during palliative stages, adapted training and activity of life guidance is possible and can facilitate the patient's remaining life.

2. Prehabilitation

Prehabilitation is the approach to start therapy shortly after definite breast cancer diagnosis to make use of the remaining time until surgery (30 ± 17 days) or other medical treatments are planned. Prehabilitation has been able to improve bodily functions, shoulder range of motion (ROM), activities of daily life (ADL), and led to a shorter recovering period after surgery [5]. Acknowledging the fact that patients' activities will inevitably diminish post-surgery, by employing prehabilitation, women can guarantee that the percentage change will be of lesser consequence. Physical as well as psychological parameters can be improved during the weeks until the therapy starts.

To achieve this, patients are encouraged to take longer walks or go for Nordic walking (30–60 min) at an average or higher walking speed (4–5,5 km/h) on flat ground and even on gradient tracks. This leads to better oxygen uptake and cardiopulmonary function. They are instructed to do specific shoulder exercises to enhance a) shoulder ROM and b) shoulder girdle muscle strength by resistance training [6]. The training furthermore affords an opportunity to distract patients from disease-centered thoughts and can divert constant and circulating worries. It should, therefore, be complemented by an easy-to-learn kind of relaxation therapy, for example, deep breathing exercises [7] or Jacobson's progressive relaxation.

3. Postoperative phase

Out-of-bed mobilization starts on post-surgery day one for BCS and mastectomy. With certain reconstructive breast surgeries, this is delayed for one or two more days. Early mobilization improves patients' independence for basic ADLs and protects against deep vein thrombosis. In a short time, patients are independent to use the toilet, to take meals at the table or to perform basic body hygiene for themselves.

Patients should train and/or walk two times a day for overall 10–20 minutes with an assured blood pressure of a minimum of 105/70 to a maximum of 150/90 and a heart rate of (180 minus age minus 10%). The walking speed is set at 60–80 steps per minute, which corresponds to a low intensity of 25–50 Watts. A recumbent bike can be used after removing urinary catheter and drains. When using the (new) BORG Scale as an intensity level parameter, patients should specify their personal level of exhaustion at 1–2/10 during training sessions.

Patients are educated to perform their own breathing exercises and thrombosis prophylaxis, that is, calf-muscle pump, by moving and circling their ankles. In their own interest, this should be done every hour with 20–30 repetitions and 2–3 sets. While lying or sitting upright in bed or in a buxton chair in their room, the pursed-lips technique is used for exhaling combined with a deep breathing technique, preferably through the nose, while inhaling. The breathing is guided to the thoracic flank, the abdominal region, or the pulmonal apex region stimulated by the patient's own hands. From 12 to 15 breathing cycle repetitions are necessary for three series, interrupted by 30–60 sec breaks. Breathing exercises can also be combined with low-level shoulder exercises [8], such as shoulder shrugs, shoulder circles, arm flexion, and arm abduction.

Patients are lying supine in bed, and the affected side's arm is supported by one or more pillows to ensure low pain levels and to enhance lymphatic flow. A heart-shaped pillow placed in the axillary region can reduce pain and muscle tension after axillary lymphadenectomy. Patients are provided with such a pillow as an individual present at the ward. For reconstructive breast surgery, such as the DIEP flap or the TRAM flap, even more pillows or a positioning block is needed to support the calves/legs to relieve the abdominal region from exorbitant scar tension.

Arm exercises at the wrist and elbow level also start on day one. This improves wound healing, pain, and quality of life [9–11]. Shoulder exercises start on day three for BCS, but are restricted to 90° flexion and abduction and should respect lower levels if patients report pain [12]. Starting too early or in a too progressive regime could lead to an enhanced risk of seroma formation [13], lymphedema, or higher fluid drainage [8]. Mastectomy patients should wait with shoulder exercises until day 5 to diminish the risk of bleeding [14]. Arm lever, and therefore, weight during shoulder exercises, should be reduced in the beginning by maximal elbow flexion, which places the fingers at the corresponding shoulder. To remember these exercises correctly, patients are receiving a written information leaflet with precise instructions and further precaution measures to be taken in the following weeks and months.

After removing surgery drains [15], which is approximately on day 2–6 for breast and axillary drains, respectively, with the axillary drain normally remaining longer than the breast drain, the physiotherapist (PT) can induce passive and passive-assisted hands-on techniques in different directions. This will enhance scapular and humerus movements and can reduce excessive muscular tensions, for example, in the rhomboid or trapezius muscle and therefore pain (cp. **Figure 1**).

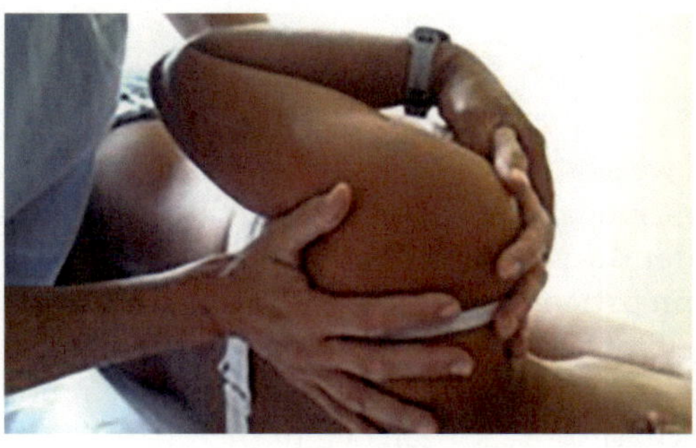

Figure 1.
Scapular movements: Cranial/caudal; ventral/dorsal and in diagonal shape (anterior elevation/posterior depression).

The patient is discharged from the hospital on days 2–14, depending on type of surgery (longer for several breast reconstructions), eventual complications, and personal wound healing. Given this possible short in-patient time, it is crucial to ensure that patients are provided with all information necessary and behavior tips to pay attention to after discharge. This can be supplemented by a list of available outpatients' services if they are in need of further therapy or advice. The wound and the scar need support and protection for at least 4–6 weeks. Exercises started during the in-patient period are to be prolonged for the following weeks and maybe even months depending on the individual symptoms. In case of breast and trunk, RT thorax stretching and breathing exercises are recommended for several months to counteract tissue fibrosis.

4. Rehabilitation

Rehabilitation for breast cancer survivors can be very heterogenous [3] depending on the different complaints and symptoms. It aims at restoring the best possible state of health, in a somatic as well as a psychic manner. In the first weeks after surgery, some precautionary measures have to be taken to not impede proper wound healing. This includes not carrying or lifting heavy weights or children with the affected arm and avoiding exhausting household tasks, such as vacuum cleaning, window cleaning, lawn mowing, snow shoveling, or lifting out heavy cooking pots. On the other hand, women are encouraged to use their arms increasingly, for example, body hygiene, such as teeth brushing or hair combing or easy household tasks, for example, dusting off. This is relevant to not becoming accustomed to prolonged "cradling of the arm" protectively against the body, which compromises shoulder ROM and/or arm swing during walking and furthermore affects posture badly.

In case of long-lasting side effects, patients should be taught compensatory mechanisms and ways to improve and economize their ADLs. This also includes supplying the patient with several necessary tools, for example, a long-handled reacher.

Even in the case of cancer recurrence, with improved medical possibilities and treatments, many patients are facing several years of life to come. This shows the need for body-oriented therapies and approaches to improve patients' symptoms and facilitate the patients' ongoing life in the aspect of mobility, edema, or pain. These recommendations should be considered even if disease progression is complicating therapy application increasingly [16]. If necessary, relatives or other caregivers should be involved in the therapy procedure to facilitate ADLs and transfers. In palliative contexts, this not only empowers and strengthens these people but also simplifies the relationship between the patient and her caregiver at home.

4.1 Shoulder joint

During the second week after surgery and after suture removal, shoulder joint mobility progresses without any limit [11] to reach high ROM as soon as possible. This is not only important for the patient herself, but is also paramount for starting an RT, which requires a certain patient position with maximal arm flexion and/or abduction to reach the axillary region. Otherwise, the RT could be delayed with unfavorable patients' outcomes [17]. Therefore, it is recommended to employ several techniques and exercises. Patients have already been taught their individualized home exercise program, which they should apply at least three times a week but better daily for 3 more months [15] with 10–20 repetitions for each exercise. Flexion, abduction, and external rotation are the most limited shoulder movements, so the focus lies on these motions. Scar treatment and muscle stretching are in close connection with shoulder ROM and complete the program enriched by relaxation techniques.

While exercising, patients are lying supine or sideward, sitting on a stool, or are standing securely on even ground. Exercise and stretching can induce a certain feeling of discomfort but should not trigger pain. If so, this exercise has to be finished or slightly varied until the pain subsides. Patients are using their own arm weight as a means of resistance or easily available tools, such as a rubber band, little hand weights or dumbbells, a broomstick, a towel, or filled small mineral water bottles as a weight substitute.

External rotation can be exercised with a yellow or later red rubber band fixed on a door handle while standing. The patient is holding her arm in a neutral position and the elbow close to the trunk with a 90° elbow flexion and is holding the loose end. She is then pulling against the rubber band resistance for the maximal possible external rotation and slowly easing back, which induces both concentric and excentric muscle activities.

For the so-called "elbow clam exercise" to enhance shoulder abduction, the patient is lying supine, both hands are crossed behind the head, and elbows together in front of the face. Now, the patient is abducting her arms, ideally, until the elbows touch the ground, left, and right (cp. **Figure 2**). She is holding this final position for at least 10 seconds, breathing steadily, and then moves slowly back.

Flexion can be enhanced, for example, with the "cleaning the door exercise." The patient stands facing the door, and the hand of the affected arm is resting on the door

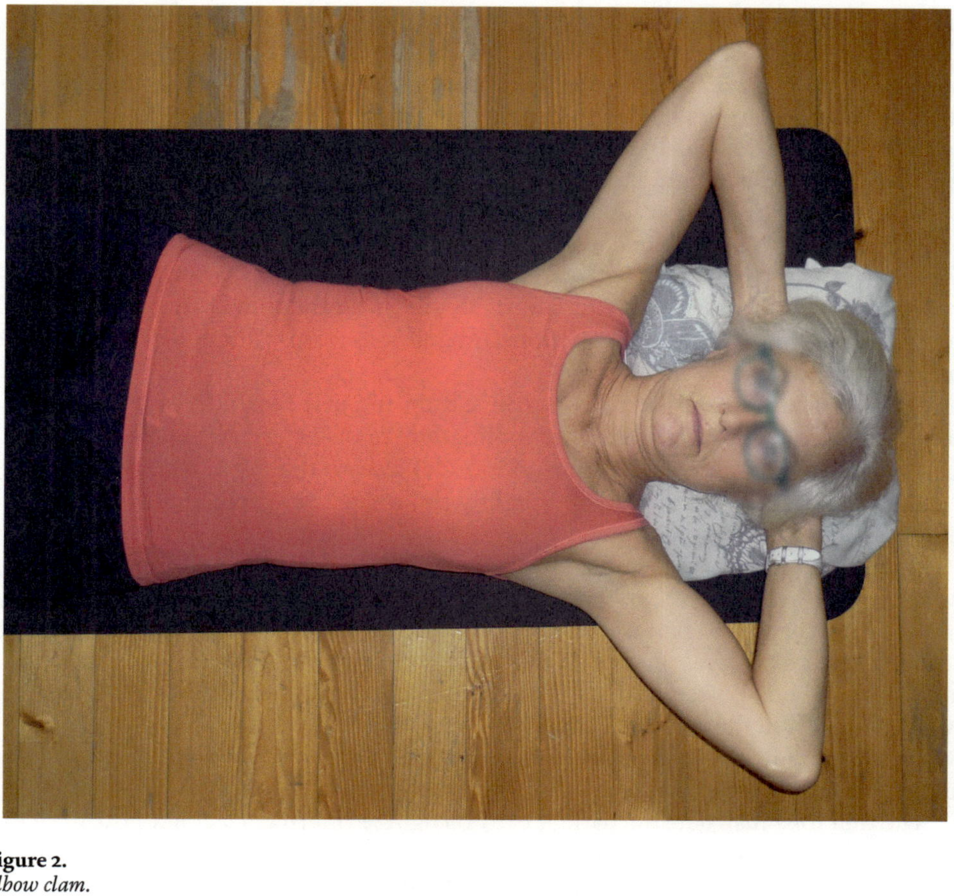

Figure 2.
Elbow clam.

panel with a small cloth in between. Now the arm is slowly gliding upward as high as possible at the time given and back to breast level. The arm's weight is resting partially on the door. During the exercise, the patient is instructed to maintain an upright body posture and not to lean back as a form of compensatory movement. Arm flexion is combined with inhaling and extension with exhaling.

4.2 Posture

Out of 82% women, after breast cancer surgery, only 35% of women develop a bad body posture [18]. This includes shoulder elevation, shoulder protraction, subacromial space reduction, trunk rotation, head rotation, and thoracic spine kyphosis [19–21]. Explainable reasons for these are pain, high muscle tension, axillary seroma, and a disproportional weight distribution after mastectomy without a breast prosthesis or a heavy-weight external prosthesis. The kyphosis also correlates with a kind of "startle pattern" so as not to show the missing/operated breast to their surroundings. The misguided postures lead to prolonged shoulder immobility, as the humerus cannot glide freely. Furthermore, muscle tension triggered pain [22] or even gait changes can follow.

Remedies are the bilateral arm exercises with the proprioceptive neuromuscular facilitation (PNF) concept [23]. This combines shoulder flexion, abduction, and external rotation with rubber-band resistance. Besides shoulder ROM improvement, trunk erection is also involved (cp. **Figure 3**). The patient is sitting on a stool, with her feet fixing both loose ends on the floor. The band is then crossed at lower legs height and fixed around both palms. In the beginning, the left hand is resting on the right knee and *vice versa*. She then starts the movement by lifting, abducting, and rotating both her arms, which inhibits unwarranted trunk movements until her maximal shoulder position is possible. The tension at the final position is to beheld for a few seconds, then the movement is slowly reversed back until both hands are resting on the knees as in the beginning.

While executing the so-called popular PT exercise "block game," the sitting patient is taught to actively feel, correct, and erect her three blocks, that is, the head, the trunk, and the pelvis in a vertical axis, one on top of the other. She then stabilizes and strengthens the now erect trunk by deploying both abdominal and back musculatures by moving the trunk slightly forward and backward without leaving the erect spine position.

Self-mobilizing exercises with the arm resting on a soft flexible ball while sitting sideward to a table correct the humerus direction caudal by activating the scapula (rhomboid muscle, transverse trapezius muscle) toward the spine, while simultaneously giving pressure on the ball and slightly abducting the arm by rolling the ball sideward (cp. **Figure 4**).

Humerus correction direction dorsal is achieved by the patient while standing with the face toward a wall. Both arms are lifted to 90° arm flexion, elbows 90° flexed, and the lower arms and hands in connection with the wall. She then approaches the sternum toward the wall slightly for correcting the humerus position, because the humerus is gliding posterior at this very moment. Secondly, she pushes her trunk slightly back from the wall. The latter also strengthens the serratus anterior muscle, which is sometimes weakened because of the possible corresponding nerve damage during surgery (cp. **Figure 5**).

The therapist instructs the patient to a) recognize and b) correct her posture. This can involve lowering the shoulder, straightening up, and de-rotating the trunk and/or head. In most cases, the trunk is pathologically rotated with the operated side moving

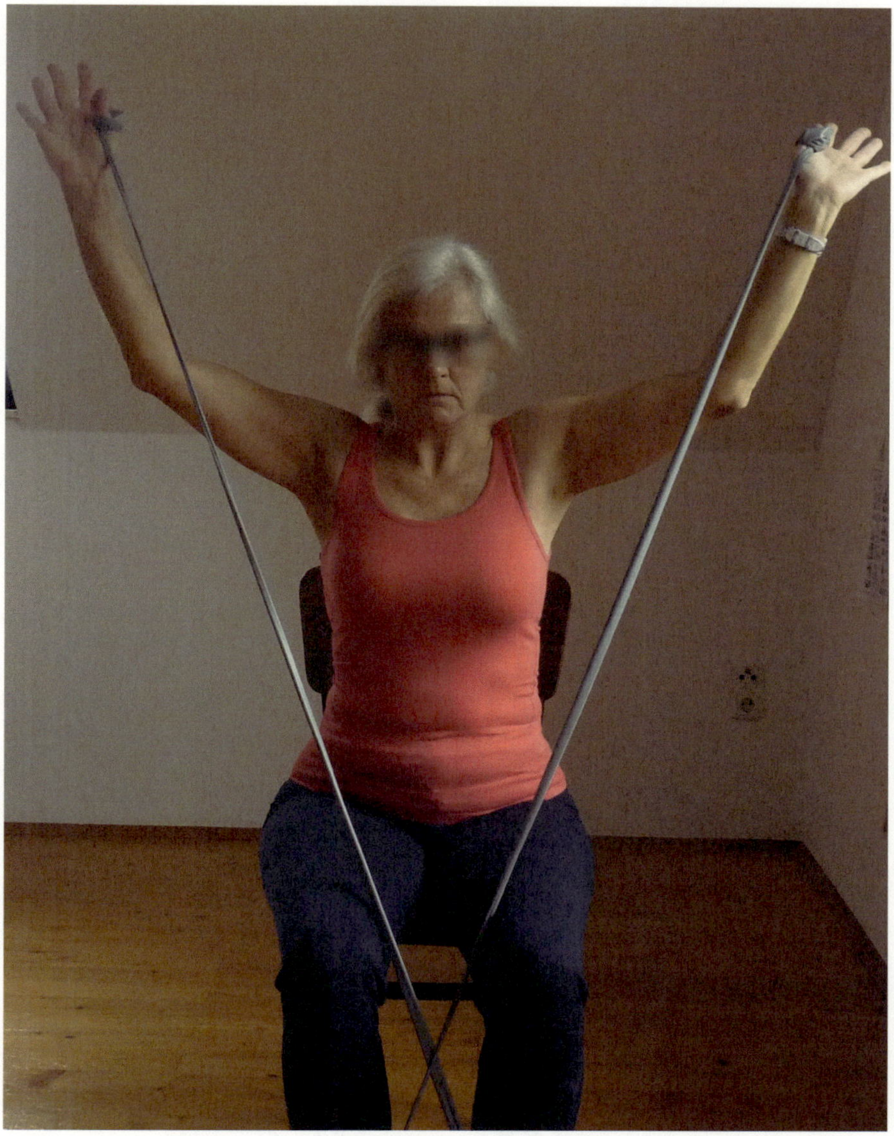

Figure 3.
PNF arm flexion/abduction/external rotation with a rubber band.

forward, while the head is rotated backward in the other direction to keep clear sight in front of the head. A mirror helps the patient to control herself and adjust her position accordingly.

4.3 Muscle stretching and strength

Different muscles incline to shorten, above all the pectoralis major and minor and the latissimus dorsi muscle because of pain, RT, or non-usage. Stretching is possible as a hands-on (cp. **Figure 6**) and a hands-off procedure by the patient herself. Other muscles, such as the trapezius, levator scapulae, or deltoid muscle [24], but also the rectus capitis or semispinalis capitis muscle [25] tend to develop an often painful

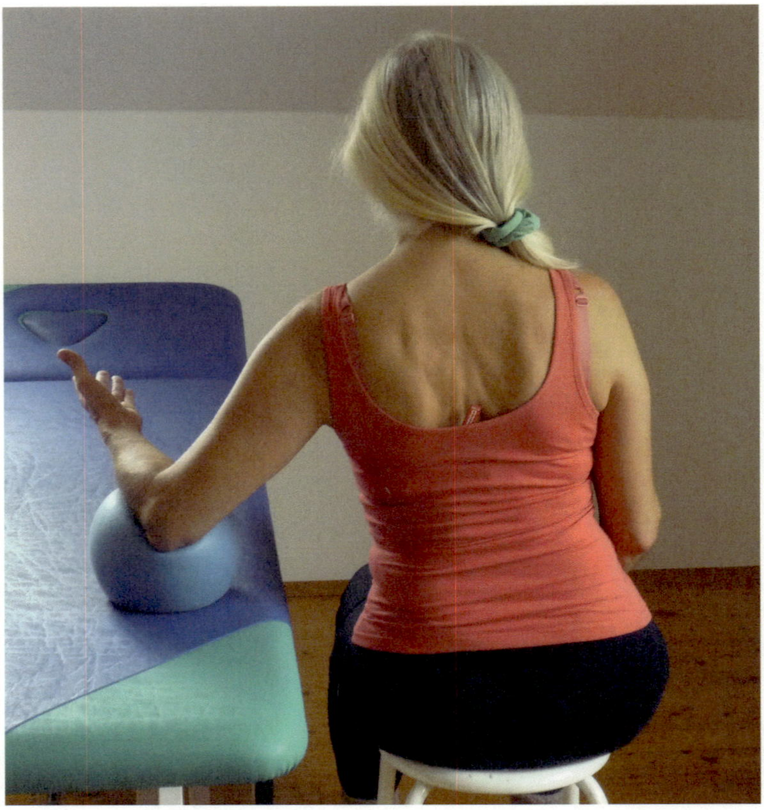

Figure 4.
Self-mobilizing humerus caudal.

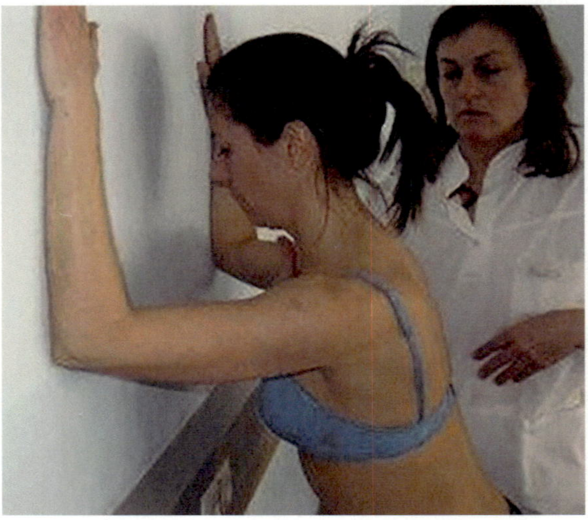

Figure 5.
Self-mobilizing humerus dorsal.

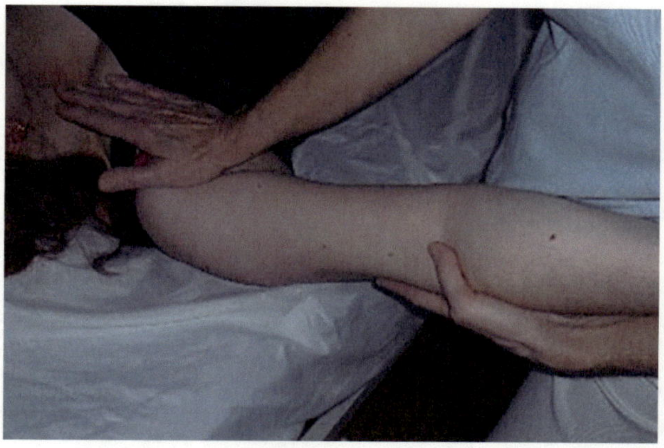

Figure 6.
Therapeutic pectoralis major stretching.

hypertonus. Pain and the described "arm-cradling" imply muscle weakness. The overall loss of strength lies at 25% with an incidence of 18–23% [15], all of which can lead to shoulder instability [26] and even rotator cuff dysfunctions [19].

For auto-stretching, yoga exercises are appropriate means. The "Crocodile position," that is, "Makarasana" is an ideal exercise to stretch the pectoralis muscle and secondly to induce a deep breathing cycle at the affected trunk side. This is also important to counteract possible RT skin and lung and connective tissue side effects, such as long-term fibrosis. The arm position can be varied according to the patient's shoulder ROM and possible lymphedema. A pillow should then ensure that the arm is supported and that the hand is in the highest position that facilitates lymphatic flow.

Another yoga asana is the adapted "Cow face" or "Gomukhasana." With the aid of a towel or a belt, one arm is extended behind the back, while the other one is flexed over the head, both with flexed elbows, holding the towel/belt with both hands. The goal is for both hands to reach out to one another as close as possible. The healthy arm is supporting the affected arm by a pull on the before-mentioned belt or towel. This enhances flexion, extension, and both in- and outward rotations.

Strength training should be focused on but not limited to the affected arm, but also include the trunk for posture, the other arm for symmetry, and the lower limbs for easier ADLs. To combine upper limb strength training with additional balance training, patients should assume a standing position while exercising with both upper and lower limbs simultaneously. One can eventually combine a) squats and double-sided elbow flexion aggravated by hand weights (0.5–1.5 kg; cp. **Figure** 7), or b) "good morning" exercises, that is, bending the trunk forward by flexing the hip combined with horizontal abduction of both arms while both hands are behind the head, or c) lower limb lunges with both arms shoulder extension aggravated by hand weights.

4.4 Lymphedema

About 20–25% of women after axillary lymph node dissection [27] and about 5% after sentinel lymph node biopsy [28] develop lymphedema (LE), most of them within the first 2–3 years [29]. As an incurable condition, LE has grave consequences

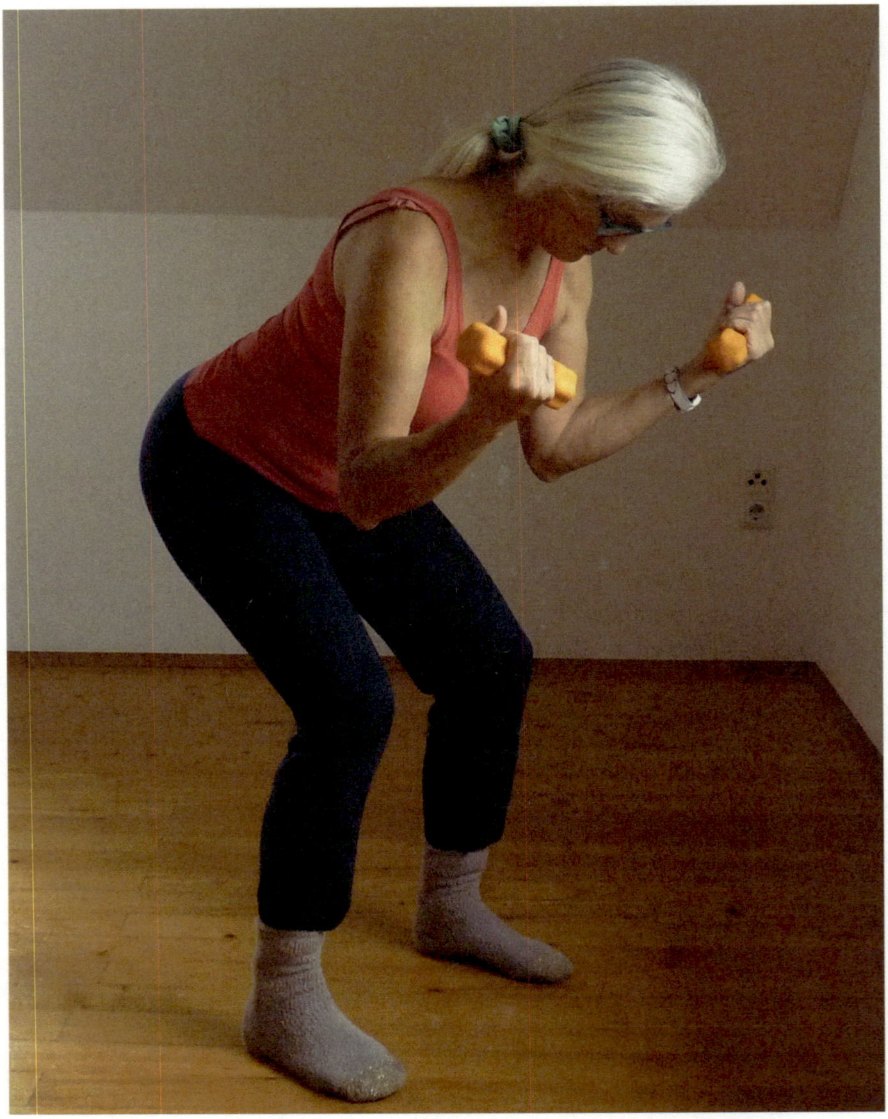

Figure 7.
Combined squats and resisted elbow flexion.

for patients' physical and psychic quality of life. LE is divided into four stages: 0 = subclinical; I = pitting edema; II = non-pitting edema, and III = elephantiasis. LE can possibly be preceded by an axillary web syndrome, also called cording, with visible and palpable cords in the middle of the axilla and the upper arm. Other early factors proved to contribute to LE formation are high BMI ($\geq$26), skin puncture, mastectomy, RT, or wound infection [30–32]. Taxan-based CT can furthermore compromise lymphangiomotoric function, that is, lymphatic contractions [33]. To capture LE early, a preoperative circumference or volume assessment is recommended. For high-risk patients, post-surgery indocyanine green lymph scintigraphy can be indicated. Women should be educated on early symptoms and how to perform regular self-measurements (pitting test, stemmer's test, and arm circumference with a one-hand tape measure). Measurements should be taken for at least one, better three-year post-surgery [34]. The gold standard for measuring and capturing LE is perometry or the water displacement method. Overall, arm edema incidence is reclining, whereas breast edema incidence is inclining [35]. Therefore, medical staff should be familiar with the corresponding symptoms and signs and be attentive.

The standard treatment for LE is complex decongestional therapy (CDT), which consists of manual lymphatic drainage (MLD) [36], compression therapy (CT), exercises, skin maintenance, patient education, and if necessary, dietary programs. CDT is divided into two phases, that is, intensive and maintenance phase. If primary edema volume exceeds 40%, in comparison with the healthy arm, patients are asked to complete first an inpatient rehabilitation continued afterward with phase II at home. MLD is a very gentle kind of massage, with the intention to redirect lymphatic fluid to non-compromised body quadrants by using accessory lymph paths. These are the non-affected axilla *via* ventral and dorsal, the neck and the ipsilateral inguinal region by improving lymphangiomotoricity. A thorough MLD includes treatment of the neck, the unaffected breast and back, the affected breast and back, and the whole of the arm, including the fingers. Afterward, in phase I, the patient is provided with a multi-layer compression bandaging inclusive of extended padding. In phase II, a customized compression sleeve and/or bra is prescribed to be worn daily from morning till evening. The most prescribed upper limb compression is class II, which ranges from 23 to 32 mmHg. If a glove is also necessary for finger or hand edema, this should be separated from the sleeve for easier donning. In lymphedema stage I, the patient is instructed to adopt elevated arm positions while resting; later on, this has no effect on the now chronic edema. Patient's adherence to CT is crucial for therapy success [37], which makes patient information and education even more important.

Exercises consist of a) endurance exercises and b) resistance exercises. The compression must be worn during these exercises to avoid lymphatic backflow. Possibilities are fist-pumping exercises or squeezing a little ball with the hand (30 repetitions, 3 series) [38] or moving a hand ergometer at 10–25 Watts [15], or any other exercise which incorporates parts of the arm musculature. If possible, the arm exercises should be combined with high arm positioning. Nordic walking [39] is also recommended as a whole-body endurance therapy and for achieving an upright walking posture. Enhanced breathing during this endurance training leads to a suction of the lymph fluid from the thoracic duct into the central veins (subclavian, jugular internal vein).

For skin maintenance, the patient applies suitable moisturizers or lotions on their arm after doffing the compression sleeve and before going to bed. While doing this, she should always distribute the lotion by stroking from the distal hand to the proximal arm. Keeping healthy and well-nourished skin is paramount for erysipelas prophylaxis. Patients should further carry along a little bottle of disinfectant at all times. In case of little wounds, for example, insect stings, thorn injury, the disinfectant should be applied immediately to protect against bacteria and secondly, erysipelas.

Patient education can be administered single-wise or group-wise [40]. Patients are learning to interpret early symptoms [41], do their self-assessments as mentioned before, and learn about arm mobility, everyday behavior, hygiene, erysipelas and lymphedema prophylaxis, wound-healing, and scar formation [42]. All these measures improve patients' health literacy [43] and facilitate ongoing shared decision-making.

Dietary measures are important if patients are overweight, that is, have a BMI exceeding 26. A correlation has been established between this high BMI and the lymphedema stage, so patients are advised to maintain or reach a healthy body weight [31]. This is achieved by a) diet and b) sports therapy.

4.5 Sports therapy

Women should be encouraged to start or re-start sporting activities. This is rewarded by easier ADLs, a better quality of life, better coping with the disease, and a better adherence to ongoing cancer therapies. Furthermore, women can reach a reduction of overall and disease-specific mortality as well as an extended recurrence-free time [44].

In the beginning, an oncologic physician's assessment to evaluate heart and kidney condition by taking the blood pressure, ECG, echocardiography, and fitness level is indispensable. A 6-minute-walk-test supports in assessing the patient's actual fitness level and is afterward used to define her walking speed during walking exercises. Lastly, a multiple repetition maximum test determines the possible repetitions for resistance exercises within different muscles/muscle groups. Sports therapy can be conducted during and after oncologic treatment with certain adaptations and precautionary measures. All in all, 150 minutes of activities per week with a level of 3–6 METs (metabolic equivalent of tasks) are recommended [45]. For example, brisk walking takes place at an intensity of approximately 5 METs. To ensure safety, patients should wear a portable heart rate monitor or watch. If dyspnea has to be taken into consideration, also, oxygen saturation should be measured during the training session and be constant above 90%. During all kinds of exercises, the compression sleeve should be worn [46]. The most popular sports after breast cancer surgery are gymnastics, walking, Nordic walking, and swimming. Women should be discouraged from dangerous and arm-exhausting sports such as judo or climbing. Other precautions are necessary in case of a port-a-cath or a PICC (peripherally inserted central catheter), which should not be under local mechanical pressure, or get dislocated or wet.

No sports therapy can be executed on the day of CT and the following day, even if patients are feeling well. There is too high risk of cardiotoxicity and nephrotoxicity. Afterward, the highest possible heart rate should be set between 40 and 60% maximal heart rate if patients still are in between chemo-cycles. Training should of course be postponed if patients have fever, are dizzy, or feel otherwise unwell.

It is possible to start with sports therapy about 4–6 weeks after BCS and 6–8 weeks after mastectomy. In the beginning, types of movement, which focus motoric load on lower limbs, such as walking or stationary cycling, are to be preferred. A combination of endurance training and resistance training promises optimized outcomes in terms of patient-reported outcomes and overall fitness [47].

In the case of bone metastases, training is only possible supervised in not metastasis-affected body regions, For example, the patient can train with the lower limbs if metastases were detected in the humerus. Moreover, the radiologist or oncologist has to give her/his approval if the bones are robust enough for the training. The training focus should have lain on activities of daily life promoting exercises. The potential benefits and harms must be weighed for each individual patient [48]. Manual techniques that rely on heavy stretching or give lots of pressure, resistance, or vibrations on the tissue are contraindicated for these patients because of possible pathological fractures.

4.5.1 Endurance training

Endurance training (ET) takes place if a minimum of 1/6–1/7 of the whole-body musculature is involved in the training. Breast cancer patients are advised to perform ET because their average activity level is about 30% less than that of age-wise comparable inactive women without breast cancer [12]. ET can have positive effects on the cardiopulmonary capacity, for example, heart muscle contractility, quality of life (QoL), and sleeping quality, and can be a means to control the patients' BMI. Furthermore, it was suggested that ET fosters cerebral plasticity in the case of "chemobrain" [12], and therefore, cognitive functions can improve.

Training is possible during as well as after CT, many training regimes are combined interventions of ET and strength training (ST) [49]. Outdoor activities are recommended for better mental health and an increase in vitamin D levels [50]. As previous or ongoing CT can change heart rate, heart rhythm, and cardial function, the usage of the heart rate as an intensity parameter has to be interpreted with caution. Alternatively, the VO2-max or lactate levels can be determined.

The ideal training type is interval endurance training, as it turns out to be less exhausting and is also feasible in patients with other co-morbidities. One- to two-minute intervals interchange with 30–60 seconds active breaks. The whole training session should last 10–15 minutes at a minimum (training and break minutes added) with an intended increase of 30 minutes over time. Training heart rate is set between 60–80% of maximum heart rate. As the training proceeds, training intervals are intensified, that is, prolonged, as breaks are shortened or even omitted. Recent research was able to demonstrate that even high-intensity interval training, a time-efficient method for improving cardiovascular capacity, is possible in breast cancer patient cohorts, but should be supervised [51]. In high intensity interval training (HIIT) patients are exercising short periods at high intensity (i.e. > 75% VO2 max), followed by low-to-moderate intensity recovery periods (40–50% VO2 max). However, HIIT did not improve outcome when compared with regular ET [52]. While exercising, patients should determine their subjective exhausting level, that is, rate of perceived exertion or BORG Scale with 4–5.5/10 (i.e., moderate). To enhance patient's motivation, the type of ET, for example, walking, running, cycling, and cross-country-skiing, needs to be matched with her preferences and experiences. Overweight women should possibly select a training style with reduced body weight for the lower limbs, that is, (stationary) cycling or swimming to protect the limbs' joints.

4.5.2 Strength training

Strength training is recommended because inactivity, fatigue, cancer cachexia, and CT side effects on protein synthesis deteriorate muscle strength [53]. ST is capable to increase fast twitch muscle fibers type II, improving posture, ROM, coordination, and by facilitating ADL, it secondly optimizes QoL [54]. It can be performed in supervised and unsupervised settings, provided that patients are instructed properly. In former years, strength training was mainly avoided out of concern of triggering lymphedema, a hypothesis that was falsified [55]. Strength training should involve both upper and lower limbs, and a great effect size (ES = 0.99) can be expected [56]. Low-intensity strength training implies an intensity of 30–40% 1-RM (repetition maximum) with 15–30 repetitions or 40–60% with 10–15 repetitions. An increase to 50–80% 1-RM with 8–12 repetitions, that is, moderate intensity is possible [55]. Two or three sets of each exercise incorporating various muscle groups for an overall 30–45 minutes are recommended. The multiple repetition maximum test defines the exact individual training capacity while avoiding the hazards of a real 1-RM test.

A warm-up phase (5–10 minutes light endurance exercise on the treadmill or stationary bike) in advance as well as a cool-down phase (stretching exercises, relaxation) afterward is mandatory. Strength training is recommended two times a week with a minimum of 48 hours in between to recover. If adherence to this training frequency is problematic, even a once-a-week ST could show an increase in muscle strength and could therefore be an alternative for frail patients [57]. ST can be performed with free weights or rubber bands, own body weight, or strength-training machines. Changing body positions can facilitate or aggravate the training intensity by implementing or eliminating gravity and/or balance and coordination. ST should be postponed if thrombocyte counting is less than 20.000, if hemoglobin falls short of 8 g/dl or if the patient is suffering from arterial hypertension as well as on the days of CT and the following day.

Specific exercises, including arm flexion, above head height should not be implemented for three-month post-surgery. The patient is supposed to maintain steady breathing through all kinds of exercise to avoid a Valsalva mechanism and therefore high intrathoracic pressure. Common exercises are the seated row, leg extension, chest press, or the latissimus pull-down, when exercising with machines. Body weight-driven exercises are squats or lunges, combined with shoulder press, arm abduction, or resisted upper arm curls (cp. **Figure** 7).

Most efficient exercises involve muscles with trunk-associated insertion to furthermore improve spine bone density. This is of special interest in the case of (hormone therapy-associated) osteoporosis. To enhance this effect, patients are exercising while standing, also combined with an unstable surface, such as a balance pad or a tightly rolled-up gymnastic mat.

4.6 Cancer-related fatigue syndrome

Cancer-related fatigue syndrome (CRF) is one of the most troublesome symptoms after cancer and/or its treatments and is often present even after years [58]. Firstly, the patient should keep the so-called "energy-diary" for at least 14 days. Therein, low- and high-exhausting activities and the state of exhaustion should be noted with a numeric rating scale (1–10). This serves to identify energy-robbing activities, which should be avoided, if possible, or split up into smaller segments.

Exercise has been proven to be an efficient means of CRF, and it enhances QoL and depression [59, 60]. Low endurance training [61], that is, 40–60% of the heart rate maximum is recommended, that is, (treadmill) walking at a speed of 4–5 km/h or stationary cycling. Additionally, low-level resistance training with incorporating great muscle groups is indicated. Patients start with only a 5-minute sequence, subsequently increasing the session up to 30 minutes over weeks and months. Concerning endurance training, interval training, that is, alternating training and resting intervals suit these patients' demands better. They start with a 30–60 seconds training period, followed by 60–120 seconds resting period, representing a 1:2 frequency. Training time can be divided into two sessions per day. Patients should assess their personal rate of perceived exertion (BORG Scale) with "very easy" to "easy" (1–2/10). Strength exercises should be chosen with particular consideration of functional ADLs.

Relaxation training is another important part of CRF treatment. It aims at diminishing fear, depression, or sleeping problems. Jacobson's progressive muscle relaxation [62] or very gentle yoga exercises [63], for example, the "Dead Men's Position," "Shavasana," or the "The lying Butterfly," "Supta Baddha Konasana" are recommended in these circumstances. In each of these, the patient is concentrating on her own body, its' functions, and her personal breathing cycle. The positions can be practiced for up to 7–10 minutes. Alternatively, the patient can try a verbally guided relaxation exercise, which takes her to a virtually preferred environment, such as a gentle tropical beach or a lush-green forest surrounding.

4.7 Chemotherapy-induced polyneuropathy

Chemotherapy-induced polyneuropathy (CIPN) affects approximately 30–60% of patients. It affects sensory, motoric, and autonomous nervous system and deteriorates QoL. As a consequence, patients suffer from pain, paresthesia, and tingling sensations. They are furthermore at a high risk of falling [64]. Upper limb ADL dexterity problems, for example, closing buttons, counting coins, or holding cutlery are equally common. Training is even more effective if it is launched in advance of the symptom onset of CIPN [65]. Patients are advised to start walking training [66] and balance training on even and uneven grounds, for example, a rolled-up gymnastic mat, a balance pad, gravel underground, or a soft forest surface. Different standing positions with normal to small-positioned feet, semi-tandem and tandem stance as well as squats or lunges are practiced. If necessary and to ensure safety, patients can grasp a wall or a table. To enhance the exercises' difficulty, patients can close their eyes during exercise or add other motor or cognitive tasks simultaneously [67], for example, open or close a zip while walking, counting while stepping, etc. Furthermore, electric vibration plates can be used combined with different positions, for example, standing, sitting, or bridging the tool with the feet while lying supine with bent legs.

For upper limb and hand, sensory functions patients can exercise using a "hedgehog ball" or a spiked acupuncture massage ball, which they move around in their palm. They practice finger dexterity by picking up small objects such as coins, pens, and marbles. Therapists can give patients a hand massage to relieve numbness and pain by increasing blood circulation.

4.8 Scar therapy

Scarring in breast cancer patients is not only a cosmetic issue but can affect patients' physical as well as psychological well-being [68]. Scars can induce pain and additionally impede shoulder joint and thoracic mobility. Furthermore, they can be an obstacle for lymphatic flow [69]. Scar formation in deeper layers can even lead to muscle weakness. Patients can report pruritus and feelings of disfigurement. A well-healed scar is thin and flat, showing a similar color to the surrounding skin. On the contrary, hypertrophic scars are red or pink and raised, while keloids are beyond the original scar region. After the wound-healing process is completed, the scar tissue is manually mobilized, massaged, and stretched by both the PT and the educated patient. The patient cares for the scar by applying special moisturizers. This is even important after RT, which induces skin and tissue fibrosis [70], followed by a deteriorated ROM. Starting too early, on the other hand, would have deleterious effects, for example, aberrant wound healing, such as hypertrophic scarring or even keloids, because of an ongoing inflammation process [71].

Different physiotherapeutic techniques, such as massage, manual lymphatic drainage, connective tissue massage, acupuncture massage, or compression therapy, can be employed to improve the before-mentioned symptoms [72]. Silicone-based wound dressings are recommended for scar management. They ensure hydration and reduce inflammation. Additionally, patients should avoid excessive sun exposure. Scar therapy is possible as a self-treatment after accordingly instruction for five to ten minutes daily. This aims to loosen agglutinated connective fibers, to improve the scar pliability, the itching sensations, the cosmetic outcome, the aberrant color, and the pain [72]. Lymph vessel growth should be induced by stretching the skin during MLD, which is supposed to release vascular endothelial growth factor VEGF-c [73]. Evidence suggests that the activation of lymphatic vessels is correlated with anti-inflammatory mechanisms [74]. Therefore, it can be hypothesized that regenerated lymphatic function in scar tissue can avoid excessive scarring and scar-associated lymphedema.

It should be mentioned that clearly defined therapy regimes concerning duration, direction, frequency, or intensity are lacking until now [75]. In addition to that, robust scar treatment trials and therapy should utilize validated scar measurement tools.

4.9 Radiation-induced lung injury

Radiation-induced lung fibrosis is a long-term side effect after RT with an incidence of 1–5% in breast cancer patients. RT-induced tissue damages are followed by inflammation processes of the alveoli and lung fibrosis at the final stages. The patient suffers from dyspnea, chest pain or tightness, a dry cough, and low cardiopulmonary function [76]. All in all, this represents a restrictive lung syndrome with reduced lung volumes, lung compliance, gas diffusion, and decreased mucociliary clearance. The patient's dyspnea can be disproportionately in comparison with the radiation dose she was exposed to. The diaphragm's workload during inspiration is intensified because the lung's expansion is more difficult than in healthy conditions.

The compromised oxygen uptake capacity can be enhanced through endurance training (cp. chapter 4.5.1). The patient is educated the learn active diaphragmatic breathing techniques and different lung stretching positions, for example, the "moon position" (the body is forming a "C-shape" in a supine position, arms stretched over the head). Diaphragmatic breathing is facilitated by gravity if patients exercise in a vertical position, that is, sitting [77] and is guided by the hands lying on the abdomen. Additional oxygen can be prescribed for symptomatic relief. Self-mobilizing techniques for the diaphragm while lying supine with one's own fingers reaching up to the diaphragm *via* the short ribs can be taught. Airway secretion mobilization is crucial to avoid high bacterial load and concurrent infections. This includes postural drainage, the instruction of effective coughing techniques, and chest percussions by the therapist's cupped hand or massage machines to induce vibration [78].

5. Conclusion

Breast cancer patients are present with a multitude of complaints and symptoms according to their type of surgery, oncologic treatment, and ongoing behavior. Physiotherapy, as a body- and patient-oriented approach, offers a wide range of hands-on and hands-off treatment modalities and techniques to enhance patients´ physical and psychological well-being. It is the therapists' task to a) assess the patient thoroughly, b) evolve a suitable therapy plan, c) implement, and d) evaluate this plan for effectiveness. Physiotherapy guides the patient from early postoperative mobilization back to daily independence, social participation, and better awareness of a healthy lifestyle and their own bodies. Physiotherapy is a means to complete state-of-the-art medical cancer treatment.

Conflict of interest

The author declares no conflict of interest.

Author details

Margit Eidenberger
Bachelor Programme Physiotherapy, University of Applied Sciences for Health Professions Upper Austria, Steyr, Austria

*Address all correspondence to: margit.eidenberger@fhgooe.ac.at

References

[1] Sancho-Garnier H, Colonna M. Breast cancer epidemiology. Presse Médicale. 2019;**48**(10):1076-1084. DOI: 10.1016/j.lpm.2019.09.022

[2] American Society of Plastic Surgeons. Evidence-Based Clinical Practice Guideline: Breast Reconstructions with Expanders and Implants. Arlington Heights: American Society of Plastic Surgeons; 2013

[3] Olsson Möller U et al. A comprehensive approach to rehabilitation interventions following breast cancer treatment - a systematic review of systematic reviews. BMC Cancer. 2019;**19**(1):472. DOI: 10.1186/s12885-019-5648-7

[4] Cheng KKF et al. Home-based multidimensional survivorship programmes for breast cancer survivors. Cochrane Database of Systematic Reviews. 2017;**8**(8):CD011152. DOI: 10.1002/14651858.CD011152.pub2

[5] Yang A, Sokolf J, Gulati A. The effect of preoperative exercise on upper extremity recovery following breast cancer surgery: A systematic review. International Journal of Rehabilitation Research. 2018;**41**(3):189-196. DOI: 10.1097/MRR.0000000000000288

[6] Lokapavani Y, Ragava Krishna S, Madhavi K. Influence of pre-operative physical therapy education and exercise on post-operative shoulder range of motion and functional activities in subjects with modified radical mastectomy. International Journal of Physiotherapy. 2014;**1**(4):170-177. DOI: 10.15621/ijphy/2014/v1i4/54556

[7] Mulhaeriah AY, Engkus KA, Moh SS. Effectiveness of relaxation breathing exercise on fatigue in gynecological cancer patients undergoing chemotherapy. International Journal of Nursing Science. 2018;**5**(4):331-335. DOI: 10.1016/j.ijnss.2018.09.004

[8] Galantino ML, Stout NL. Exercise interventions for upper limb dysfunction due to breast cancer treatment. LEAP. 2014;**93**(10):1291-1295. DOI: 10.2522/ptj.20120049

[9] Bendz I, Fagevik OM. Evaluation of immediate versus delayed shoulder exercises after breast cancer surgery including lymph node dissection – A randomized controlled trial. Breast. 2002;**11**(3):241-248. DOI: 10.1054/brst.2001.0412

[10] Loh SY, Musa AN. Methods to improve rehabilitation in patients following breast cancer surgery: A review of systematic reviews. Breast Cancer: Targets and Therapy. 2015;7:81-98. DOI: 10.2147/BCTT.S47012

[11] Bruce J et al. Exercise versus usual care after non-reconstructive breast cancer surgery (UK- PROSPER): Multicentre randomised controlled trial and economic evaluation. BMJ. 2021;**375**:e066542. DOI: 10.1136/bmj-2021-066542

[12] Casla S et al. Running away from side effects: Physical exercise as a complementary intervention for breast cancer patients. Clinical & Translational Oncology. 2014;**17**(3):180-196. DOI: 10.1007/s12094-014-1184-8

[13] Shamley D et al. Delayed versus immediate exercises following surgery for breast cancer: A systematic review. Breast Cancer Research and Treatment. 2005;**90**:263-271. DOI: 10.1007/s10549-004-4727-9

[14] De Lorenzi F. How to manage complications in breast reconstruction. In: Veronesi U, Goldhirsch A, Veronesi P, Gentilini OD, Leonardi MC, editors. Breast Cancer. Innovations in Research and Management. 1st ed. Berlin: Springer International Publishing; 2017. pp. 521-532. DOI: 10.1007/978-3-319-48848-6

[15] Kärki A. Physiotherapy for the Functioning of Breast Cancer Patients [Thesis]. Jyväskyla: University of Jyväskyla. Faculty of Sport and Health Sciences; 2005

[16] Groen WG et al. Feasibility and outcomes of a goal-directed physical therapy program for patients with metastatic breast cancer. Support Care Cancer. 2021;**29**(6):3287-3298. DOI: 10.1007/s00520-020-05852-9

[17] Yuste Sanchez MJ et al. Health related quality of life improvement in breast cancer patients: Secondary outcome from a simple blinded, randomised clinical trial. The Breast. 2015;**24**:75-81. DOI: 10.1016/j.breast.2014.11.012

[18] Malicka I et al. Body posture of women after breast cancer treatment. Ortopedia, Traumatologia, Rehabilitacja. 2010;**12**(4):353-361

[19] Ebaugh D, Spinelli B, Schmitz KH. Shoulder impairments and their association with symptomatic rotator cuff disease in breast cancer survivirs. Medical Hypothesis. 2011;**77**:481-487. DOI: 10.1016/j.mehy.2011.06.015

[20] Barbosa Jde A et al. Evalution of body posture in women with breast cancer. Revista Brasileira de Ginecologia e Obstetrícia. 2013;**35**(5):215-220. DOI: 10.1590/s0100-72032013000500005

[21] Atanes Mendes Peres AC et al. Body posture after mastectomy: Comparison between immediate breast reconstruction versus mastectomy alone. Physiotherapy Research International. 2017;**22**(1):e1642. DOI: 10.1002/pri.1642

[22] Warpenburg MJ. Deep friction massage in treatment of radiation-induced fibrosis: Rehabilitative Care for Breast Cancer Survivors. Integrative Medicine (Encinitas). 2014;**13**(5):32-36

[23] Ha KJ et al. Synergistic effects of proprioceptive neuromuscular facilitation and manual lymphatic drainage in patients with mastectomy-related lymphedema. Frontiers in Physiology. 2017;**8**:959. DOI: 10.3389/fphys.2017.00959. eCollection 2017

[24] Galiano-Castillo N et al. Altered pattern of cervical muscle activation during performance of a functional upper limb task in breast cancer survivors. American Journal of Medical Rehabilitation. 2011;**90**(5):349-355. DOI: 10.1097/PHM.0b013e318214e406

[25] Torres Lacomba M et al. Incidence of myofascial pain syndrome in breast cancer surgery: A prospective study. The Clinical Journal of Pain. 2010;**26**(4):320-325. DOI: 10.1097/AJP.0b013e3181c4904a

[26] Leonardis JM et al. Functional integrity of the shoulder joint and pectoralis major following subpectoral implant breast reconstruction. Journal of Orthopaedic Research. 2019;**37**(7):1610-1619. DOI: 10.1002/jor.24257

[27] Di Sipio T et al. Incidence of unilateral arm lymphoedema after breast cancer: A systematic review and meta-analysis. The Lancet Oncology. 2013;**14**(6):500-515. DOI: 10.1016/S1470-2045(13)70076-7

[28] Liu S et al. Using the axillary reverse mapping technique to screen breast cancer patients with a high risk of lymphedema. World Journal of Surgical

Oncology. 2020;**18**(1):118. DOI: 10.1186/s12957-020-01886-9

[29] Garza R et al. A comprehensive overview on the surgical management of secondary lymphedema of the upper and lower extremities related to prior oncologic therapies. BMC Cancer. 2017;**17**(1):468. DOI: 10.1186/s12885-017-3444-9

[30] Kilbreath SL et al. Risk factors for lymphoedema in women with breast cancer: A large prospective cohort. The Breast. 2016;**28**:29-36. DOI: 10.1016/j.breast.2016.04.011

[31] Yusof K et al. Assessment of potential risk factors and skin ultrasound presentation associated with breast cancer-related lymphedema in long-term breast cancer survivors. Diagnostics. 2021;**11**:1303. DOI: 10.3390/diagnostics11081303

[32] Basta MN et al. A propensity-matched analysis of the influence of breast reconstruction on subsequent development of lymphedema. Plastic and Reconstructive Surgery. 2015;**136**(2):134e-143e. DOI: 10.1097/PRS.0000000000001417

[33] Tokumoto H et al. Investigation of the association between breast cancer-related lymphedema and the side effects of Taxane-based chemotherapy using Indocyanine green Lymphography. Lymphatic Research and Biology. 2022. DOI: 10.1089/lrb.2021.0065 [Epub ahead of print]

[34] Armer JM et al. Best practice guidelines in assessment, risk reduction, management, and surveillance for post-breast cancer lymphedema. Current Breast Cancer Report. 2013;**5**(2):134-144. DOI: 10.1007/s12609-013-0105-0

[35] Young-Afat DA et al. Breast edema following breast-conserving surgery and radiotherapy: Patient-reported prevalence, determinants, and effect on health-related quality of life. JNCI Cancer Spectrum. 2019;**3**(2):pkz011. DOI: 10.1093/jncics/pkz011

[36] Shao Y, Zhong DS. Manual lymphatic drainage for breast cancer-related lymphoedema. European Journal of Cancer Care (Engl). 2017;**26**(5):e12517. DOI: 10.1111/ecc.12517

[37] Vignes S et al. Long-term management of breast cancer-related lymphedema after intensive decongestive physiotherapy. Breast Cancer Research and Treatment. 2007;**101**(3):285-290. DOI: 10.1007/s10549-006-9297-6

[38] Olszewski WL. Contractility patterns of human leg lymphatics in various stages of obstructive lymphedema. Annals of the New York Academy of Sciences. 2008;**1131**:110-118. DOI: 10.1196/annals.1413.010

[39] Fischer MJ et al. Stick together: A Nordic walking group intervention for breast cancer survivors. Journal of Psychosocial Oncology. 2015;**33**(3):278-296. DOI: 10.1080/07347332.2015.1020465

[40] Omidi Z et al. Effect of lymphedema self-management group-based education compared with social network-based education on quality of life and fear of cancer recurrence in women with breast cancer: A randomized controlled clinical trial. Quality of Life Research. 2020;**29**:1789-1800. DOI: 10.1007/s11136-020-02455-z

[41] Svensson BJ et al. Screening for breast cancer-related lymphoedema: Self-assessment of symptoms and signs. Screening for breast cancer-related lymphoedema: Self-assessment of symptoms and signs. Support Care Cancer. 2020;**28**(7):3073-3080. DOI: 10.1007/s00520-019-05083-7

[42] Shaitelman SF et al. Recent progress in the treatment and prevention of cancer-related lymphedema. CA: a Cancer Journal for Clinicians. 2015;**65**(1):55-81. DOI: 10.3322/caac.21253

[43] Soliman GH, El Gahsh NF, Shehata OSMH. Effect of a planned educational programme regarding post mastectomy exercises on living activities among breast cancer patients. National Journal of Advanced Research. 2018;**4**(1):1-11

[44] Friedenreich CM et al. Physical activity and mortality in cancer survivors: A systematic review and meta-analysis. JNCI Cancer Spectrum. 2019;**4**:pkz080. DOI: 10.1093/jncics/pkz080

[45] Jung AY et al. Pre- to postdiagnosis leisure-time physical activity and prognosis in postmenopausal breast cancer survivors. Breast Cancer Research. 2019;**21**(1):117. DOI: 10.1186/s13058-019-1206-0

[46] Godoy M et al. Synergic effect of compression therapy and controlled exercises using a facilitating device in the treatment of arm lymphedema. International Journal of Medical Sciences. 2012;**9**(4):280-284. DOI: 10.7150/ijms.3272

[47] An KY et al. Effects of exercise dose and type during breast cancer chemotherapy on longer-term patient-reported outcomes and health-related fitness: A randomized controlled trial. International Journal of Cancer. 2020;**146**(1):150-160. DOI: 10.1002/ijc.32493

[48] Weller S et al. Exercise for individuals with bone metastasis: A systematic review. Critical Reviews in Oncology/Hematology. 2021;**166**:103433

[49] Gebruers N et al. The effect of training interventions on physical performance, quality of life, and fatigue in patients receiving breast cancer treatment: A systematic review. Support Care Cancer. 2019;**27**(1):109-122. DOI: 10.1007/s00520-018-4490-9

[50] Rafie C et al. Impact of physical activity and sleep quality on quality of life of rural residents with and without a history of cancer: Findings of the day and night study. Cancer Management and Research. 2018;**10**:5525-5535. DOI: 10.2147/CMAR.S160481

[51] Tsuji K, Matsuoka YJ, Och E. High-intensity interval training in breast cancer survivors: A systematic review. BMC Cancer. 2021;**21**(1):184. DOI: 10.1186/s12885-021-07804-w

[52] Mugele H et al. High-intensity interval training in the therapy and aftercare of cancer patients: A systematic review with meta-analysis. Journal of Cancer Survivorship. 2019;**13**(2):205-223. DOI: 10.1007/s11764-019-00743-3

[53] Klassen O et al. Muscle strength in breast cancer patients receiving different treatment regimes. Journal of Cachexia, Sarcopenia and Muscle. 2017;**8**(2):305-316. DOI: 10.1002/jcsm.12165

[54] Cešeiko R et al. The impact of maximal strength training on quality of life among women with breast cancer undergoing treatment. Experimental Oncology. 2019;**41**(2):166-172. DOI: 10.32471/exp-oncology.2312-8852.vol-41-no-2.13249

[55] Montaño-Rojas LS et al. Resistance training in breast cancer survivors: A systematic review of exercise programs. International Journal of Environmental Research and Public Health. 2020;**17**(18):6511. DOI: 10.3390/ijerph17186511

[56] Speck RM et al. An update of controlled physical activity trials in cancer survivors: A systematic review and meta-analysis. Journal of Cancer Survival. 2010;**4**(2):87-100. DOI: 10.1007/s11764-009-0110-5

[57] Dos Santos WDN et al. Once a week resistance training improves muscular strength in breast cancer survivors: A randomized controlled trial. Integrative Cancer Therapies. 2019;**18**:1534735419879748. DOI: 10.1177/1534735419879748

[58] Chinapaw MJM et al. Alpe d'HuZes cancer rehabilitation (A-CaRe) research: Four randomized controlled exercise trials and economic evaluation in cancer patients and survivors. International Journal of Behavioral Medicine. 2012;**19**:143-156. DOI: 10.1007/s12529-011-9158-5

[59] Mustian KM et al. Comparison of pharmaceutical, psychological, and exercise treatments for cancer-related fatigue: A meta-analysis. JAMA Oncology. 2017;**3**(7):961-968. DOI: 10.1001/jamaoncol.2016.6914

[60] Tomlinson D et al. Effect of exercise on cancer-related fatigue: A meta-analysis. American Journal of Physical Medicine & Rehabilitation. 2014;**93**(8):675-686. DOI: 10.1097/PHM.0000000000000083

[61] Cramp F, Byron-Daniel J. Exercise for the management of cancer-related fatigue in adults. Cochrane Database of Systematic Reviews. 2012;**11**:CD006145. DOI: 10.1002/14651858.CD006145.pub3

[62] Kapogiannis A, Tsoli S, Chrousos G. Investigating the effects of the progressive muscle relaxation-guided imagery combination on patients with cancer receiving chemotherapy treatment: A systematic review of randomized controlled trials. Explore (New York, N.Y.). 2018;**14**(2):137-143. DOI: 10.1016/j.explore.2017.10.008

[63] Dong B et al. Yoga has a solid effect on cancer-related fatigue in patients with breast cancer: A meta-analysis. Breast Cancer Research and Treatment. 2019;**177**(1):5-16. DOI: 10.1007/s10549-019-05278-w

[64] Müller J et al. Out of balance - postural control in cancer patients before and after neurotoxic chemotherapy. Gait & Posture. 2020;**77**:156-163. DOI: 10.1016/j.gaitpost.2020.01.012

[65] Zhang S. Chemotherapy-induced peripheral neuropathy and rehabilitation: A review. Seminars in Oncology. 2021;**48**(3):193-207. DOI: 10.1053/j.seminoncol.2021.09.004

[66] Kleckner IR et al. Effects of exercise during chemotherapy on chemotherapy-induced peripheral neuropathy: A multicenter, randomized controlled trial. Support Care Cancer. 2018;**26**(4):1019-1028. DOI: 10.1007/s00520-017-4013-0

[67] Kneis S et al. It's never too late - balance and endurance training improves functional performance, quality of life, and alleviates neuropathic symptoms in cancer survivors suffering from chemotherapy-induced peripheral neuropathy: Results of a randomized controlled trial. BMC Cancer. 2019;**19**:414. DOI: 10.1186/s12885-019-5522-7

[68] Lee KC et al. Burns objective scar scale (BOSS): Validation of an objective measurement devices based burn scar scale panel. Burns. 2020;**46**(1):110-120. DOI: 10.1016/j.burns.2019.05.008

[69] Warren AG, Slavin SA. Scar lymphedema: Fact or fiction? Annals of Plastic Surgery. 2007;**59**(1):41-45. DOI: 10.1097/01.sap.0000258449.23979.3f

[70] Wei J et al. Radiation-induced skin reactions: Mechanism and treatment. Cancer Management and Research. 2018;**11**:167-177. DOI: 10.2147/CMAR.S188655

[71] Ogawa R. Keloid and hypertrophic scars are the result of chronic inflammation in the reticular dermis. International Journal of Molecular Sciences. 2017;**18**(3):606. DOI: 10.3390/ijms18030606

[72] Deflorin C et al. Physical Management of Scar Tissue: A systematic review and meta-analysis. Journal of Alternative and Complementary Medicine. 2020;**26**(10):854-865. DOI: 10.1089/acm.2020.010

[73] Planas-Paz L, Lammert E. Mechanosensing in developing lymphatic vessels. Advances in Anatomy, Embryology, and Cell Biology. 2014;**214**:23-40. DOI: 10.1007/978-3-7091-1646-3_3

[74] Dieterich LC, Seidel CD, Detmar M. Lymphatic vessels: New targets for the treatment of inflammatory diseases. Angiogenesis. 2014;**17**:359-371. DOI: 10.1007/s10456-013-9406-1

[75] Zhang YT, Li-Tsang CWP, Au RKC. A systematic review on the effect of mechanical stretch on hypertrophic scars after burn injuries. Hong Kong Journal of Occupational Therapy. 2017;**29**(1):1-9. DOI: 10.1016/j.hkjot.2016.11.001

[76] Huang Y et al. The cellular and molecular mechanism of radiation-induced lung injury. Medical Science Monitor. 2017;**23**:3446-3450. DOI: 10.12659/msm.902353

[77] Hellyer NJ et al. Comparison of diaphragm thickness measurements among postures via ultrasound imaging. PMR. 2017;**9**(1):21-25. DOI: 10.1016/j.pmrj.2016.06.001

[78] Giridhar P et al. Radiation induced lung injury: Prediction, assessment and management. Asian Pacific Journal of Cancer Prevention. 2015;**16**(7):2613-2617. DOI: 10.7314/apjcp.2015.16.7.2613

Chapter 18

Antibody Drug Conjugates

Farah Raheem and Vishal Shah

Abstract

Antibody drug conjugates (ADCs) continue to change the treatment paradigm of breast cancer and recent regulatory approvals of next generation ADCs are shifting how breast cancer is classified and treated. ADCs combine precision targeting with traditional cytotoxic treatment allowing for the delivery of highly potent chemotherapeutic agents to malignant cells. This chapter will cover ADCs used for the treatment of breast cancer including pharmacology, novel mechanism of action, pharmacokinetic and pharmacodynamic properties, clinical outcomes and role in breast cancer therapy, key toxicities and monitoring.

Keywords: breast cancer, antibody drug conjugates, ADC, bystander effect, HER2 low, ado-trastuzumab emtansine, fam-trastuzumab deruxtecan, sacituzumab govitecan

1. Introduction

Antibody drug conjugates (ADCs) continue to change the treatment paradigm of breast cancer and recent regulatory approvals of next generation ADCs are shifting how breast cancer is classified and treated. ADCs combine precision targeting with traditional cytotoxic treatment allowing for the delivery of highly potent chemotherapy to malignant cells. There are three U.S. Food and Drug Administration (FDA) approved ADCs in breast cancer including ado-trastuzumab emtansine (T-DM1), fam trastuzumab deruxtecan (T-Dxd), and sacituzumab govitecan (SG). The 3 approved ADCs in breast cancer are summarized in **Table 1**. T-DM1 is approved for the treatment of human epidermal growth factor receptor 2 positive (HER2+) early breast cancer (EBC) and advanced, recurrent or metastatic breast cancer (MBC). T-Dxd is approved for the treatment of HER2+ MBC and hormone receptor positive (HR+), HER2 low MBC. HER2 overexpression or HER2+ is defined as having immunohistochemistry (IHC) 3+ or IHC 2+ with positive HER2 gene amplification measured by in situ hybridization (ISH) [1]. Approximately, 15–20% of breast tumors are HER2+ [2]. HER2 low is defined as IHC 1+ or IHC 2+ and ISH negative [1]. Approximately, 50–55% of HR+, HER2 negative breast cancer is HER2-low [3]. HER2-low breast tumors do not respond to trastuzumab or T-DM1 [4, 5].

SG is approved for the treatment of metastatic triple negative breast cancer (TNBC) and HR+ MBC after progressing on prior lines of chemotherapy. Both SG and T-Dxd have a topoisomerase I inhibitor cytotoxic payload, which presents a clinical challenge in terms of how to best sequence these two agents when used for the treatment of HR+ MBC. In this chapter, we will describe ADCs pharmacology,

IntechOpen

Drug	mAb	Linker	Target antigen	Payload	Payload mechanism of action	DAR
T-DM1	IgG1	Non-cleavable (4-MCC)	HER2	DM1	Microtubule inhibitor-inhibit tubulin polymerization	3.5
T-Dxd	IgG1	Cleavable peptide linker	HER2	Dxd	Topoisomerase 1 inhibitor	8
SG	IgG1	Cleavable hydrolysable linker	Trop-2	SN-38	Topoisomerase 1 inhibitor	7.6

Abbreviations: ADCs, antibody drug conjugates; DAR, Drug-to-antibody ratio; FDA, U.S. Food and Drug Administration; HER2, human epidermal growth factor receptor 2; IgG, immunoglobulin G; mAb, monoclonal antibody; MMC, maleimidomethyl cyclohexane-1-carboxylate; SG, sacituzumab govitecan; T-DM1, ado-trastuzumab emtansine; T-Dxd, fam-trastuzumab deruxtecan.

Table 1.
Approved ADCs in breast cancer [14–16].

pharmacokinetic and pharmacodynamic properties, pharmacogenomic implications, clinical outcomes and place in breast cancer therapy, safety and monitoring.

2. Pharmacology

ADCs allow for a targeted delivery of cytotoxic chemotherapy agents that are too potent to be given in a similar fashion to traditional chemotherapy agents [6]. An advantage of the novel design of ADCs is the efficient delivery of highly toxic chemotherapy afforded by the high specificity of the antibody to the target antigen that is usually highly expressed on cancer cells. ADCs consist of a monoclonal antibodies (mAb) and a cytotoxic payload covalently attached to the mAb via a chemical linker [6].

Designing a successful ADC depends on various factors and properties of each individual component of the ADC [7]. In order to be safe and effective, an ADC needs to be chemically stable in circulation until it reaches the target cancer cell where it will be internalized followed by degradation of the linker or the mAb and subsequent release of the cytotoxic payload in the cell and adjacent cancer cells [7]. Each ADC component plays an important role and should be taken into consideration when designing and developing ADCs. Desired characteristics of ADCs are summarized in **Table 2**.

2.1 The target antigen

Binding of the antibody to the target antigen is needed to gain access into the cancer cells. This process is referred to as internalization, which occurs via endocytosis [8]. Internalization is required before releasing the cytotoxic payload. It is also desired that the target is an extracellular antigen in order to be recognized by the corresponding antibody. Additionally, the antigen should be non-secreted to prevent ADC binding outside of the tumor vicinity [9]. Secreted antigen in the bloodstream can also lead to significant increase in toxicities. Lastly, the ideal target antigen is highly expressed on cancer cells with minimal to no expression on healthy cells to reduce off-target toxicity [10]. This makes HER2 a great target antigen for T-DM1 and

Antigen selection	Antibody	Linker	Payload
High expression on tumor cells	Target specificity	Stable to avoid release of cytotoxic drug to an off-target tissue	High stability in plasma
Low to no expression on healthy cells	Target binding affinity	Maintain inactive state while being bound to antibody	Cell membrane permeable
Displayed on the surface of tumor cells (i.e., extracellular)	Good retention to payload and long half-life	Ability to unleash cytotoxic drug once internalized	Small molecular weight
Internalization properties	Low immunogenicity	Hydrophilic	High drug to antibody ratio

Table 2.
Desired characteristics of ADCs [6].

T-Dxd [6]. Trophoblast cell-surface antigen 2 (Trop2) is a transmembrane glycoprotein that is highly and differentially expressed in certain solid tumors including breast cancer making it an ideal target antigen for SG [6].

2.2 The monoclonal antibody

Ideal characteristics of mAbs used in ADCs include high affinity to the target antigen, efficient internalization upon binding to the antigen, low immunogenicity, and long plasma half-life [11]. Immunogenicity was a significant challenge associated with mouse-derived antibodies leading to serious adverse events [12]. Current technology employes humanized and fully human mAbs with reduced immunogenicity [11]. The most commonly utilized mAb is immunoglobulin G (IgG) antibody, and specifically IgG1, which exhibits long half-life and can induce antibody-dependent cell-mediated cytotoxicity, phagocytosis, and complement dependent cytotoxicity [13]. The mAb component of T-DM1, T-Dxd and SG is humanized, IgG1 mAb [14–16].

2.3 The linker

The linker is the chemical bond that connects the cytotoxic payload to the antibody of ADCs. The linker is important to maintain stability of ADCs in plasma and to control the release of payload in the desired tumor site [6]. The linker can be cleavable or non-cleavable. Cleavable linkers are designed to be sensitive to the tumor environment where they can be chemically (hydrazone and disulfide based) or enzymatically degraded (glucuronide and peptide based) to release the payload [17]. Hydrazone-based linkers are acid sensitive or pH dependent [18]. These bonds are stable in plasma but hydrolyze in the lysosome and endosome where $pH < 7$ [18]. SG utilizes an acid sensitive, carbonate linker that is cleavable at low pH [19]. The most commonly utilized linker is the peptide linker, which is cleaved via lysosomal proteases such as cathepsin B that are typically overexpressed in cancer cells [20, 21]. This type of bond is employed in T-Dxd [22].

Non cleavable linkers such as thioether based linkers are more stable compared to cleavable linkers leading to less off-target toxicity. These bonds are not sensitive to the enzymatic and chemical environment of the tumor [23, 24]. When non-cleavable linkers are utilized, such as in T-DM1, the release of the cytotoxic agent takes place after catabolism of the antibody component whereas enzymatic or chemical degradation of the linker releases the payload when cleavable linkers are utilized such as in T-Dxd and SG [25].

2.4 The cytotoxic payload

The novel design of ADCs allows for use of potent cytotoxic agents with half-maximal inhibitory concentrations in nano and picomolar range [26]. High potency of the payload is required since only a small fraction of the ADC reaches the tumor site [27]. As previously mentioned, internalization of the ADC is the first step required for release of the cytotoxic payload followed by linker or mAb degradation in cleavable and non-cleavable linkers-based ADCs, respectively. Other desired characteristics of the cytotoxic payload include stability in physiological conditions, ability to chemically conjugate with the antibody and cell membrane permeability [28]. Currently, the majority of approved ADCs utilize one of three pharmacologic categories of payloads including tubulin inhibitors, DNA damaging agents, and immunomodulators [29].

Tubulin inhibitors can be classified either as tubulin polymerization promoters (e.g., auristatin derivatives monomethyl auristatin E and monomethyl auristatin F) or tubulin polymerization inhibitors (e.g., maytansinoid derivatives DM1 and DM4) [30, 31]. Tubulin inhibitors halt cell division by interfering with mitosis and are considered cell-cycle specific [30]. T-DM1 was the first FDA approved ADC with a maytansinoid derivative cytotoxic payload [14].

The mechanism of action of DNA damaging agents include: DNA alkylation (e.g., duocarmycins), DNA double strand break (e.g., calicheamicins), DNA crosslink (e.g., pyrrolobenzodiazepines), and DNA intercalation (e.g., topoisomerase I inhibitors) [32]. DNA damaging agents are not cell-cycle specific and can be relatively more potent than tubulin inhibitors [32]. The payloads utilized in T-Dxd and SG are topoisomerase I inhibitors [33, 34]. The cytotoxic payload of SG is SN-38, which is the active metabolite of irinotecan. Dxd is the paylaod of T-Dxd, which is an exatecan derivative [33, 34]. It is reported that Dxd has potency that is 10-fold higher than SN-38 [5].

Drug-to-antibody ratio (DAR) is another important characteristic of ADCs that impacts efficacy and safety. DAR refers to the average number of cytotoxic molecules conjugated to the mAb [35]. Low DAR can negatively impact efficacy and high DAR can affect stability, antigen binding ability, and clearance [36]. DAR is also used to determine the therapeutic index of ADCs [35]. DAR values vary among ADCs, and low values can result in reduced potency and efficacy. Initially developed ADCs have a DAR average of 2–4 [37]. T-Dxd and SG have higher DAR values at 8:1 and 7.6:1, respectively compared to T-DM1 that has DAR of 3.5:1 [38].

2.5 The bystander effect

The bystander effect is described with certain ADCs that exhibit an antitumor activity against cancer cells located near those expressing the targeted antigen [39, 40]. In other words, the cytotoxic payload can diffuse through the target cell membrane to and kill adjacent cancer cells that are antigen negative. Properties that allow for bystander effect include having cleavable linkers and cell membrane permeable cytotoxic payload. These properties allow the payload to diffuse to neighboring cells. ADCs with bystander effect may not require high expression of the target antigen to be effective. Due to having cleavable linkers and membrane permeable payloads, both T-Dxd and SG exhibit bystander effect. Conversely, T-DM1 does not exhibit the bystander effect. The release of payload in T-DM1 requires complete digestion of trastuzumab followed by release of the metabolite, lysine-MCC-DM1, which is charged under physiologic pH and thus is not cell membrane permeable. Therefore, T-DM1 can only exert cytotoxic effect against antigen positive cancer cells (i.e., HER2 positive cells) [6]. Unlike T-DM1, T-Dxd has demonstrated efficacy in both HER2 overexpressing cancer cells as well as cells that are HER2 low due to the bystander effect [41, 42].

3. Pharmacokinetics and pharmacodynamics

Pharmacokinetic (PK) properties of T-DM1, T-Dxd, and SG including metabolism and elimination are described in **Table 3**. The mAb component is expected to be catabolized into small peptides and amino acids via the same pathways used to degrade endogenous IgG monoclonal antibodies [14–16].

3.1 T-DM1

Based on population PK studies, covariates that can impact T-DM1 clearance include body weight, albumin, AST, and baseline trastuzumab concentrations. However, with the exception of weight, other covariates are unlikely to have meaningful impact on clearance. Exposure to T-DM1 was not shown to be affected by mild (CrCl 60–89 mL/min) or moderate (CrCl 30–59 mL/min) renal impairment. Patients with severe renal impairment (CrCl <30 mL/min) were not included in clinical trials. Therefore, no renal dose adjustment is required, but no recommendations can be made for use of T-DM1 in severe renal impairment due to lack of data in this patient population [14].

DM1 is primarily hepatically metabolized via CYP3A4 and to a lesser extent by CYP3A5. Serum concentrations of DM1 in patients with mild (Child-Pugh A) and moderate (Child-Pugh B) hepatic impairment were comparable to those achieved in patients with normal liver function. T-DM1 was not studied in patients with severe hepatic impairment (Child-Pugh C). Based on this, no dose adjustment is required in mild or moderate hepatic impairment and no recommendations can be made for patients with severe hepatic impairment.

Drug	Substrate of	Payload metabolism	Elimination
T-DM1	CYP3A4 (minor), P-gp	DM1 undergoes hepatic metabolism via CYP3A4/5	DM1 half-life ~4 days
T-Dxd	BCRP, CYP3A4 (minor), OATP1B1/1B3, P-pg (minor)	Dxd undergoes hepatic metabolism via CYP3A4	Dxd half-life ~5.4 to 6.1 days
SG	UGT1A1	SN-38 is metabolized via UGT1A1 to the inactive glucuronide metabolite (SN-38G)	SG half-life ~23.4 h; free SN-38 ~ 17.6 h

Abbreviations: ADCs, antibody drug conjugates; BCRP, breast cancer resistance protein; OATP, organic anion transporting polypeptides; P-gp; p-glycoprotein; SG, sacituzumab govitecan; T-DM1, ado-trastuzumab emtansine; T-Dxd; fam-trastuzumab deruxtecan; UGT1A1, UDP glucuronosyltransferase 1 family, polypeptide A1.

Table 3.
ADCs pharmacokinetic properties [14–16].

In a population-based PK study, age and race had no clinically meaningful impact on T-DM1 exposure. While there are no safety studies of T-DM1 in pregnant women, cases of oligohydramnios presenting as pulmonary hypoplasia, skeletal abnormalities, and neonatal death are reported with use of trastuzumab [14]. Given the mechanism of action of DM1 and sensitivity of rapidly dividing cells to its cytotoxic antimicrotubular effect, animal studies suggest that T-DM1 has the potential to cause embryotoxicity and teratogenicity [14]. Women of childbearing age should be tested for pregnancy prior to initiating treatment. Women of childbearing age and men with female partners of reproductive potential should use effective contraception during treatment and for 7 months and 4 months after the last dose of T-DM1, respectively. Women should also be advised to avoid breastfeeding during treatment and for 7 months after the last dose of T-DM1 [14].

3.2 T-Dxd

Based on population PK studies, there was no difference observed in exposure to Dxd in patients with mild (CrCl 60–89 mL/min) or moderate (CrCl 30–59 mL/min) renal impairment. Patients with severe renal impairment (CrCl <30 mL/min) were not included in clinical trials. Patients with moderate renal impairment should be monitored for interstitial lung disease more frequently. No recommendations can be made for use of T-Dxd in patients with severe renal impairment due to lack of data in this patient population [15].

T-Dxd is primarily hepatically metabolized via CYP3A4. There was no difference in exposure to T-Dxd in patients with mild hepatic impairment (total bilirubin ≤ ULN and any AST > ULN or total bilirubin >1 to 1.5 times ULN and any AST) compared to patients with normal hepatic function. PK of T-Dxd in patients with moderate to severe hepatic impairment is not known. T-Dxd dose adjustment is not required in patients with mild to moderate hepatic impairment, but these patients need to be monitored more closely for adverse events related to Dxd. No significant difference in exposure to Dxd was observed for age or race [15].

Given the known risk of the trastuzumab component of T-DXd to the fetus as described above and Dxd cytotoxic effect on actively diving cells, T-Dxd is considered genotoxic. Women of childbearing age should be tested for pregnancy prior to initiating treatment. Women of childbearing age and men with female partners of reproductive potential should use effective contraception during treatment and for 7 months and 4 months after the last dose of T-Dxd, respectively. Women should also avoid breastfeeding during treatment and for 7 months after the last dose of T-Dxd [15].

3.3 SG

SN-38 is metabolized via uridine diphosphate glucuronosyltransferase 1A1 (UGT1A1) to the inactive glucuronide metabolite, SN-38G, which is then eliminated by biliary excretion [43]. Based on population PK studies, there was no difference observed in exposure to SN-38 in patients with mild or moderate renal impairment, and renal elimination of SN-38 is found to be minimal [16]. Therefore, no renal dose adjustment is required for SG for mild or moderate renal function impairment. No recommendations can be made for use of SG in severe renal impairment due to lack of data in this patient population [16]. There is no difference in exposure to SG between patients with mild hepatic impairment compared to patients with no hepatic impairment. SG PK is not known for patients with severe hepatic impairment [16].

Drug	Indications	Dose and administration
T-DM1	Early, HER2+ breast cancer*adjuvant for residual disease Metastatic, recurrent HER2+ breast cancer	3.6 mg/kg IV every 3 weeks for 14 cycles (adjuvant) or until disease progression (metastatic)
T-Dxd	Metastatic, recurrent HER2+ breast cancer Metastatic, recurrent HER2 low breast cancer	5.4 mg/kg IV every 3 weeks until disease progression
SG	Metastatic, recurrent TNBC after ≥2 chemotherapy Metastatic, recurrent HR+, HER2 negative or low after progression on endocrine therapy and chemotherapy	10 mg/kg on days 1 and 8 of a 21-day cycle until disease progression

Abbreviations: HER2, human epidermal growth factor receptor 2; HR+, hormone receptor positive; IV, intravenous; SG, sacituzumab govitecan; T-DM1, ado-trastuzumab emtansine; T-Dxd; fam-trastuzumab deruxtecan; TNBC, triple negative breast cancer.

Table 4.
Dose and administration [14–16].

There was no significant impact of age or race on PK properties of SG and exposure to SN-38 [16]. Given the mechanism of action of SN-38 and its effect on rapidly dividing cells, SG is considered teratogenic and genotoxic [16]. Women of childbearing age should be tested for pregnancy prior to initiating treatment. Women of childbearing age and men with female partners of reproductive potential should use effective contraception during treatment and for 6 months and 3 months after the last dose of SG, respectively. Women should also avoid breastfeeding during treatment and for 1 months after the last dose of SG (**Table 4**) [16].

4. Drug-drug interactions

4.1 T-DM1

There are no formal drug interaction studies with DM1. DM1 is extensively metabolized by CYP3A4, and it is anticipated that strong CYP3A4 inhibitors can increase DM1 concentrations and toxicity. Therefore, it is recommended that concomitant use of strong CYP3A4 inhibitors with T-MD1 is avoided. If concomitant use cannot be avoided, closely monitor for T-DM1 toxicities [14]. However, a phase I study evaluated the safety and efficacy of T-DM1 in combination with tucatinib, which is a strong CYP3A4 inhibitor revealed that DM1 concentration was similar to those reported in studies of T-DM1 monotherapy suggesting lack of clinically meaningful interactions [44]. The impact of strong CYP3A4 on T-DM1 has not been evaluated to date. DM1 does not inhibit or induce major CYP450 enzymes [14].

4.2 T-DXd

Dxd is a substrate of OATP1B1/3, MATE2-K, P-gp, MRP1, and BCRP. Coadministration of strong CYP3A4 inhibitors increased Dxd area under the curve (AUC) by 18%, and that was not considered clinically meaningful [15]. Coadministration of ritonavir, dual inhibitor of CYP3A4 and OATP1B increased Dxd AUC by 22%. The impact was not clinically significant. According to in vitro studies, DXd does not inhibit CYP1A2, CYP2B6, CYP2C8, CYP2C9, CYP2C19, CYP2D6, and

CYP3A nor induce CYP1A2, CYP2B6, or CYP3A [15]. Dxd has low potential to inhibit OAT1/3, OCT1/2, OATP1B1/3, MATE1/2-K, P-gp, BCRP, and BSEP transporters [15].

4.3 SG

No formal drug interaction studies were conducted with SG or SN-38 [16]. Given metabolism and clearance mechanism of SN-38 via UGT1A1, UGT1A1 inhibitors may increase the concentration and toxicity of SN-38 and thus coadministration should be avoided. Additionally, UGT1A1 inducers may decrease exposure to SN-38 and its efficacy [16].

There are challenges with drug interaction assessment with ADCs. There is no specific guidance from regulatory bodies on how to formally evaluate drug interactions with cytotoxic payloads. There is an unmet need for understanding how cytotoxic payloads will be affected by oxidative enzymes and drug transporters. It is speculated that given the low systemic exposure, cytotoxic payload molecules are unlikely to cause clinically meaningful interactions but can be significantly affected by enzymes and transporters. Unique considerations may be needed when designing PK studies to evaluate interactions with cytotoxic payloads [45].

5. Pharmacogenomics

The cytotoxic payload, SN-38 in SG is metabolized via UGT1A1 to an inactive metabolite. The genetic variant UGT1A1*28 has reduced enzyme activity. Patients who are homozygous (UGT1A1*28/*28; diminished enzyme activity) and heterozygous (UGT1A1*28/*1; reduced enzyme activity) are at increased risk for neutropenia, febrile neutropenia, anemia, and other toxicities due to increased exposure to SN-38 compared to wild type (UGT1A1*1/*1; normal enzyme activity) [16, 46]. There are no known pharmacogenomics implications for T-DM1 and T-Dxd [14, 15].

The frequency of having homozygous UGT1A1*28 allele varies with about 20% of the Black population, 10% of the White population, and 2% of the East Asian population are homozygous for the UGT1A1*28 allele [47]. Approximately, 40% of Black, 50% of White, and 25% of East Asian population are heterozygous for the UGT1A1*28 allele [47].

Patients presenting with acute-onset, severe neutropenia and anemia may indicate reduced UGT1A1 enzyme activity. The median time to neutropenia and febrile neutropenia was 9 days in patients who are homozygous for UGT1A1*28 allele, 15 days in patients who are heterozygous for the allele, and 20 days who are wild type for UGT1A1* [16]. The median time to anemia in patients homozygous for UGT1A1*28, heterozygous for UGT1A1*28, and homozygous for wild type UGT1A1* was 21 days, 25 days, and 28 days, respectively [16].

In a safety analysis from phase III, randomized clinical trial of SG in metastatic TNBC, the impact of UGT1A1 polymorphism was evaluated. In patients treated with SG, UGT1A1 genotype was known for 250 patients. Of 250 patients, 113 (44%), 96 (37%), and 34 (13%) were homozygous for the wild type UGT1A1 (*1/*1), heterozygous (*1/*28), and homozygous (*28/*28) [48]. Patients with homozygous *28 genotype had comparable grade 3/4 neutropenia (59%) to those with heterozygous *28 (47%) or wild type (53%), but the rate of febrile neutropenia was higher (18% vs. 5% and 3%, respectively). Grades 3/4 anemia (15% vs. 6% and 4%, respectively) and diarrhea (15% vs. 9% and 10%, respectively) occurred more frequently in patients with homozygous

UGT1A1*28 genotype compared to those with heterozygous and wild type genotypes. Treatment discontinuation due to adverse events was also more common in patients with homozygous UGT1A1*28 genotype compared to heterozygous *28 and wild type genotypes (6%, 1%, and 2%, respectively). Other adverse events including nausea, vomiting, fatigue and alopecia were not impacted by UGT1A1 genotype [48].

Increased risk for severe adverse reactions including neutropenia and febrile neutropenia with irinotecan in patients with reduced UGT1A1 activity is attributed to its active metabolite, SN-38, which is the cytotoxic payload of SG [49, 50]. While the FDA recommends reducing the starting dose of irinotecan in patients with colorectal cancer and known UGT1A1*28/*28 status [50], there are currently no guidelines for SG dosing recommendations for patients who have known UGT1A1*28/*28 genotype. The FDA only recommends SG dose modification or discontinuation based on tolerance [16].

6. Clinical outcomes of ADC in breast cancer treatment

6.1 T-DM1

T-DM1 was evaluated in the phase III, randomized clinical trial EMILIA, which enrolled 991 patients with metastatic, HER2+ breast cancer with disease progression after first line trastuzumab plus taxane based chemotherapy for metastatic disease or with disease recurrence during or within six months of completing adjuvant therapy [51]. Patients were randomized 1:1 to T-DM1 or lapatinib and capecitabine. The co-primary endpoints were progression free survival (PFS) and overall survival (OS). Most patients (88%) received prior chemotherapy for metastatic disease with a median of 3 prior lines of treatment. PFS was significantly improved with median PFS of 9.6 months in the T-DM1 arm versus 6.4 months in the control arm [hazard ratio (HR), 0.65; 95% CI, 0.55–0.77; $p < 0.0001$]. Overall survival was also significantly improved with median OS of 30.9 months in the T-DM1 arm vs. 25.1 months in the control arm (HR, 0.68; 95% CI, 0.55–0.85; P, 0.0006). Based on the results of this study, T-DM1 was FDA approved for the treatment of HER2+ metastatic breast cancer after progression on first line therapy, and T-DM1 became the standard second line treatment in this patient population until recent findings from DESTINY-Breast03 that demonstrated superiority of T-Dxd over T-DM1 as second line treatment for metastatic, HER2+ breast cancer [41].

Adjuvant T-DM1 for early stage, HER2+ breast cancer and residual disease post taxane and trastuzumab based neoadjuvant chemotherapy was evaluated in the KATHERINE trial, a randomized, phase III study [52]. The study enrolled 1486 patients who were randomized 1:1 to adjuvant T-DM1 or trastuzumab for 14 cycles. The primary outcome was invasive disease free survival (IDFS), which was defined as the time from randomization to first local or regional breast cancer recurrence, distant recurrence, or death from any cause. Key secondary outcomes were PFS and OS. Most patients (77%) received anthracycline based neoadjuvant chemotherapy, and 20% of patients received additional anti-HER2 therapy, 94% of which was pertuzumab. At a median follow up of 40 months, IDFS was significantly improved with T-DM1 versus adjuvant trastuzumab (HR, 0.50; 95% CI, 0.39–0.64; $P < 0.001$). The 3-year IDFS rate was 88.3% in the T-DM1 group and 77.0% in the trastuzumab group. The results of this study led to the FDA approval of T-DM1 as an adjuvant therapy for patients with early stage, HER2+ breast cancer with residual disease after neoadjuvant chemotherapy and surgery and has established adjuvant T-DM1 as a standard therapy in this patient population [2].

6.2 T-Dxd

T-Dxd was first FDA approved based on results from the single arm, multicenter, phase II DESTINY-Breast 01 trial that enrolled patients with HER2+ metastatic breast cancer who progressed on prior chemotherapy including T-DM1 [53]. The median number of prior lines of treatment was 6 (range, 2–27). T-Dxd was associated with an objective response rate of 60.9% (95% CI, 53.4–68.0) in a heavily pre-treated population. The benefit of T-Dxd for the treatment of HER2+ metastatic breast cancer after progression on T-DM1 was confirmed in the phase III, randomized clinical trial, DESTINY-Breast02 that demonstrated significant improvement in PFS and OS when compared to chemotherapy [54].

The clinical trial that changed practice when choosing a second line treatment for patients with HER2+, metastatic breast cancer whose disease progressed after first line anti-HER2 therapy plus taxane chemotherapy was the DESTINY-Breast03 trial, which was a randomized, phase III study that compared T-Dxd to T-DM1 in the second line setting [41, 55]. A total of 524 patients were randomized in 1:1 to T-Dxd or T-DM1. The primary endpoint of PFS was significantly improved with median PFS of 28.8 months with T-Dxd vs. 6.8 months with T-DM1 (HR, 0.33; P < 0.000001). Overall survival was significantly improved with T-Dxd with the median not reached in either treatment arm although the risk of death was reduced by 36% with T-Dxd (HR, 0.64; P, 0.0037) demonstrating superiority of T-Dxd and establishing its role as a preferred second line treatment in this patient population [2].

DESINY-Breast 04 (DB-04), a phase III randomized clinical trial, has transformed the way breast cancer is categorized and treated [42]. Through demonstrating superior efficacy of T-Dxd in breast cancer cells that has reduced HER2 expression (previously categorized as HER2 negative), DB-04 provided clinical evidence that the bystander effect is an important characteristic of ADCs. Up to 60% of HER2 negative breast cancer cells express low levels of HER2, and more than 50% of HR+ breast cancer is HER2 low making the findings from DB-04 clinically relevant [56, 57]. In DB-04, patients with metastatic, recurrent HER2-low breast cancer defined as IHC 1+ or IHC 2+/ISH- were randomized 2:1 to T-Dxd or chemotherapy (capecitabine, eribulin, gemcitabine, paclitaxel, or nab-paclitaxel). More than 70% of patients with HR+ disease received prior CDK4/6 inhibitors and more than 99% of patients progressed on 1 line of prior chemotherapy. T-Dxd was associated with significant improvement in PFS and OS in the HR+ cohort and all patients. The median PFS in the HR+ cohort was 10.1 vs. 5.4 months (HR, 0.51; 95% CI, 0.40–0.64 P < 0.001) and in HR-negative was 8.5 vs. 2.9 months (HR, 0.46; 95% CI, 0.24–0.89). Median OS in the HR+ cohort was 23.9 vs. 17.5 months (HR, 0.64; P, 0.003) and in HR-negative was 18.2 vs. 8.3 months (HR, 0.48; 95% CI, 0.24–0.95). Benefit was observed across all subgroups including HER2 IHC 1+ and IHC 2+/ISH negative [42]. For patients with HR+ metastatic breast cancer and visceral crisis or with endocrine resistant disease, the National Comprehensive Cancer Network (NCCN) guidelines list T-Dxd as a preferred, category 1 treatment in the second line setting [2]. The NCCN guidelines list SG as a preferred, category 1 option in the second line setting for this patient population if not candidate for T-Dxd. For TNBC with HER2-low, T-Dxd is listed as preferred, category 1 treatment option in the second line setting [2].

6.3 SG

SG is the first approved ADC targeting Trop-2 [58]. SG was evaluated in the ASCENT, a phase III, randomized clinical trial in patients with metastatic TNBC who progressed after at least two lines of chemotherapy, one of which had to be for metastatic disease [59]. Patients (N = 529) were randomized 1:1 to SG or chemotherapy (eribulin, capecitabine, gemcitabine, or vinorelbine). The primary efficacy outcome was PFS in patients without brain metastases. Key secondary outcomes were PFS in all patients and OS. SG was associated with significant improvement in PFS and OS. In patients without brain metastases, median PFS in SG was 5.6 months vs. 1.7 months with chemotherapy (HR, 0.41; 95% CI, 0.32–0.52; P < 0.001). The median OS was 12.1 with SG vs. 6.7 months with chemotherapy (HR, 0.48; 95% CI, 0.38–0.59; P < 0.001). A total of 61 patients had stable, treated brain metastases at baseline, 32 of which were treated with SG. In a subgroup analysis, patients with stable baseline brain metastases treated with SG had median PFS of 2.8 months compared to1.6 months in patients treated with chemotherapy (HR, 0.65; 95% CI, 0.35–1.22). This analysis is exploratory and limited by small sample size [60]. The NCCN lists SG as a preferred, category 1 treatment option in the second line setting for patients with metastatic TNBC who progressed on at least 2 prior chemotherapy lines, at least one of which for metastatic disease [2].

SG was also evaluated in the TROPiCS-02, a phase III, randomized clinical trial evaluating SG in 543 patients with HR+, HER2 negative or low who have progressed on the following: a CDK 4/6 inhibitor, endocrine therapy, and a taxane and at least two prior chemotherapies in the metastatic setting [61]. The primary outcome of PFS was statistically significant with median PFS of 5.5 in the SG arm vs. 4 months in the chemotherapy arm (HR, 0.661; 95% CI, 0.529–0.826; P, 0.0003). The median OS was also significantly improved in these heavily pretreated patients with endocrine resistant disease with median OS of 14.4 in the SG arm vs. 11.2 months in the chemotherapy arm (HR, 0.789; 95% CI, 0.646–0.964; P, 0.020) [62].

7. Adverse events and monitoring

7.1 T-DM1

The most common adverse events associated with T-DM1 were musculoskeletal pain (37.9%), nausea (40.6%), thrombocytopenia (45.7%), constipation (26.9%), fatigue (38.8%), and transaminitis (36.8%). T-DM1 has a low emetic risk [2]. T-DM1 is not associated with alopecia. Due to hepatotoxicity, it is recommended to monitor bilirubin and transaminases before each dose of T-DM1.

Decreased left ventricular ejection fraction (LVEF) has been observed with anti-HER2 therapies including T-DM1 (2–3%). Patients with history of significant cardiac disease and those with baseline LVEF <50% were excluded from clinical trials. It is recommended to monitor left ventricular ejection fraction (LVEF) before initiating T-DM1 and throughout treatment [14]. In clinical practice, LVEF is typically monitored prior to initiating treatment with T-DM1 and every 3 months thereafter.

7.2 T-Dxd

The most common hematologic adverse events associated with T-Dxd were decrease in hemoglobin (66%), white blood cells (71%), neutrophil (65%), platelets (47%), and lymphocyte (55%). The most common non-hematologic adverse events were fatigue, increase in aminotransferases, constipation, vomiting, decreased appetite, musculoskeletal pain, diarrhea, and hypokalemia [15]. T-Dxd is considered highly emetogenic [2]. T-Dxd is associated with alopecia (21 to 46%). An increased incidence of interstitial lung disease (ILD)/pneumonitis including fatal events were observed in clinical trials (all grade, 15.4%; grades 1/2,11.9%; grades 3/4,1.3%; grade 5 or death, 2.2%). Median time to onset is approximately 5.4 months (range, <0.1–46.8 mo). Risk factors include moderate to severe kidney impairment, having pulmonary comorbidities at baseline (i.e., asthma, prior ILD, radiation pneumonitis), time since initial cancer diagnosis >4 years, age <65 years, baseline oxygen saturation < 95%, and T-Dxd dose >6.4 mg/kg. No consensus guidelines exist on type and frequency of monitoring besides symptoms assessment. High resolution chest computed tomography (CT) was obtained every 6 weeks in clinical trials investigating T-Dxd. Frequent imaging mimicking clinical trials may not be feasible in clinical practice for reasons such as cost and insurance coverage. As a result, frequent monitoring for ILD symptoms in patients receiving T-Dxd is imperative. Similarly to T-DM1, LVEF reduction was reported with T-Dxd (3–8%; mostly asymptomatic) it is recommended to monitor LVEF before starting and periodically thereafter [15]. In clinical practice, LVEF is typically monitored prior to initiating treatment with T-Dxd and every 3 months thereafter.

7.3 SG

The most common adverse events associated with SG were febrile neutropenia (6%), vomiting (5%), diarrhea (4%), dyspnea (3%), nausea (3%), and anemia (2%). It is recommended to monitor patients for severe neutropenia with known reduced activity of UGT1A1 (see pharmacogenomics for details) [16].

8. ADCs in development

Datopotamab deruxtecan (DS-1062) or Dato-Dxd is a Trop2 ADC with a topoisomerase I inhibitor payload (Dxd). Dato-Dxd is comprised of a humanized IgG1 mAb conjugated to the cytotoxic payload via a cleavable, tetrapeptide based linker, and it has an average of 4 DAR with demonstrated bystander effect [63]. Dato-Dxd is being investigated in ongoing clinical trials in solid tumors including breast cancer [64].

Dato-Dxd is being investigated in heavily pretreated patients with metastatic TNBC in the TROPIONPanTumor01 trial (NCT03401385) and has demonstrated encouraging results with an objective response rate of 34% in all patients and 52% in patients who are treatment-naïve to topoisomerase I inhibitor-based therapies [64]. Most common adverse events reported with Dato-Dxd were stomatitis (all grade, 73%; grade 3, 11%), nausea (all grade, 66%; grade 3, 2%), and vomiting (all grade, 39%; grade 3, 5%). The incidence of alopecia was 36% (grade 2, 14%) [64].

Dato-Dxd is also being investigated in the TROPION-Breast01 (NCT05104866), an ongoing randomized, phase III trial that enrolled 700 patients with metastatic, HR+ HER2 negative breast cancer. Patients are randomized 1:1 to Dato-Dxd or chemotherapy (eribulin, capecitabine, vinorelbine, or gemcitabine). Included patients had to have progressed on endocrine therapy and 1–2 prior lines of chemotherapy [65]. Results are not yet reported.

9. Conclusion

ADCs combine precision targeting with traditional cytotoxic treatment allowing for the delivery of highly potent chemotherapeutic agents to malignant cells. Recent regulatory approvals of next generation ADCs have changed how breast cancer is classified and treated. There are three approved ADCs for the treatment of breast cancer to this dare, and more ADCs are currently in development.

Conflict of interest

The authors declare no conflict of interest.

Author details

Farah Raheem and Vishal Shah*
Mayo Clinic, Phoenix, USA

*Address all correspondence to: shah.vishal@mayo.edu

References

[1] Wolff AC, Hammond MEH, Allison KH, Harvey BE, Mangu PB, Bartlett JMS, et al. Human epidermal growth factor receptor 2 testing in breast cancer: American Society of Clinical Oncology/College of American Pathologists Clinical Practice Guideline Focused Update. Journal of Clinical Oncology. 2018;**36**(20):2105-2122. DOI: 10.1200/JCO.2018.77.8738. Epub 2018 May 30

[2] NCCN Clinical Practice Guidelines in Oncology (NCCN Guidelines®). Breast Cancer [Internet]. 2023. Available from: https://www.nccn.org/professionals/physician_gls/pdf/breast.pdf [Accessed: February 19, 2023]

[3] Gampenrieder SP, Rinnerthaler G, Tinchon C, Petzer A, Balic M, Heibl S, et al. Landscape of HER2-low metastatic breast cancer (MBC): Results from the Austrian AGMT_MBC-Registry. Breast Cancer Research. 2021;**23**(1):112. DOI: 10.1186/s13058-021-01492-x

[4] Fehrenbacher L, Cecchini RS, Geyer CE Jr, Rastogi P, Costantino JP, Atkins JN, et al. NSABP B-47/NRG oncology phase III randomized trial comparing adjuvant chemotherapy with or without Trastuzumab in high-risk invasive breast cancer negative for HER2 by FISH and with IHC 1+ or 2. Journal of Clinical Oncology. 2020;**38**(5):444-453. DOI: 10.1200/JCO.19.01455. Epub 2019 Dec 10

[5] Ogitani Y, Aida T, Hagihara K, Yamaguchi J, Ishii C, Harada N, et al. DS-8201a, a novel HER2-targeting ADC with a novel DNA topoisomerase I inhibitor, demonstrates a promising antitumor efficacy with differentiation from T-DM1. Clinical Cancer Research. 2016;**22**(20):5097-5108. DOI: 10.1158/1078-0432.CCR-15-2822. Epub 2016 Mar 29

[6] Fu Z, Li S, Han S, Shi C, Zhang Y. Antibody drug conjugate: The "biological missile" for targeted cancer therapy. Signal Transduction and Targeted Therapy. 2022;**7**(1):93. DOI: 10.1038/s41392-022-00947-7

[7] Khongorzul P, Ling CJ, Khan FU, Ihsan AU, Zhang J. Antibody-drug conjugates: A comprehensive review. Molecular Cancer Research. 2020;**18**(1):3-19. DOI: 10.1158/1541-7786.MCR-19-0582. Epub 2019 Oct 28

[8] Donaghy H. Effects of antibody, drug and linker on the preclinical and clinical toxicities of antibody-drug conjugates. MAbs. 2016;**8**(4):659-671. DOI: 10.1080/19420862.2016.1156829. Epub 2016 Apr 5

[9] Ritchie M, Tchistiakova L, Scott N. Implications of receptor-mediated endocytosis and intracellular trafficking dynamics in the development of antibody drug conjugates. MAbs. 2013;**5**(1):13-21. DOI: 10.4161/mabs.22854. Epub 2012 Dec 6

[10] Damelin M, Zhong W, Myers J, Sapra P. Evolving strategies for target selection for antibody-drug conjugates. Pharmaceutical Research. 2015;**32**(11):3494-3507. DOI: 10.1007/s11095-015-1624-3. Epub 2015 Jan 15

[11] De Cecco M, Galbraith DN, McDermott LL. What makes a good antibody-drug conjugate? Expert Opinion on Biological Therapy. 2021;**21**:1-7

[12] Hock MB, Thudium KE, Carrasco-Triguero M, Schwabe NF.

Immunogenicity of antibody drug conjugates: Bioanalytical methods and monitoring strategy for a novel therapeutic modality. The AAPS Journal. 2015;**17**(1):35-43. DOI: 10.1208/s12248-014-9684-6. Epub 2014 Nov 8

[13] Natsume A, Niwa R, Satoh M. Improving effector functions of antibodies for cancer treatment: Enhancing ADCC and CDC. Drug Design, Development and Therapy. 2009;**3**:7-16

[14] Kadcyla Prescribing Information [Internet]. 2022. Available from: https://www.gene.com/download/pdf/kadcyla_prescribing.pdf [Accessed: February 19, 2023]

[15] Enhertu Prescribing Information [Internet]. 2022. Available from: https://daiichisankyo.us/prescribing-information-portlet/getPIContent?productName=Enhertu&inline=true [Accessed: February 19, 2023]

[16] Trodelvy Prescribing Information [Internet]. 2023. Available from: https://www.gilead.com/-/media/files/pdfs/medicines/oncology/trodelvy/trodelvy_pi.pdf [Accessed: February 19, 2023]

[17] Bargh JD, Isidro-Llobet A, Parker JS, Spring DR. Cleavable linkers in antibody-drug conjugates. Chemical Society Reviews. 2019;**48**(16):4361-4374. DOI: 10.1039/c8cs00676h

[18] Nolting B. Linker technologies for antibody-drug conjugates. Methods in Molecular Biology. 2013;**1045**:71-100

[19] Cardillo TM, Govindan SV, Sharkey RM, Trisal P, Arrojo R, Liu D, et al. Sacituzumab Govitecan (IMMU-132), an anti-Trop-2/SN-38 antibody-drug conjugate: Characterization and efficacy in pancreatic, gastric, and other cancers. Bioconjugate Chemistry. 2015;**26**(5):919-931. DOI: 10.1021/acs.bioconjchem.5b00223. Epub 2015 May 8

[20] Doronina SO, Bovee TD, Meyer DW, Miyamoto JB, Anderson ME, Morris-Tilden CA, et al. Novel peptide linkers for highly potent antibody-auristatin conjugate. Bioconjugate Chemistry. 2008;**19**(10):1960-1963. DOI: 10.1021/bc800289a. Epub 2008 Sep 20

[21] Gondi CS, Rao JS. Cathepsin B as a cancer target. Expert Opinion on Therapeutic Targets. 2013;**17**(3):281-291. DOI: 10.1517/14728222.2013.740461. Epub 2013 Jan 8

[22] Yver A, Agatsuma T, Soria JC. The art of innovation: Clinical development of trastuzumab deruxtecan and redefining how antibody-drug conjugates target HER2-positive cancers. Annals of Oncology. 2020;**31**(3):430-434. DOI: 10.1016/j.annonc.2019.11.019. Epub 2019 Dec 11

[23] Kovtun YV, Audette CA, Ye Y, Xie H, Ruberti MF, Phinney SJ, et al. Antibody-drug conjugates designed to eradicate tumors with homogeneous and heterogeneous expression of the target antigen. Cancer Research. 2006;**66**(6):3214-3221. DOI: 10.1158/0008-5472.CAN-05-3973

[24] Erickson HK, Widdison WC, Mayo MF, Whiteman K, Audette C, Wilhelm SD, et al. Tumor delivery and in vivo processing of disulfide-linked and thioether-linked antibody-maytansinoid conjugates. Bioconjugate Chemistry. 2010;**21**(1):84-92. DOI: 10.1021/bc900315y

[25] Girish S, Gupta M, Wang B, Lu D, Krop IE, Vogel CL, et al. Clinical pharmacology of trastuzumab emtansine (T-DM1): An antibody-drug conjugate in development for the treatment

of HER2-positive cancer. Cancer Chemotherapy and Pharmacology. 2012;**69**(5):1229-1240. DOI: 10.1007/s00280-011-1817-3. Epub 2012 Jan 20

[26] Zhao P, Zhang Y, Li W, Jeanty C, Xiang G, Dong Y. Recent advances of antibody drug conjugates for clinical applications. Acta Pharmaceutica Sinica B. 2020;**10**(9):1589-1600. DOI: 10.1016/j.apsb.2020.04.012. Epub 2020 Apr 24

[27] Beck A, Goetsch L, Dumontet C, Corvaïa N. Strategies and challenges for the next generation of antibody-drug conjugates. Nature Reviews. Drug Discovery. 2017;**16**(5):315-337. DOI: 10.1038/nrd.2016.268. Epub 2017 Mar 17

[28] Birrer MJ, Moore KN, Betella I, Bates RC. Antibody-drug conjugate-based therapeutics: State of the science. Journal of the National Cancer Institute. 2019;**111**(6):538-549. DOI: 10.1093/jnci/djz035

[29] Diamantis N, Banerji U. Antibody-drug conjugates—An emerging class of cancer treatment. British Journal of Cancer. 2016;**114**(4):362-367. DOI: 10.1038/bjc.2015.435. Epub 2016 Jan 7

[30] Kaur R, Kaur G, Gill RK, Soni R, Bariwal J. Recent developments in tubulin polymerization inhibitors: An overview. European Journal of Medicinal Chemistry. 2014;**87**:89-124. DOI: 10.1016/j.ejmech.2014.09.051. Epub 2014 Sep 16

[31] Walczak CE. Microtubule dynamics and tubulin interacting proteins. Current Opinion in Cell Biology. 2000;**12**(1):52-56. DOI: 10.1016/s0955-0674(99)00056-3

[32] Cheung-Ong K, Giaever G, Nislow C. DNA-damaging agents in cancer chemotherapy: Serendipity and chemical biology. Chemistry & Biology. 2013;**20**(5):648-659. DOI: 10.1016/j.chembiol.2013.04.007

[33] Kawato Y, Aonuma M, Hirota Y, Kuga H, Sato K. Intracellular roles of SN-38, a metabolite of the camptothecin derivative CPT-11, in the antitumor effect of CPT-11. Cancer Research. 1991;**51**(16):4187-4191

[34] Meddahi A, Lemdjabar H, Caruelle JP, Barritault D, Hornebeck W. FGF protection and inhibition of human neutrophil elastase by carboxymethyl benzylamide sulfonate dextran derivatives. International Journal of Biological Macromolecules. 1996;**18**(1-2):141-145. DOI: 10.1016/0141-8130(95)01074-2

[35] Wakankar A, Chen Y, Gokarn Y, Jacobson FS. Analytical methods for physicochemical characterization of antibody drug conjugates. MAbs. 2011;**3**(2):161-172. DOI: 10.4161/mabs.3.2.14960. Epub 2011 Mar 1

[36] Hamblett KJ, Senter PD, Chace DF, Sun MM, Lenox J, Cerveny CG, et al. Effects of drug loading on the antitumor activity of a monoclonal antibody drug conjugate. Clinical Cancer Research. 2004;**10**(20):7063-7070. DOI: 10.1158/1078-0432.CCR-04-0789

[37] Tang Y, Tang F, Yang Y, et al. Real-time analysis on drug-antibody ratio of antibody-drug conjugates for synthesis, process optimization, and quality control. Scientific Reports. 2017;**7**(1):7763. DOI: 10.1038/s41598-017-08151-2

[38] Corti C, Giugliano F, Nicolò E, Ascione L, Curigliano G. Antibody-drug conjugates for the treatment of breast cancer. Cancers (Basel). 2021;**13**(12):2898. DOI: 10.3390/cancers13122898

[39] Giugliano F, Corti C, Tarantino P, Michelini F, Curigliano G. Bystander effect of antibody-drug conjugates: Fact or fiction? Current Oncology Reports. 2022;**24**(7):809-817. DOI: 10.1007/s11912-022-01266-4. Epub 2022 Mar 19

[40] Singh AP, Sharma S, Shah DK. Quantitative characterization of in vitro bystander effect of antibody-drug conjugates. Journal of Pharmacokinetics and Pharmacodynamics. 2016;**43**(6):567-582. DOI: 10.1007/s10928-016-9495-8. Epub 2016 Sep 26

[41] Cortés J, Kim SB, Chung WP, Im SA, Park YH, Hegg R, et al. Trastuzumab Deruxtecan versus Trastuzumab Emtansine for breast cancer. The New England Journal of Medicine. 2022;**386**(12):1143-1154. DOI: 10.1056/NEJMoa2115022

[42] Modi S, Jacot W, Yamashita T, Sohn J, Vidal M, Tokunaga E, et al. Trastuzumab deruxtecan in previously treated HER2-low advanced breast cancer. The New England Journal of Medicine. 2022;**387**(1):9-20. DOI: 10.1056/NEJMoa2203690. Epub 2022 Jun 5

[43] Takano M, Sugiyama T. UGT1A1 polymorphisms in cancer: Impact on irinotecan treatment. Pharmacogenomics and Personalized Medicine. 2017;**10**:61-68. DOI: 10.2147/PGPM.S108656

[44] Borges VF, Ferrario C, Aucoin N, Falkson C, Khan Q, Krop I, et al. Tucatinib combined with ado-trastuzumab emtansine in advanced ERBB2/HER2-positive metastatic breast cancer: A phase 1b clinical trial. JAMA Oncology. 2018;**4**(9):1214-1220. DOI: 10.1001/jamaoncol.2018.1812

[45] Li C, Menon R, Walles M, Singh R, Upreti VV, Brackman D, et al. Risk-based pharmacokinetic and drug-drug interaction characterization of antibody-drug conjugates in oncology clinical development: An international consortium for innovation and quality in pharmaceutical development perspective. Clinical Pharmacology and Therapeutics. 2022;**112**(4):754-769. DOI: 10.1002/cpt.2448. Epub 2021 Nov 23

[46] Fenn KM, Kalinsky K. Sacituzumab govitecan: Antibody-drug conjugate in triple-negative breast cancer and other solid tumors. Drugs Today (Barc). 2019;**55**(9):575-585. DOI: 10.1358/dot.2019.55.9.3039669

[47] PharmGKB. UGT1A1 [Internet]. 2023. Available from: https://www.pharmgkb.org/gene/PA420/prescribingInfo [Accessed February 19, 2023]

[48] Rugo HS, Tolaney SM, Loirat D, Punie K, Bardia A, Hurvitz SA, et al. Safety analyses from the phase 3 ASCENT trial of sacituzumab govitecan in metastatic triple-negative breast cancer. NPJ Breast Cancer. 2022;**8**(1):98. DOI: 10.1038/s41523-022-00467-1

[49] Dean L. Irinotecan therapy and UGT1A1 genotype. In: Pratt VM, Scott SA, Pirmohamed M, Esquivel B, Kattman BL, Malheiro AJ, editors. Medical Genetics Summaries [Internet]. Bethesda (MD): National Center for Biotechnology Information (US); 2012

[50] Camptosar Prescribing Information [Internet]. 2014. Available from: https://www.pfizermedicalinformation.com/en-us/camptosar/highlights [Accessed: February 19, 2023]

[51] Verma S, Miles D, Gianni L, Krop IE, Welslau M, Baselga J, Pegram M, Oh DY, Diéras V, Guardino E, Fang L, Lu MW, Olsen S, Blackwell K; EMILIA Study Group. Trastuzumab emtansine for

HER2-positive advanced breast cancer. New England Journal of Medicine. 2012;367(19):1783-1791. doi: 10.1056/NEJMoa1209124. Epub 2012 Oct 1. Erratum in: New England Journal of Medicine 2013;**368**(25):2442

[52] von Minckwitz G, Huang CS, Mano MS, Loibl S, Mamounas EP, Untch M, et al. Trastuzumab emtansine for residual invasive HER2-positive breast cancer. The New England Journal of Medicine. 2019;**380**(7):617-628. DOI: 10.1056/NEJMoa1814017. Epub 2018 Dec 5

[53] Modi S, Saura C, Yamashita T, Park YH, Kim SB, Tamura K, et al. Abstract PD3-06: Updated results from DESTINY-breast01, a phase 2 trial of trastuzumab deruxtecan (T-DXd) in HER2 positive metastatic breast cancer. Cancer Research. 2021;**81**(Suppl. 4):PD3-06

[54] Krop I, Park YH, Kim S-B, et al. Trastuzumab deruxtecan vs physician's choice in patients with HER2+ unresectable and/or metastatic breast cancer previously treated with trastuzumab emtansine: Primary results of the randomized phase 3 study DESTINY-Breast02. In: San Antonio Breast Cancer Symposium. Presented at: SABCS; December 6-10, 2022; San Antonio, TX. Abstract GS2-01

[55] Hurvitz SA, Hegg R, Chung WP, Im SA, Jacot W, Ganju V, et al. Trastuzumab deruxtecan versus trastuzumab emtansine in patients with HER2-positive metastatic breast cancer: Updated results from DESTINY-Breast03, a randomised, open-label, phase 3 trial. Lancet. 2023;**401**(10371):105-117. DOI: 10.1016/S0140-6736(22)02420-5. Epub 2022 Dec 7. Erratum in: Lancet 2023 Feb 18;401(10376):556

[56] Schettini F, Chic N, Brasó-Maristany F, Paré L, Pascual T, Conte B, et al. Clinical, pathological, and PAM50 gene expression features of HER2-low breast cancer. NPJ Breast Cancer. 2021;7(1):1. DOI: 10.1038/s41523-020-00208-2

[57] Tarantino P, Hamilton E, Tolaney SM, Cortes J, Morganti S, Ferraro E, et al. HER2-low breast cancer: Pathological and clinical landscape. Journal of Clinical Oncology. 2020;**38**(17):1951-1962. DOI: 10.1200/JCO.19.02488. Epub 2020 Apr 24

[58] Bardia A, Mayer IA, Vahdat LT, Tolaney SM, Isakoff SJ, Diamond JR, et al. Sacituzumab Govitecan-hziy in refractory metastatic triple-negative breast cancer. The New England Journal of Medicine. 2019;**380**(8):741-751. DOI: 10.1056/NEJMoa1814213

[59] Bardia A, Tolaney SM, Loirat D, Punie K, Oliveira M, Rugo HS, et al. LBA17 ASCENT: A randomized phase III study of sacituzumab govitecan (SG) vs treatment of physician's choice (TPC) in patients (pts) with previously treated metastatic triple-negative breast cancer (mTNBC). Annals of Oncology. 2020;**31**:S1149-S1150

[60] Diéras V, Weaver R, Tolaney SM, Bardia A, Punie K, Brufsky A, et al. Abstract PD13-07: Subgroup analysis of patients with brain metastases from the phase 3 ASCENT study of sacituzumab govitecan versus chemotherapy in metastatic triple-negative breast cancer. Cancer Research. 2021;**81**(Suppl. 4): PD13-07

[61] Rugo HS, Bardia A, Marmé F, Cortes J, Schmid P, Loirat D, et al. Primary results from tropics-02: A randomized phase 3 study of sacituzumab govitecan (SG) versus treatment of Physician's choice (TPC) in patients (PTS) with hormone receptor–positive/HER2-negative

(HR+/HER2-) advanced breast cancer. Journal of Clinical Oncology. 2022;**40**(Suppl. 17). DOI: 10.1200/jco.2022.40.17_suppl.lba1001

[62] Rugo HS, Bardia A, Marmé F, Cortes J, Schmid P, Loirat D, et al. LBA76 overall survival (OS) results from the phase III TROPiCS-02 study of sacituzumab govitecan (SG) vs treatment of physician's choice (TPC) in patients (pts) with HR+/HER2-metastatic breast cancer (mBC). Annals of Oncology. 2022;**33**:S1386

[63] Okajima D, Yasuda S, Maejima T, Karibe T, Sakurai K, Aida T, et al. Datopotamab Deruxtecan, a novel TROP2-directed antibody-drug conjugate, demonstrates potent antitumor activity by efficient drug delivery to tumor cells. Molecular Cancer Therapeutics. 2021;**20**(12):2329-2340. DOI: 10.1158/1535-7163.MCT-21-0206. Epub 2021 Aug 19

[64] Krop I, Juric D, Shimizu T. Datopotamab deruxtecan (Dato-DXd) in advanced/metastatic HER2 negative breast cancer: Triple negative breast cancer results from the phase 1 TROPION-PanTumor01 study. In: San Antonio Breast Cancer Symposium. San Antonio, TX; 2021

[65] Bardia A, Kalinsky K, Tsurutani J, Hamilton EP, Johnston S, Sohn J, et al. 274TiP Datopotamab deruxtecan (Dato-DXd), a TROP2 antibody-drug conjugate, vs investigators' choice of chemotherapy (ICC) in previously-treated, inoperable or metastatic hormone-receptor (HR) positive, HER2-negative (HR+/HER2–) breast cancer: TROPION-Breast01. Annals of Oncology. 2022;**33**:S663